ALWAYS
DELICIOUS

Also by David Ludwig, MD, PhD

ALWAYS HUNGRY?:
Conquer Cravings, Retrain Your Fat Cells,
and Lose Weight Permanently

ENDING THE FOOD FIGHT:
Guide Your Child to a Healthy Weight in a
Fast Food/Fake Food World

ALWAYS DELICIOUS

Over 175 Satisfying Recipes to Conquer Cravings, Retrain
Your Fat Cells, and Keep the Weight Off Permanently

DAVID LUDWIG, MD, PhD,
and DAWN LUDWIG

Foreword by Mark Hyman, MD

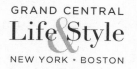

GRAND CENTRAL
Life & Style
NEW YORK · BOSTON

Grand Central Life & Style
Hachette Book Group
1290 Avenue of the Americas, New York, NY 10104
grandcentrallifeandstyle.com
twitter.com/grandcentralpub

First Edition: March 2018

Grand Central Life & Style is an imprint of Grand Central Publishing. The Grand Central Life & Style name and logo are trademarks of Hachette Book Group, Inc.

The publisher is not responsible for websites (or their content) that are not owned by the publisher.

The Hachette Speakers Bureau provides a wide range of authors for speaking events. To find out more, go to www.hachettespeakersbureau.com or call (866) 376-6591.

Library of Congress Cataloging-in-Publication Data

Names: Ludwig, David, 1957– author. | Ludwig, Dawn, author.
Title: Always delicious : over 175 satisfying recipes to conquer cravings,
    retrain your fat cells, and keep the weight off permanently / David
    Ludwig, MD, PhD, and Dawn Ludwig.
Description: First edition. | New York : Grand Central Life & Style, [2018] |
    Includes bibliographical references and index.
Identifiers: LCCN 2017039689| ISBN 9781478947776 (hardcover) | ISBN
    9781478947769 (audio downloadable) | ISBN 9781478947783 (ebook)
Subjects: LCSH: Reducing diets—Recipes. | Weight loss. | LCGFT: Cookbooks.
Classification: LCC RM222.2 .L737 2018 | DDC 641.5/635—dc23
LC record available at https://lccn.loc.gov/2017039689

ISBNs: 978-1-4789-4777-6 (hardcover), 978-1-4789-4778-3 (ebook)

Printed in the United States of America

LSC-C

10 9 8 7 6 5 4 3 2 1

To the members of our Facebook community and our wonderful moderators.
We are honored to travel along this (tasty) path of healing with you!

Note to Readers

All personal stories in this book are real and represent the authentic experience of our Facebook community* members. Each of these members provided permission to include his or her actual first name, last initial, age, and place of residence. Stories have been edited for grammar and brevity.

Contents

	Foreword	xi
Chapter 1:	Welcome to *Always Delicious*!	1
Chapter 2:	The Science of *Always Delicious*	11
Chapter 3:	Becoming an *Always Delicious* Chef	28
Chapter 4:	Do It Yourself (DIY)	53
Chapter 5:	Breakfasts	81
Chapter 6:	Entrées	110
Chapter 7:	Chickpea Flour & Revisionist Foods	195
Chapter 8:	Side Dishes	211
Chapter 9:	Soups, Salads & Buddha Bowls	238
Chapter 10:	Snacks & Appetizers	270
Chapter 11:	Sauces, Rubs & Marinades	283
Chapter 12:	Beverages & Desserts	308
	Acknowledgments	327
	Appendix	329
	Notes	336
	Index	339
	About the Authors	351

Foreword

Knowing what to eat is not so easy in a world of conflicting nutrition science and confusing guidelines. The truth is that not all science is equal. And not all diet recommendations are based on great science. Harder still is to know how to prepare and enjoy food that will bring us joy, pleasure, and health. *Always Delicious* solves all these problems.

In *Always Delicious*, David and Dawn Ludwig have done something remarkable. They created a guide and manual that explains both why we are sick and overweight (now 70 percent of Americans are overweight) and how to choose and prepare amazing food that you love and that loves you back.

I have known Dr. Ludwig for twenty years. I have been inspired and enlightened by his groundbreaking research at Harvard. And by his scientific integrity. He once was invited to give a talk to CEOs of major food companies. They wanted to pay his expenses and an honorarium. Dr. Ludwig attended the meeting at his own expense, and has never taken money from the food industry.

Industry-funded studies are many times more likely to show benefit for the company or organization that funded the research. If the National Dairy Council funds a study on milk, guess what? It shows that dairy has benefits. If the soda industry funds studies on obesity, that research almost always acquits soda as a cause of obesity, despite mountains of evidence to the contrary. Dr. Ludwig's research is published in the world's top medical journals, meticulously designed and executed, and has made major contributions to scientific knowledge.

Applying his findings in my medical practice has led to extraordinary outcomes. One recent patient had type 2 diabetes, which was completely out of control despite multiple medications and insulin. After just a few months, her blood sugars were normal and she got off all insulin and medications. This is not a rare occurrence, but commonplace when I have applied Dr. Ludwig's research and dietary recommendations. Patients reverse chronic disease and lose weight effortlessly and sustainably. All without starving or eating tasteless foods.

The principles of Dr. Ludwig's book *Always Hungry?* and the companion *Always Delicious* are based on the most compelling and credible science (much of it done by Dr. Ludwig himself), simple principles that profoundly change our view of how to eat for health and weight loss. First and most important, all calories are not equal. Weight loss isn't about eating less and exercising more. That will just make you cranky and irritable or "hangry." You can white-knuckle it for a bit, but then you rebound and gain all the weight and more, messing up your metabolism. Being on a low-calorie diet fails over and over.

There is an entirely new approach to eating and food. *Always Delicious* lays it out in a simple, beautiful, doable, delicious way. So, if all calories are not equal, which ones should you eat? The ones that make you feel full, speed up your metabolism, help release calories from your fat cells, increase your energy, and taste great. Those calories importantly include good, savory, yummy, satisfying fats. Not all the low-fat processed starches (and sugars) we have been told were good for us.

The failure of conventional low-fat diets is that they focus on calories. It's all about moderation, and if you can't control yourself at the dinner table (or snack cupboard), and if you can't exercise enough, then it's your fault. You are just a lazy glutton. Sounds right. Except for one thing: It's not true. Yet it is still the recommendation of most nutritionists, doctors, and public health associations responsible for guiding our eating choices. It only helps perpetuate the pervasive processed-food industry. If soda calories or cereal calories are the same as almond or avocado calories, then as long as you stay in balance it doesn't matter what you eat. Not only is that wrong. It defies common sense.

In *Always Delicious* you will learn that *what* we eat is far more important than *how much* we eat, that choosing the right foods will lead to spontaneous changes in your hormones, immune system, and metabolism that drive health and weight loss without struggle or effort. This way, you replace deprivation and tasteless food with abundance and deliciousness.

I have been to dinner at Dawn and David's house and I promise you that the meals were extraordinary adventures in taste, pleasure, and joy. With this cookbook, you also get to have dinner with them. Getting healthy and losing weight is just a nice side effect.

Mark Hyman, MD
Director, Cleveland Clinic Center for
Functional Medicine
December 14, 2017

ALWAYS
DELICIOUS

CHAPTER 1

Welcome to Always Delicious!

In 2016, our book *Always Hungry?* introduced a three-phase weight loss program based on a radical idea:

> Overeating doesn't make you gain weight—the process of gaining weight makes you overeat.

In other words, hunger and overeating are symptoms of an underlying problem. Although this idea may sound counterintuitive, it's supported by a century of research that shows body weight is controlled more by biology than willpower over the long term. It means that your weight problem isn't your fault. And it means you can solve your weight problem with a satisfying, delicious diet and a sustainable lifestyle plan!

WHY CONVENTIONAL LOW-CALORIE DIETS FAIL

You've heard it a thousand times: "All calories are alike." To lose weight, just eat less and move more. It sounds so simple, anyone should be able to do it. But there are a few problems with this *calories in, calories out* approach to weight control.

First, it doesn't work, not for most people over the long term. Sure, you can lose weight for a short while, but after a few weeks or months, the weight usually comes racing right back. Researchers analyzed low-calorie diet studies published in the *New England Journal of Medicine* and *JAMA*, two of the world's most prestigious medical journals.[1] Overall, participants in these studies lost a maximum of just 10 pounds—a small portion of their excess weight—and most regained much of the weight after one year. How many times has this happened to you?

How about exercise? Although physical activity has many important benefits, for most people, weight loss isn't one of them. Scientific studies have consistently concluded that exercise by itself is not effective as a treatment for obesity.

Sadly, fewer than 1 in 5 people with excessive weight in the United States has ever lost just 10 percent of their weight and kept it off for just one year using standard approaches to diet and exercise.[2] And this finding, based on self-reported data, is likely to be overstated, as many people tend to think they're a little taller and a little lighter than they really are.

The second problem with the calories in, calories out approach is that it's actually impossible to do in real life. Even nutrition experts can't accurately determine their energy balance to within 300 calories a day—just one extra muffin. A daily excess of that magnitude would cause massive weight gain. For that matter, if calorie counting were critical to weight control, how did humans ever maintain a healthy body weight before the very notion of the calorie was invented?

And the third problem with calories in, calories out is that it implicitly blames overweight people. If losing weight is simply a matter of eating less and moving more, then everyone with excess weight must lack discipline, self-respect, or even proper values. This way of thinking explains why you might be blamed for being overweight in ways that would never occur with other medical problems. In a thousand ways, our culture says, "It's your fault you're fat." Unfortunately, many people have internalized these beliefs. One survey found that a substantial proportion of adults would rather be infertile or die ten years earlier than be obese.[3] And these attitudes begin very early in life, as demonstrated by one famous study. When children were shown images of other kids with various ailments—including one in a wheelchair, one on crutches, one with a facial disfigurement, one with no left hand, and one with obesity—they chose the heavy child for a friend last.[4]

Though pervasive, weight prejudice simply isn't justified. Studies show that people with obesity aren't any different from the general population when it comes to personal characteristics like discipline, values, and morals.[5]

In fact, the calories in, calories out approach fails not for lack of effort or willpower, but because it ignores the biological systems that control body weight.

THE NEW SCIENCE OF WEIGHT CONTROL WITHOUT HUNGER

When you cut back calories, of course you'll lose weight—it's a basic law of physics. But the body fights back, with rising hunger, slowing metabolism, and release of stress hormones that break down lean tissue. That's the starvation response, and it primes your body to regain weight.

Think about it. People overeat mainly because of hunger. What happens when you eat less? You get even hungrier! Are you supposed to spend the rest of your life feeling that way? And even if you could, your body has other tricks, like slowing down your metabolism. This is a battle very few of us can ultimately win.

It's like trying to treat a fever with an ice bath. Sure, you can force body temperature down for a short while, but your body would fight back, with severe shivering and blood vessel constriction—and you'd feel miserable. Treat the *cause* of the fever, and your body temperature decreases naturally. Treat the *cause* of obesity, and your weight decreases with your body's cooperation, not with your body kicking and screaming.

What is the cause of obesity? As we'll explore in chapter 2, the primary problem is fat cells stuck in calorie-storage overdrive. The low-fat, carbohydrate-laden diet we've been told to eat for forty years has raised levels of the hormone insulin, triggering our fat cells to hoard too many calories. Consequently, there are too few calories circulating in the bloodstream to satisfy the needs of the brain and the rest of the body. That's why we get hungry, our metabolism slows down, and we gain weight. Cutting back on calories only makes this situation worse—creating a battle between mind and metabolism we're destined to lose.

The solution is a diet and lifestyle plan that lowers insulin levels and calms chronic inflammation (insulin's twin troublemaker). As insulin levels drop, fat cells settle down and release their excess calories back into the body. When that happens, hunger decreases, cravings vanish, metabolism speeds up, and you lose weight without the struggle. This marks the transition from the *Always Hungry* Vicious Cycle of weight gain to the *Always Delicious* Victorious Cycle of weight control (see the Figures in chapter 2, pages 25 and 26).

THE THREE-PHASE PROGRAM

The quickest, easiest, and most delicious way to lower insulin levels is to substitute luscious high-fat foods for all those processed carbohydrates that invaded our diet during the low-fat craze. Since this approach works with your body, not against it, you'll eat until satisfied, snack when hungry, and never count calories again. (For further explanation of the program, see *Always Hungry?*)

You'll enjoy nuts and nut butters, full-fat dairy, rich sauces and spreads, savory proteins (with vegetarian alternatives), and real dark chocolate. But this isn't an Atkins-type very-low-carbohydrate diet either—you can have a range of natural carbohydrates.

Phase 1: *Jump-start weight loss.* For just weeks, you'll give up grain products, potatoes, and added sugar. But with these luscious high-fat foods, you won't crave the processed carbs at all. (Approximately 50 percent fat, 25 percent protein, and 25 percent carbohydrate.)

Phase 2: *Reach your new body weight "set point."* You can add back whole-kernel grains, like steel-cut oats, brown rice, buckwheat, millet, and quinoa. You can also include nonstarchy vegetables like yam, sweet potato, and squash—just no white potato for now. You can even have a touch of added sugar. You'll stay in this phase as you lose weight, until reaching a stable plateau— your new lower body weight set point. For people with relatively little weight to lose, that may take just a few weeks or months; for others, many months. (Approximately 40 percent fat, 25 percent protein, and 35 percent carbohydrate.)

Phase 3: *Design your personalized prescription for life.* You can mindfully add back modest amounts of more processed carbohydrates, according to your body's ability to handle them, creating an individualized plan that's right for you. (Approximately 40 percent fat, 20 percent protein, and 40 percent carbohydrate.)

In addition, the program includes three "Life Supports"—quality sleep, stress relief, and enjoyable physical activities. These important practices work with diet to help fat cells calm down and release their stored calories back into the body.

We especially recommend a daily *passeggiata*—the Italian word for a relaxing walk after dinner. The goal isn't to burn off a lot of calories. Instead, the *passeggiata* provides an enjoyable opportunity to improve metabolism and control blood sugar, while preparing your body for a restorative night's sleep (see *Always Hungry?*, page 124).

OUR COMMUNITY

Even the best possible diet will miss the mark if people don't feel motivated and empowered to follow it. We live in what has been termed a "toxic environment," surrounded by cheap junk foods and other harmful influences. For many of us, resisting these ubiquitous temptations and finding more healthful alternatives takes support—and that's the power of community.

Prompted by our readers, we formed the Official *Always Hungry?* Book Community on Facebook in early 2016. Our goal was to provide a noncommercial and nonjudgmental space for people to ask questions, receive support, and travel together along the path of healing and wellness. With guidance from several dozen phenomenal volunteer moderators, the community has now grown to more than ten thousand members and counting. Since then, we've been honored to follow the experiences of readers as they've struggled with almost every imaginable health problem, encountered obstacles, and achieved success. (You'll find the authentic stories of community members throughout this book.)

Since *Always Hungry?*—called *"AH"* in our Facebook group—is a "diet book," many people were initially focused on losing weight, but the group evolved into much more. Without calorie restriction, weight loss may not be a sensational 30 pounds in 30 days. But without hunger and deprivation, it's more sustainable.

For example, Charlotte A., age 52, from Charlotte, North Carolina, posted: "Sometimes people who have a lot of weight to lose look longingly at stomach surgery as the quick solution. I understand that. Last year, a friend and I who both work in healthcare were at a similar crossroads with our weight. The week I started *AH*, she had a vertical sleeve gastrectomy. Initially, she lost weight more quickly. But to date, she's down 50 pounds, and I'm down 60 pounds—and 8 inches from my natural waist. Weight loss on this program may not be fast, but it's steady and requires no anesthesia!"

Regardless of weight loss, members often relate "non-scale victories" (NSVs)—our term for benefits beyond weight loss involving physical, emotional, or mental health. Reports of diabetes resolution, better blood pressure, lower cholesterol, less "brain fog," and improvement in chronic inflammatory conditions emphasize how powerful the combination of diet and community can be.

Billy W., age 35, from Clarksville, Tennessee, wrote: "Last November, I went to the doctor with frequent urination and excessive thirst. They discovered my hemoglobin A1c was 11.0 percent and my blood sugar was over 500! My doctor recommended *Always Hungry?* and I started the next week. Now, less than 4 months later, my Hemoglobin A1c level is down to 6.6 percent and blood sugar is averaging 109 to 117—without insulin! My blood pressure went from 150/90 to 115/70. I have energy I've never had, and I'm the happiest I have ever been. This program is helping save my life!"

Jennifer H., age 52, of Easton, Pennsylvania, posted: "My biggest NSV was totally unexpected: almost complete cessation of gastroesophageal reflux disease. I have a large hiatal hernia, for which I'd been taking proton pump inhibitors for more than a decade. Even with the treatment, I'd still wake up vomiting at least two nights a week. The doctors had recommended surgery, which I was putting off. Within a few months on *AH*, I realized I was no longer waking up at night. In consultation with my doctor, I was able to wean myself from the medication altogether. My quality of life has increased tremendously."

And Amy T., age 43, of Toronto, Canada, reported: "I have endometriosis (among other things), and usually mid-month I have a few days of unrelenting pain. Then, right before my time, I break out like crazy. Since starting *AH*, the mid-month issues have really quieted down and my skin is amazing."

Some of the most inspiring stories from our community chronicle an evolving relationship with food and triumph over addictive tendencies. As fat cells calm down and the body enjoys a more stable food supply, people often feel less obsessed with eating, more in control, and a natural desire for more nourishing foods.

Annette C., age 51, from Livingston, Scotland, wrote: "I've been reading posts in this group for a while, and I'm glad to say it's a really supportive and safe place to talk about our weight loss and health journeys. Because of this, I wanted to share my biggest NSV. I had a very traumatic and difficult childhood and upbringing. I resorted to 'comfort eating' and started to gain weight from the age of nineteen. I'd punished myself by eating until I felt sick—sort of like bulimia without throwing up.

I had some success in structured weight loss programs, but they never fully rid me of my compulsion. I started to feel different on *AH* around day three; my husband was working and I was on my own at night, a common trigger for extreme overeating. But this time I was able to ask myself, 'Are you really hungry?' and the answer was no! By the end of the fortnight I realized that I had had no bingeing episodes. Although I had assumed that my eating compulsion was emotional, it had actually been driven by cravings due to my low-fat, high-carb diet. I likened it to radio interference. As I eradicated the white noise of cravings, I was able to genuinely hear what my body was saying. For the first time in my life I feel normal. This isn't a diet or an eating plan: If I never lost another pound or inch, it wouldn't matter. I have gained so much more."

And Trish M., age 42, from Vancouver, Washington, said: "For much of my life, I experienced hunger as a stress and could barely cope. I feared that if I didn't eat, I would lose my usually cool head. When out running errands, even just ten minutes away from home, I'd feel compelled to stop for fast food if I got hungry…and I was always hungry! Now I've realized that 'hunger' was really a powerful addiction to sugar and grains. With *AH*, I notice my hunger and rationally think that it's time to go home and make something to eat. This is huge for me! The palate adjustment has allowed me to enjoy fruits and berries more, and all the sweetness in natural foods. With every new recipe, I joyfully think, 'Yep, I'm not suffering. This is SO GOOD!' There is satisfaction in knowing that this food will help keep me healthy and active so that I can pursue my life goals. This life is so brief and I want to wring as much enjoyment out of it as possible."

We've also seen frequent reports of improved energy level and physical fitness.

Kim G., age 28, from Davie, Florida, announced: "Huge NSV today! I am a freelance musician and work late hours that mess up my schedule. When I have to teach early, I roll out of bed and barely make it where I need to be. This morning, not only did I wake up early without trouble, I had time for my morning routine and a proper breakfast. AND after teaching four hours in a row, I miraculously did not feel remotely in need of a nap, which would've been guaranteed before. One of the greatest benefits of *AH* has been my increased energy levels, and the consistency of that energy. My stress levels seem way down. I'm able to get to sleep easier, stay asleep, and wake up without feeling like death warmed over. The weight loss is great, too, but I have to say, this is the big one for me!!"

And Sandy H., age 51, of Jefferson City, Missouri, wrote: "Yesterday I took a half-mile hike through the woods and up a hill. That may not seem like much, but a month ago, even thinking about doing that would have worn me out. Although I have lost 18 pounds on *AH*, there's still a long way to go, so hauling my 300-plus-pound body up a hill is quite a big deal for me. It was beautiful up there!"

Others, like Paula T., age 61, of Sully, Iowa, experienced relief from anxiety or depression and a sense of internal peace: "*AH* has set me free! Free...from counting calories, from constant gnawing hunger, from weakness and fatigue, from fearing food. It's been about forty-two years since I've known this kind of freedom and joy! Another benefit of this way of eating is a new calmness. My anxiety levels are practically nonexistent these days. I'm not afraid to eat anymore!"

We've also been privileged to extend our community outside the United States, including through a collaboration with the Centre for Hospitality and Culinary Arts at George Brown College (GBC), the largest culinary school in Canada. Working with the GBC Culinary Management Nutrition faculty, we helped create a recipe development course based on *Always Hungry?* guidelines. The first class of eighty students produced an amazing variety of delicious Phase 1 and 2 recipes for their final projects—you'll find several of these featured in this book (and more on our blog, www.drdavidludwig.com). To change the food culture, we need a new generation of chefs with a vision for truly health-supportive cuisine.

Ultimately, the power to affect fundamental social change rests with community. After healing ourselves and our families, we can join together to help make the world a healthier place for everyone. In addition to the human toll, diseases of poor nutrition affect us all, through higher insurance costs, increasing Medicare spending, and the massive drag on our economy from lost productivity. Together, we can help create a society in which healthful foods and lifestyle choices are also convenient and affordable (see the Epilogue of *Always Hungry?* for our ten-point plan to make healthy food a national priority). Especially for the sake of our children, we must ensure that public health takes precedence over special interest and the short-term profits of the food industry.

WHY *ALWAYS DELICIOUS?*

One of the most frequent requests in our Facebook community is for new recipes... and you'll find more than 175, ranging from appetizers to desserts, in chapters 4 through 12—each adapted to all three program phases. In addition, many members have described overcoming a lifelong fear of the kitchen as they discovered the joys and rewards of home cooking. In chapter 3, Chef Dawn shares her secrets for how anyone can become a confident, competent home chef the *Always Delicious* way.

But first, we'll explode the forty-year low-fat diet myth that has caused so much suffering. Chapter 2 takes a deep dive into the fascinating science of hunger, cravings, food addiction, and taste. You'll learn how a luscious higher-fat diet reprograms fat cells *and* taste buds, so that nutritious foods become delicious and junk foods lose their hold on us.

And as you get started, please keep our motto in mind:

Forget calories.
Focus on food quality.
And let your body do the rest!

My *Always Delicious* Story

1 month: I've eaten dark chocolate for years, usually a large bar at a time. This evening, it tasted completely differently. Same chocolate bar, but now it tastes like *food*: I can taste minerals, sense complexity in it, notice a texture, enjoy the smell of it. Before, it was something I craved instead of enjoyed. Tonight, I had less than an ounce and almost didn't finish it. I really enjoyed it, but didn't crave or need it. I'm fairly certain an alien has taken over my body.

4 to 5 months: I've been adding NSVs to a list whenever I notice a new one. Just added one more and have tears in my eyes. (Oh, and I've lost 24 pounds—that's not even on the list!):

- Blood pressure lower
- Knees don't hurt anymore
- Sleeping more soundly
- Mood more stable
- Don't get upset about small things
- More serene, like someone installed a Zen monk in my brain
- Depression lifted
- More confident in the future
- Energy level higher and stable, not up and down
- Mental fog lifted; less trouble retrieving words
- Mental focus better; many fewer typing mistakes
- Concentrate longer periods of time

- No more zombie-walking into pantry
- Don't spend much time thinking about/craving foods
- Don't eat and eat when already full; eat what I want to, then stop
- Food tastes better; notice subtle tastes more
- Reflux now quite rare
- Psoriasis on elbows nearly gone

10 months: To anyone new to the program with aspirations for improving your situation, I was like you ten months ago. I had (and have) very little self-discipline. And I wasn't sure if this plan would work. Guess what: It did work! I'm nearly 50 pounds lighter, and I feel better than I've felt in years. Even with poor self-discipline, I'm happy enough on the plan to execute it quite well. You can do this. Give it a chance.

14 months: I've lost 55 pounds and my waist is down 7.5 inches. I've been rapidly descending into menopause during this time, which I thought meant weight loss would be difficult. Two people have recently said, "You are *half* the woman you used to be!" People think if I lost this much weight, I must have really suffered. But I'm no hero! I wasn't deprived, and I wasn't hungry. I'm eating delicious food that I love. This is the opposite of deprivation—it's a naughty romp through the food forest!

—Mary M., age 50, Dallas, Texas

CHAPTER 2

The Science of Always Delicious

Why do overweight people overeat?

More than any other, this question bewilders experts in nutrition and the public alike. One common explanation is that people with excess weight lack willpower, discipline, and motivation. In a world with ubiquitous tasty foods, they simply succumb to temptation too easily, too often.

To address this perceived deficiency, conventional obesity treatment typically focuses on psychological techniques to help people control their behavior. Cut back on fat, which contains twice as many calories per gram as carbohydrate or protein. Eat on a small plate to make your meal seem larger. When hungry, distract yourself with an activity. Get up an hour earlier to make time for exercise. Find other sources of pleasure in life than food.

The problem is, these methods rarely result in lasting weight loss. Unfortunately, the mind-set they reflect regularly causes suffering, by reinforcing the view of obesity as a personal failing. If losing weight is simply a matter of self-control, then everyone should be able to do it. Anyone who can't must lack basic knowledge or have a serious character flaw.

But as we'll explore here, this way of thinking is completely wrong. Obesity is more about biology than willpower. *The essential problem is too little enjoyment from food, not too much*. The solution is to break the vicious cycle of hunger, cravings, and overeating and instead create a victorious cycle of pleasure and long-lasting satisfaction from truly nourishing foods. We call this *Always Delicious*.

My *Always Delicious* Story

I hate to be clichéd, but I used to feel...always hungry! When I was being "bad," I would eat quickly, hoping to finish before my guilt or my attention would catch up. I justified eating junk food because I felt like I deserved it. When I was being "good," I felt like I had to white knuckle it to stay in my calorie range every day. I counted calories obsessively for over 365 days straight. Often, I found myself making less nutritious choices, just because they were lower in calories and I could then eat more. I rarely felt satisfied with the low-fat processed carbohydrates I ate and felt sorry for myself that I would always have to stay below 1,500 calories a day. This tug of war between good and bad made my weight seesaw radically. I was either gaining or losing and had lost all hope of ever being at peace with food or maintaining a healthy weight without a ton of willpower and effort.

Since starting the *Always Hungry?* program, I have felt truly nourished and satiated for the first time in my life. I have learned to relax into eating and listen to my body. I don't feel like I'm fighting against my body anymore. My hunger has calmed down tremendously from being urgent and frantic, to a milder interest and pleasure when it is time to eat again. I don't feel like I need to muster up willpower to continue to eat this way—it is simply a part of who I am now! I am now close to my goal weight, and even if it takes another year to reach it, I am not worried because I wouldn't change a thing about my new way of life.

—Keri R., age 41, Round Rock, Texas

HUNGER

Considering the importance of weather to the Inuit peoples of the Arctic, it's not surprising that they have at least fifty names for snow.[1] Along the same lines, we'd argue that all languages need several words to describe hunger.

One kind of hunger actually feels pleasant—the stimulating sensations that heighten anticipation and enjoyment of a good meal. Some cultures, such as the French, embrace and prolong those sensations as a daily practice before dinner. An entirely different experience is feeling ravenous and in desperate need for food. More than any other factor, that kind of overwhelming hunger drives overeating and dooms weight loss diets.

So why do many people become ravenously hungry after just a few hours without food, especially when trying to cut calories, whereas others cruise along comfortably, even when skipping meals? The answer can be found in our fat cells.

All except the thinnest among us have enough calories stored in fat cells to supply the needs of the body for many weeks, reserves that helped our ancestors survive famine. Under normal conditions, hormones and other biological influences precisely control the size and number of our fat cells. After we eat, calorie-rich fuels in the form of glucose, amino acids, and fats flood into the bloodstream, and hormonal signals tell fat cells to store the excess. A few hours later, after the meal has been digested, other signals instruct fat cells to release some of their calories, providing energy until the next meal. Our brain, monitoring this process, then makes us feel hungry, and we eat just enough to replenish the fuel supply, keeping body weight in a healthy range. That's why humans—for example, in the United States from the end of the Great Depression to the 1970s—could live amid an abundance of food and maintain stable body weight across the population, without counting calories. However, this carefully controlled system has recently been thrown out of balance.

As we explored in *Always Hungry?*, something has triggered our fat cells to hoard too many calories, leaving too few for the rest of the body. Although we typically view obesity as a state of excess, it's also a matter of starvation—not enough calories in the bloodstream to meet the needs of the brain and other organs. That's why we get *so hungry, so soon* after eating, and why metabolism slows. It's a distribution problem, like having a clogged fuel line in your car. No matter how much gasoline you put into the tank, the engine will be starved for fuel and won't function efficiently until the underlying problem is fixed.

What's driving our fat cells into a feeding frenzy? The clear culprit is too much of the hormone insulin. Think of insulin as Miracle-Gro for your fat cells...just not the sort of miracle you want happening in your body! Under the influence of insulin, calories check in to fat cells, but they don't check out.

Consider what happens in type 1 diabetes, a disease mainly of youth in which the body can't make enough insulin. A child with newly diagnosed type 1 diabetes will have typically lost weight, no matter how much he or she has been eating: 3,000, 5,000, or even 7,000 calories a day. Treat that child with the right amount of insulin, and body weight returns to normal. Give that child too much insulin, and excessive weight gain will predictably occur.

If you don't have diabetes, the most important influence on insulin levels is the amount and type of carbohydrate you eat.[2] Calorie for calorie, processed, fast-digesting (high-glycemic-load) carbohydrates raise blood sugar and insulin more than any other food. These include all those starchy and sugary foods that flooded our diets during the forty-year low-fat craze: white bread, white rice, potato products, cookies, crackers, chips, candy, and sugary drinks. In fact, refined starchy foods can be just as much a problem as sugar. Starches are nothing more than molecules of the sugar glucose in a long chain. Try this experiment yourself. Take a bite of a bagel and chew it thoroughly. Do you notice it begins to taste sweet? That's sugar popping off the starch under the weak effects of enzymes in saliva. Once that bagel hits the powerful enzymes lower down in the digestive track, it literally melts into glucose. By contrast, natural carbohydrates like nonstarchy vegetables, whole fruits, beans, and minimally processed grains have a much gentler effect on blood sugar and insulin.

Proteins also cause some release of insulin, but less so than most processed carbohydrates. And unlike carbohydrate, protein raises levels of the hormone glucagon, which counteracts insulin and encourages fat cells to release calories. For this reason, balanced proportions of protein play an important role in the *Always Delicious* meal plan, including vegetarian options.

The third major nutrient, dietary fat, has virtually no effect on blood sugar and insulin at all, a key point in designing a more effective approach to control hunger and lose weight. Despite what we were told during the last forty years, low-fat diets are clearly *inferior* to all higher-fat diets, such as Mediterranean diets, low-carbohydrate diets, very-low-carbohydrate diets, and ketogenic diets—the grandfather of all high-fat diets, with up to 80 percent fat![3] And as every chef knows, fat is tasty, making recipes delicious without having to resort to sugar and artificial additives. You'll find an abundance of healthy high-fat foods among the recipes—including nuts and nut butters, full-fat dairy, avocado, rich sauces and spreads, and real dark chocolate!

Dr. Ludwig's Science Bite

A High-Fat Diet: Good for Your Waist, Great for Your Heart

Let's have a look at the two biggest trials of dietary fat in the last decade. The Women's Health Initiative assigned almost fifty thousand women to a low-fat diet or a control.[4] The low-fat diet group received intensive support, with multiple individual and group sessions. The control group was just given written education materials. Despite being designed to favor the low-fat diet, that group showed no reduction in cardiovascular disease after eight years. Another low-fat diet study, the Look Ahead trial, included five thousand patients with diabetes at high risk for heart disease.[5] This study was also designed to favor the low-fat diet, because that group got more intensive support than the control group. Look Ahead closed early for "futility," when an early analysis showed no benefit of the low-fat diet and no likelihood that this diet would ever show benefit.

Unfortunately, there are no high-fat diet studies of similar size (and it's high time the government funded them). However, systematic analyses of smaller trials show consistent benefits for blood pressure, triglycerides, HDL cholesterol, and overall risk for atherosclerosis (although LDL cholesterol typically increased). Other studies highlight the potential benefits of a high-fat diet for chronic inflammation, fatty liver, and insulin resistance. These positive effects on cardiovascular disease risk factors may explain a recent dramatic finding: Adults following a high-fat/low-carbohydrate eating pattern had *lower* rates of premature death (although the types of fats consumed also had an important influence).[6]

In addition to the major nutrients, other aspects of diet influence fat cells in various ways. Micronutrients (vitamins and minerals), phytochemicals (protective plant chemicals), prebiotics (fiber), and probiotics (microbes that promote healthy gut function) can lower insulin levels, calm chronic inflammation, and directly communicate with fat cells. *Always Delicious* recipes provide a rich source of these beneficial dietary components.

Beyond diet, lifestyle has a major influence on fat cells, too, which is why the program in *Always Hungry?* includes a focus on stress relief, quality sleep, and enjoyable physical activities.

In summary, the standard "eat less, move more" approach to weight control rarely works, because it ignores the underlying problem. Sure, you can lose weight for a short while by restricting calories, but the body fights back, with rising hunger and slowing metabolism. That's a battle we're destined to lose. A better approach is to target the biological cause of excessive hunger—fat cells stuck in calorie-storage overdrive. When fat cells calm down, the cycles of ravenous hunger and overeating naturally subside, along with other remarkable changes in the body, as we shall see in the next sections.

My *Always Delicious* Story

Before starting the *Always Hungry?* program, I was starving all the time and I didn't even know it! Struggling with overeating and constant cravings felt normal because I wasn't aware of any other option. I had spent my life existing on highly processed carbohydrates and sugary foods. Every day I consumed sweeteners in drinks and packaged meals. A meal rarely left me feeling satiated longer than an hour or two unless I ate a very large quantity of food. Changing the way I eat has had a life-changing impact on my relationship with food. For the first time ever, I feel in control. I naturally eat smaller portions at meals, without feeling deprived, because the food is so filling. I often make myself snacks but end up not having them because I'm simply not hungry. Even when I get hungry, it isn't the raw, painful gnawing in my stomach that used to torment me between meals.

—Cassandra S., age 38, Des Moines, Iowa

CRAVINGS

Have you ever eaten enough to be full, but somehow still felt unsatisfied? While others contentedly sipped coffee or tea after dinner, you couldn't keep your mind off those cookies in the kitchen cabinet. You didn't need more food. You weren't even hungry. Oddly, you may not have especially *liked* those cookies before, but you *wanted* them now, and your mind wouldn't leave you alone until you succumbed.

Though we tend to associate hunger with cravings, they are quite distinct experiences controlled by different regions of the brain. Hunger comes primarily from the hypothalamus, a deep brain region that also regulates metabolism. Damage to the hypothalamus, from an injury or a tumor for example, can cause massive obesity that defies treatment. In contrast, cravings arise from dopamine-rich brain areas involved in reward and "saliency" (how important something is right now). These areas, centered around the nucleus accumbens, play a critical role in the classic addictions to alcohol, nicotine, cocaine, heroin, and even gambling.

Thousands of scientific studies have explored the psychological aspects and environmental triggers of eating. However, this research often overlooks the strong biological basis of food cravings, and without this understanding, treatment of binge eating and related conditions may miss the mark. As with hunger, cravings aren't inherently harmful. Instead, they're a signal that the body has an unmet need or is otherwise out of balance. For this reason, attempts to simply ignore or resist cravings often fail, and can actually make matters worse over the long term.

Consider what happens in Addison's disease, a hormone deficiency that causes the kidneys to lose too much sodium in the urine. People with this disease characteristically develop intense cravings for salty foods in the body's attempt to avoid dangerously low levels of sodium in the blood. Indeed, salt cravings in someone with unrecognized Addison's can be life-saving. But eating more salt will restore sodium levels and satisfy the cravings only temporarily, unless the underlying problem—loss of sodium in the urine—is corrected with replacement of the missing hormone.

So what drives food cravings? Let's have a look at three illuminating studies.

An extraordinary experiment from 1946 used somewhat unsettling methods to examine taste preferences during severe hypoglycemia.[7] The investigators examined one hundred patients receiving an intentional insulin overdose for treatment of psychiatric disease (a method abandoned by medicine decades ago). The patients were asked to sample five solutions as their blood sugar plummeted after the insulin injection, for as long as they stayed conscious and able to communicate:

1. Water
2. Water with 5 percent sugar (similar in sweetness to a sports drink)
3. Water with 30 percent sugar (extremely sweet)
4. Water with saccharin matched in sweetness to 30 percent sugar
5. Water with salt

While blood sugar remained close to normal, virtually all the patients rejected the 30 percent sugar solution as too sweet. But as hypoglycemia progressed, most reversed their preferences and chose that solution over all the others. Of particular interest, some people seemed to lose the ability to perceive the saccharin solution as sweet during hypoglycemia, suggesting that at this critical time, the body can distinguish natural sweeteners (which raise blood sugar) from artificial sweeteners (which don't).

A more recent (and perhaps more ethical) study also used insulin injections to drive down blood sugar, but this time taking precautions to ensure safety.[8] Before the insulin injection, very few subjects reported food cravings of any sort, whereas during hypoglycemia, most did. The items craved most frequently were bread, cereal, pizza, and sandwiches—that is, processed carbohydrates high in glycemic load.*

---

* Glycemic load describes how blood sugar changes after consuming typical portions of carbohydrate-containing foods. Technically, glycemic load is equal to glycemic index multiplied by amount of carbohydrate consumed (see *Always Hungry?*, pages 73–78 for details).

When subjects were given choices of high-carbohydrate, high-protein, or high-fat foods, they expressed the greatest desire for the carbohydrates.

A third study administered insulin infusions by vein under two conditions: either with enough glucose, also by vein, to keep blood sugar normal (88 milligrams per deciliter); or with somewhat less glucose, to produce slightly low blood sugar (67 milligrams per deciliter).[9] Then, scans of brain activity were done as the subjects viewed images of high-calorie foods. Under both conditions, the subjects reported liking the foods to the same degree. However, with the lower blood sugar, they reported wanting the foods more, and scans showed increased activity in the reward and addiction areas of the brain, including the nucleus accumbens.

These findings demonstrate that food craving is another trick your brain uses, in addition to hunger, to make you eat when your blood sugar is low, especially if other fuels (like fatty acids) have been locked away by high insulin levels. We specifically crave processed carbohydrates—rather than unprocessed carbohydrates like apples, fats like butter, or proteins like egg whites—because they raise blood sugar fast. The problem is, they also raise insulin the most, setting the stage for the next surge/crash cycle.

So the concept of "food addiction," often dismissed by experts,[10] may not be far-fetched after all. Fortunately, the same approach used to control hunger also calms cravings, and relief can be just one meal away!

Dr. Ludwig's Science Bite

Cravings ≠ Tastiness

Despite common misconceptions, we don't crave foods simply because of their taste. Are pretzels, popcorn, chips, and other common binge foods really so delicious? To explore this question, my colleagues and I gave twelve overweight men two different milk shakes on separate occasions, one made with a fast-digesting carbohydrate (corn syrup) and the other with a slow-digesting carbohydrate (uncooked cornstarch).[11] We adjusted the taste of the milk shakes so both would have similar sweetness. Following consumption of the fast-digesting milk shake, insulin rose twice as high compared to the slow-digesting milk shake; by four hours, blood sugar had crashed. At that time, brain scans showed one area lit up like a laser after the fast-digesting milk shake—the nucleus accumbens, ground zero for the classic addictions. These findings show that processed carbohydrates can hijack our pleasure and reward centers and cause cravings—through their effects on biology, not their taste—setting the stage for bingeing and weight gain.

My *Always Delicious* Story

Candy was my downfall. I craved it after finishing meals, especially at times of stress. I'd eat a whole bag and feel really happy for a little while, then really hungry and tired afterward. But I don't crave those bags of candy anymore. I fell in love with berries! Strawberries, blueberries, blackberries, and raspberries are so sweet and absolutely delicious! They've been my go-to dessert for eight months, and every time I eat them I can't believe how fantastic they taste. I found an amazing new sense of happiness and contentment around foods, and am never going back to the sugar and processed food addiction. *Always Hungry?* changed my life! The fact that I went from 154 to 134 pounds is honestly just icing on Chef Dawn's grain-free pancakes. The most important thing for me is, I now enjoy what I'm eating, know when I'm full, and never have cravings. And those berries . . .

—*Kimberly P., age 48, Florence, Kentucky*

SATIETY

The word "satiety" comes from the Latin *satietatem*, meaning abundance, sufficiency, and fullness.[12] Satiety, basically the opposite of hunger, refers to how long we feel full after eating, and from this perspective, the number of calories eaten at any one time doesn't tell the whole story. A 2-ounce snack of cotton candy provides fewer calories than the same amount of nuts. But if you became much hungrier much sooner after the candy, you wouldn't be better off by the end of the day—another reason why focusing exclusively on calories makes little sense.

As we considered earlier, fast-digesting carbohydrates raise insulin excessively, driving too many incoming calories into storage. Soon after eating, the body runs low on fuel, provoking hunger[13] and cravings. However, whole natural carbohydrate, healthy fats, and protein in the right proportions produce long-lasting satiety. Other aspects of food also influence satiety, such as the total volume of a meal (determined mainly by water content), fiber, the type of protein and fat, and the types and intensity of flavors. The *Always Delicious* recipes take full advantage of these effects. In addition, environmental conditions (lighting, sound, presence of others), our psychological state (relaxed or stressed), and the pace of the meal can play significant roles, underscoring the importance of mindful eating.

Beyond physical sensations of hunger and fullness, the concept of satiety gets at something broader, involving our general well-being. With every meal, hormones, metabolism, and even the expression of genes throughout the body change according to what we eat. These biological changes can make all the difference between feeling awake and alert, or sluggish and sleepy for hours to come. Have you experienced the powerful effects of food on mood, long after eating? If not, the research linking fast-digesting (high-glycemic-load) carbohydrate to physical, emotional, and mental well-being may surprise you.

In one clever study, nineteen children from an economically disadvantaged school in Wales were recruited to participate in a "breakfast club."[14] Each school day for a month, the children were given one of three different breakfasts in random order: cornflakes and a waffle with reduced-fat milk and sugar (high glycemic load, and quite typical of what many kids have for breakfast); scrambled eggs, conventional bread, jam, and yogurt (medium glycemic load); or a ham and cheese sandwich with a special reduced-carbohydrate bread (low glycemic load). Then, their behavior and cognitive performance were monitored with video games and other tests two to three hours later. The children demonstrated better memory and ability to sustain attention, fewer signs of frustration, and more time on-task working individually in class on the morning following the low-glycemic-load breakfast. However, since the meals differed in many ways, it is hard to know what specific food components contributed to the observed effects.

Another study of sixty-four elementary school students in England compared the effects of two more comparable breakfasts, high-glycemic-index Cocoa Puffs or low-glycemic-index All-Bran cereal with milk.[15] The investigators found that the children's attention and memory deteriorated throughout the morning (a phenomenon no doubt bemoaned by teachers around the world), but the declines were less severe following the low-glycemic-index breakfast.

In another study, among seventy-one adult women, memory for hard words was impaired after a high-glycemic-index compared to low-glycemic-index cereal-based breakfast.[16] As expected, this difference emerged after 2½ hours—that is, following the rise and fall in blood sugar. Similarly, executive function, selective attention, verbal memory performance, and working memory were worse among twenty-one patients with diabetes following a high-glycemic-index meal compared to a low-glycemic-index meal.[17]

Do the effects from these one-day studies persist? A clinical trial with eighty-two adults in the Seattle area suggests they do.[18] The participants received two fully prepared diets in random order, low or high glycemic index, both with the same calories, carbohydrate, protein, and fat. After four weeks, those on the high-glycemic-index diet had significantly worse scores for total mood disturbances (55 percent), depressive symptoms (38 percent), and fatigue/inertia (26 percent). During a six-month weight loss study including forty-two overweight adults, worsening mood was observed among those given a high-glycemic-load diet compared to low-glycemic-load diet—a side effect that might weaken resolve to stick with that diet.[19] Furthermore, in the Women's Health Initiative Observational Study, higher dietary glycemic index, added sugar, and refined grains were each associated with a greater risk of developing depression over three years among about seventy thousand postmenopausal women.[20] In contrast, whole fruits and vegetables were associated with lower risk.

The relationship between food and mood is, of course, complicated, and not all published studies have reached similar conclusions. But overall, the research indicates that—beyond the number of calories in a meal—the quality of those calories can help you feel full longer, have more energy, remain calm and focused, think more clearly, feel better, and be happier. As we'll see in the next section, these positive experiences can lead to a remarkable transformation of taste perceptions, making healthful foods progressively more appealing with time.

Dr. Ludwig's Science Bite

Put Metabolism to Work for You!

After significant weight loss, metabolism slows down, reducing our body's calorie requirement, even as hunger and desire for extra calories increase—making long-term weight loss exceedingly difficult. Slowing metabolism also tends to make us feel tired, weak, and disinclined to exercise, further contributing to the likelihood of weight regain. But as we've seen, these biological responses aren't set in stone.

My colleagues and I gave adults with high body weight a low-calorie diet until they had lost about 25 pounds.[21] Then we fed them weight-maintenance diets varying in glycemic load, each for a month at a time. During the critical period three to five hours after eating, the subjects had more calories in their blood and significantly faster metabolic rate following the low-glycemic-load meal compared to the high-glycemic-load meal. These results show how the right diet might help you feel more energetic after weight loss, and resist the temptation to collapse on the couch!

My *Always Delicious* Story

My entire adult life, no matter how fit I was, no matter what kind of "diet" I was on, come midafternoon, I would mentally and physically crash. I remember it as early as sitting in afternoon college classes, then in my adult career working at a desk, or as recently as playing games with my children in the afternoon as a stay-at-home mom. It was a feeling of uncontrollable and pure exhaustion. The feeling of it taking everything I had just to pry my eyes open and stay awake. I started noticing a big change two to three weeks into the *Always Hungry?* program. Now I can go straight through the afternoon without even thinking about sleep! I have gained more hours in my day to be productive and, most of all, more quality time with my family.

—*Misty Y., age 36, Amarillo, Texas*

TASTINESS

We typically think of tastiness, scientifically termed "palatability," as an inherent component of food. Some foods by their very nature seem to give us a lot of pleasure; others simply don't. Unhappily, items in the first category tend to be the most fattening. So must people with a weight problem inevitably choose between virtuous self-denial or harmful hedonism? Despite some early-life hardwiring, the answer is emphatically no.

In a classic series of studies, researchers examined the facial expressions of new-born infants in response to sweet, sour, and bitter solutions placed on their tongues. The sweet solution elicited signs of satisfaction, including licking, sucking, and a slight smile. The other solutions produced distinct grimaces.[22] These programmed preferences prime infants for breast milk (which tastes sweet) and protect them from ingesting potentially toxic substances. However, like the startle reflex, children normally outgrow this instinctual behavior, learning to like an increasingly broad range of tastes—including savory, spicy, sour, bitter, and pungent. That's why Inuit children like *muktuk* (raw blubber), Korean children like kimchi (fermented cabbage), and Mexican children like hot pepper sauce.

In fact, taste perceptions can change quickly, at any age, as the 1946 study of psychiatric disease patients on page 17 demonstrated. For a less extreme scenario, imagine you had an unexpectedly long wait at a favorite restaurant and became ravenously hungry. When you were finally seated, the waiter brought a basket of freshly baked bread to the table. How do you think it would taste? Probably delicious. Now, suppose you had a huge meal—appetizers, wine, main course, side dishes, a rich dessert—and afterward, the waiter accidentally provided another basket of the very same bread, warm from the oven. How would it taste then? Probably unappealing.

These examples demonstrate a fundamental principle: *Palatability isn't intrinsic to food—it's a response to food determined largely by our biology.* We learn to like foods that make us feel good and dislike those that don't. For this reason, many people savor beer and coffee—the pleasurable effects of alcohol and caffeine on our mood eclipse the intense bitterness of these beverages. Conversely, even a favorite food can become aversive for a long time, if we develop food poisoning soon after eating it. (From this perspective, we can also see why "forcing" kids to eat vegetables can be counterproductive, as it pairs the taste of healthful foods with the unpleasant experience of stress.)

The Standard American Diet keeps taste preferences in an infantilized state, but not because it's inherently so tasty. Do we really think America leads the world in obesity because we've got the world's most delicious diet? The French, Italians, Japanese, and others would probably beg to differ. As we learned from several studies mentioned earlier, the palatability of sugar and other processed carbohydrates increases rapidly after insulin injection as a biological response to low blood sugar. Changes in taste perception may be less dramatic if the insulin excess comes from within the body, in response to eating those fast-digesting carbohydrates in the first place, but the ultimate outcome is the same. It's the secret to the processed food industry's success—Cheetos, Froot Loops, Twinkies, Ritz Crackers, Coke, and of course Lay's ("Bet you can't eat just one") potato chips become tastier the more you eat them. The good news is that this vicious cycle can be quickly broken.

My *Always Delicious* Story

I loved sugar! I had such a sweet tooth. I especially craved homemade baked goods and candy. Cookies, cakes, and breads were my comfort foods. After being on the *Always Hungry?* program for just a few weeks, I could not believe how much my taste buds and cravings changed. Sugar now is far too sweet. I think the thing that helped me the most was indulging in fat. Growing up, we never had butter or cream in our house. It was difficult to believe that heavy cream was allowed and okay. Who knew coffee could taste so good! I have noticed that veggies taste so much sweeter and fruit is delicious. Food just tastes better. Sugar numbed my taste buds. I never thought that I would be able to give up sugar, but it is true. I will not go back to my previous eating habits.

—*Jenny D., age 48, Fargo, North Dakota*

FROM *ALWAYS HUNGRY* TO *ALWAYS DELICIOUS*

A low-fat diet high in processed carbohydrates propagates what we call the *Always Hungry* Vicious Cycle (as depicted in Figure 2.1). Soon after eating, blood sugar and insulin rise rapidly, providing intense but brief biological reward as calories flood into the body. However, the excess insulin directs too many calories into storage, especially into fat cells (promoting weight gain). About two hours later, the rest of the body starts to run low on fuel, and hunger rises. At that time, physical energy and mental abilities may wane. Craving for processed carbohydrate also occurs, making it more likely we'll make the wrong choices at the next meal or snack, setting up another binge-crash cycle.

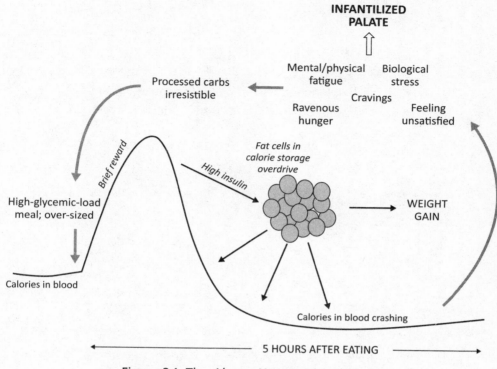

Figure 2.1: The *Always Hungry* Vicious Cycle

The solution is a higher-fat diet, with slow-acting carbohydrates and the right amount of protein to lower insulin (and reduce chronic inflammation, insulin's troublemaking twin). As insulin levels drop, fat cells calm down, releasing their pent-up calories back into the body. Hunger and cravings diminish, energy increases, well-being improves, and these enjoyable bodily experiences feed back to our taste preferences, helping them evolve spontaneously. Soon, the power of hyperprocessed products over us wanes, as we activate the *Always Delicious* Victorious Cycle (see Figure 2.2). When you reprogram your fat cells, you automatically reprogram your taste buds—resolving the conflict between nutritious and delicious once and for all.

In the next chapter, we'll prepare to put these principles into action with a step-by-step guide to becoming an *Always Delicious* chef.

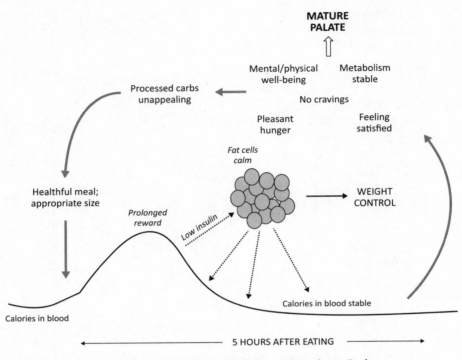

Figure 2.2: The *Always Delicious* Victorious Cycle

My *Always Delicious* Story

I have struggled with polycystic ovarian syndrome since my early twenties, which ultimately caused me to become insulin resistant, and my endocrinologist began to throw around the word "diabetes." I was told numerous times that if I could just lose weight, that would really help things. Soon after, I went to a nutritionist who gave me a low-fat diet, but I was constantly hungry and miserable. It made me want to eat more. I tried this way of eating several times, all with the same result.

Before *Always Hungry?*, I would feel shaky and anxious in between meals. I'd get brain fog and I could feel my blood sugar dropping. I'd feel an instant need to eat something right at that very moment. Then after eating, I would feel *horrible* and want to sleep. Now I can go hours in between eating. When it's time to eat, it's time to eat, but I don't get that desperate "low" feeling anymore. I don't think about food constantly. I feel "normal" for once around food; something I feared would never happen. It is such a wonderful freedom!

I used to crave sugary drinks and all sorts of processed carbohydrates. Now I crave things like full-fat Greek yogurt with strawberries and blueberries. I never thought it was acceptable to eat full-fat dairy, especially if you were trying to lose weight. That's what has been instilled in us for so long, and boy, were they wrong! The berries taste so sweet to me now. It's crazy how your palate changes!

One of my biggest rewards in following this lifestyle is peace of mind. I don't feel guilty if I have a special treat, and I have the confidence now that it won't dictate my next meal. I can't express how much this has made a positive difference in my life...

—*Lindsey C., age 32, Woburn, Massachusetts*

CHAPTER 3

Becoming an Always Delicious *Chef*

TOPICS

Think Like a Chef, *28*

Meal Planning, *29*

Recipe Planning Worksheet, *31*

Prep Day, *32*

Stock and Organize Your Kitchen, *34*

Let Your Tools Do the Work, *36*

Fresh and Seasonal Ingredients, *38*

Making the Swap: Food Substitutions, *39*

Compose a Meal Efficiently, *41*

Plan for and Use Leftovers Creatively, *43*

Obstacles and If-Then Planning, *44*

Presentation and Food Appeal, *45*

Getting Out of Cooking Ruts, *46*

Getting Started with *Always Delicious* Recipes and Meal Plans, *47*

Always Delicious Recipes and Meal Suggestions, *49*

One of our favorite comments comes from a reader who went to serve dinner and thought, "Who was the French chef who showed up in my kitchen to cook this beautiful food?" She did a double take before responding, "Oh wow! It was me!" As you transition from the *Always Hungry* Vicious Cycle to the *Always Delicious* Victorious Cycle (see chapter 2), learning to think like a chef will become more and more natural. You'll hone kitchen skills like planning, cooking, and presenting foods—and discover how easy and enjoyable this can be!

THINK LIKE A CHEF

Ultimately, the goal of a true chef is to create a positive food experience, engaging the senses with flavor, smell, texture, appearance, and ambiance. But at first, that may seem easier said than done.

28

A chef must manage all that comes before the meal, including planning the menu, knowing where to find the best ingredients, and budgeting. The chef will consider what's fresh and take advantage of special deals in the market. If something delicious becomes available at a reasonable price, he or she creates recipes incorporating it. The chef will also devise creative ways to use leftovers, preparing the same foods in interesting and different ways.

After meal planning, the actual process of cooking can be like a mini Broadway production, requiring careful timing to ensure each dish comes out ready at the right time. And to complicate matters further, the chef must consider a range of special needs and preferences. Some people may prefer less salt or more spice, or have specific food allergies or aversions. Someone may be gluten-intolerant or vegetarian. Others might like meat at most meals.

How do you accomplish all this, eating the *Always Delicious* way, without years of culinary training? That's what we'll show you in this chapter. Learning to think like a chef will help demystify the process of cooking, as you discover the sensory pleasures and creative expression that come with being in the kitchen.

MEAL PLANNING

The single most important step to improve your health, and that of your family, is to get in the kitchen. Though preparing meals at home might seem time-consuming, most *Always Delicious* dinners can be made in about thirty minutes with a bit of practice, planning, and prep—breakfast and lunch are even faster. And as some of our reader stories highlight, healthy eating saves a lot of time otherwise spent coping with fatigue and caring for chronic diseases. Improved health means more energy to enjoy the things you love in life.

First, develop a vision of the meals for the week ahead. Ask yourself these questions, then make your meal plan:

- What foods do I already have in the kitchen, either fresh or left over?
- What foods are seasonally available and affordable in the market?
- What substitutions do I have to make, considering the special needs of people sharing these meals?
- Which days of the week will I have limited time to cook?

- Do I need any special kitchen tools or devices?
- Do I want to incorporate any new ingredients or recipes to avoid falling into a rut?

Meal plans can range from a simple idea about the main dishes you'll make for the week to a detailed list of every meal for each day, including sides, desserts, and snacks—as we did with the three-week meal plan in *Always Hungry?* Some people like to leave room for spontaneity; others prefer more structure. Adapt meal planning to fit your needs and your temperament. Once you have a plan, use the Recipe Planning Worksheet on page 31 (also available online at www.drdavidludwig.com) to coordinate your shopping and Prep Day activities.

RECIPE PLANNING WORKSHEET

Use this guide to plan for the week. Decide which recipes to make, then organize shopping and prep.

Phase: _____ **Recipe:** _____ **Servings (in recipe):** _____

Servings needed for main meal: _____ Servings needed for leftovers: _____

Additional recipes to complete the meal: Parts to make ahead:

_____   _____

_____   _____

Substitutions: Ingredients to add to shopping list:

_____   _____

_____   _____

Phase: _____ **Recipe:** _____ **Servings (in recipe):** _____

Servings needed for main meal: _____ Servings needed for leftovers: _____

Additional recipes to complete the meal: Parts to make ahead:

_____   _____

_____   _____

Substitutions: Ingredients to add to shopping list:

_____   _____

_____   _____

Phase: _____ **Recipe:** _____ **Servings (in recipe):** _____

Servings needed for main meal: _____ Servings needed for leftovers: _____

Additional recipes to complete the meal: Parts to make ahead:

_____   _____

_____   _____

Substitutions: Ingredients to add to shopping list:

_____   _____

_____   _____

My *Always Delicious* Story

Today marks the one-year *"AH*-versary" for my husband and me. *Always Hungry?* has changed our lives for the better. The scale results are not earth shattering, but the NSVs (non-scale victories) are exciting! HDL up, LDL down, triglycerides way down, glucose down! My husband just can't believe how much more energy he has. No more afternoon crashes while at work.

Key to our success is the habit of weekly meal planning, which helped us stop thinking about food all the time ("What am I going to have for dinner?") and kept us on track with weekly grocery shopping. We have also managed to dine out and drink with friends with only a little detour. And we know if our detour lasts too long, we gain weight and feel tired and bloated. It's amazing how we can "hear" our bodies speaking to us!

And no more artificial anything or processed foods. We love the recipes and always have frozen meal portions at the ready in case life throws a curve. This has truly been an eye-opening journey and one we will continue for life.

Ann C., age 63, Berlin, Connecticut

PREP DAY

When a professional chef walks into the kitchen, everything is prepped, pulled out, and ready to use—a culinary concept known as *mise en place* (French for "put in place"). With this system, prep cooks organize all the ingredients of a dish so that the chef can make a fresh meal from scratch as the customer waits. Unfortunately, most of us don't have the luxury of prep cooks at home (although children or a spouse provide an affordable alternative). You can still create professional-quality meals quickly with key items prepared in advance, and Prep Day simplifies the process.

Prep Day involves setting aside a few hours once a week, typically on a weekend, to make special sauces, cook proteins, assemble casseroles, prepare whole-kernel grains, and roast nuts. If you followed the *Always Hungry?* meal plans, you already have practice with this time-saving method. Here are some efficient choices for Prep Day (a Weekly Prep Day Worksheet is available online at www.drdavidludwig.com):

- Sauces (pages 283 to 306) such as Smoked Paprika Ketchup (page 291), breakfast shakshuka sauce (page 85), and enchilada sauce for the Quinoa Enchilada

Casserole (page 183), and seasonings like All-Purpose Seasoned Salt (page 283) are nice to have ready when you need them. Also plan for sauces whose flavors improve after a few days like Sugar-Free Worcestershire Sauce (page 284) or any of the salad dressings.

- Casseroles that take time to assemble but can be baked quickly, with little oversight, like Green Chile Chicken or Beef Enchilada Casserole (page 124), Black Bean Pâté (page 274), or Sage Walnut Lentil Loaf (page 168).
- Chickpea Bread Crumbs (page 196) or other ingredients needed as components in various recipes.
- Whole grains like Cooked Quinoa (page 231) or Pressure-Cooked Brown Rice (page 226) or other grains (see Guide to Cooking Whole Grains, page 333).
- Beans to have cooked and ready to use as a side dish or in a variety of recipes (see Do-It-Yourself Beans, page 74).
- Roasted nuts for snacks (see Guide to Roasting Nuts, page 334).
- Proteins like Shredded Chicken (page 110), Shredded Beef (page 148), Baked Tofu (page 175), or ones that can be used as the basis for quick meals.
- Soups to accompany a meal, like Cuban Black Bean (page 253) or Polish White Borscht (page 246) that are even better the next day, or soups that make a complete meal with the addition of fresh greens or seafood before serving, like Portuguese Seafood Stew (page 241) or Thai Coconut Fish Soup (page 238).
- Desserts that need time to set or cool like Coconut BonBons (page 316), Chocolate Truffles (page 314), or Pumpkin Pie Tartlets (page 322).

The Secret Is the Sauce

Sauces provide a luscious, convenient source of healthy fats in many of our recipes. Making them ahead of time lets you quickly create restaurant-quality flavors with almost any dinner. But don't be intimidated. Our sauces require no special culinary skills or fancy ingredients. With an immersion blender, a jar, and a few basic ingredients, you can prepare a luscious sauce in just a few minutes—and no dishes to clean! Best of all, home-prepared sauces offer top quality at minimum cost. On a busy night, a premade sauce can mean the difference between making a simple, satisfying meal and resorting to takeout.

Prep-Ahead Mind-Set

Prepping ahead needn't happen only on Prep Day. Every time you cook, consider how to save time and effort for the future. For example, with a casserole, make an extra-large amount so that you can freeze leftovers in individual portions. On days that you lack the time or inclination to cook, simply defrost one of those premade meals for a homemade "TV dinner." This strategy works best for soups, proteins, whole grains, and other items that store well in the refrigerator or freezer. Some dishes, like soups, taste even better after flavors have had time to develop.

STOCK AND ORGANIZE YOUR KITCHEN

With any new dietary program, a well-stocked, well-organized kitchen will help keep you on track. The basic idea is to fill up the home with so much nutritious, delicious foods, there will be no room left for all those mindlessly eaten, unhealthful items.

Soon after beginning the *Always Hungry?* program, one reader was shocked to see her daughter casually pick up and eat a pear. Although this mother had always kept fresh fruit available, her children passed them by in favor of the many processed, packaged foods in the cupboards. But since the kitchen cleanout, the kids reached for fruit without thinking twice. Out of sight, out of mind. Why fight temptations when you can eliminate them?

Make a list of fresh fruits and vegetables, proteins, snacks, nonperishables, freezer items, herbs and spices, and Prep Day foods that you use most often. Having these basics on hand will let you make a meal when there's no time to shop, and protect you from the accusation that "there's nothing in the house to eat!"

My *Always Delicious* Story

After reading *Always Hungry?* on vacation last summer, my husband and I decided to implement it. We asked our fifteen-year-old daughter if she would be interested in coming along for the ride. To our surprise, she jumped on board, and the three of us began to eat the *AH* way. Fast-forward nine months: My husband is lighter than he has been since we were married, and he feels great. My daughter has lost a little weight, but more important, we can *see* the difference. Her clothing fits better. She feels nourished from breakfast until lunchtime. She feels better about her food choices and her weight. Her activity level hasn't changed drastically and she hasn't grown taller—it's what she's been eating! So happy that this method has led our family to a healthier place.

Jeanette C., age 43, Fayetteville, Pennsylvania

Spice It Up

Stock a variety of dried herbs and spices to provide flavorful alternatives to sugar and other unwholesome additives. The style of food you like most will help guide selection. Choose a few styles and then expand out from there (some spices transcend categories). Herbs and spices provide a world of flavors and a rich source of health-promoting anti-inflammatory phytochemicals.

Mexican-style seasonings—Fresh, dried, or powdered chiles (ancho, chipotle, or any other favorites), cumin, garlic powder, paprika, and Mexican oregano (a spicier alternative to traditional oregano).

Italian seasonings—Basil, marjoram, thyme, oregano, rosemary, and plenty of garlic.

French seasonings—Any of a variety of fresh herbs, especially tarragon, chives, dill, shallots, parsley, sage, thyme, rosemary, and bay leaf. (Herbes de Provence is a common mixture that includes a bit of lavender.)

Asian spices—Most often used fresh or refrigerated, including ginger, garlic, cilantro, and dried or ground chiles or chile pastes. (An Asian pantry may also include soy sauce, a sweet cooking wine called mirin, miso, unseasoned rice vinegar, sesame seeds, toasted sesame oil, and specialty mushrooms like shiitake or maitake.)

Indian spices—Cumin, ginger, powdered chiles, ground turmeric, coriander, fennel seed, aniseed, garlic, and cilantro, with much variation by geographic region (also try spice mixtures such as garam masala).

Middle Eastern, Moroccan, North African—Cumin, ginger, paprika, aniseed, coriander, sumac, various sweet spices or spice blends (such as za'atar, ras el hanout, or baharat), and fresh ingredients like lemon, tahini, garlic, olives, mint, pomegranate, coconut milk, and spicy chile pastes (harissa).

Chiles—Versatile ingredients that transcend borders, with many different flavors and levels of heat. Try Korean pepper (in dried or fermented forms, in pastes, or even the probiotic-rich kimchi), New Mexico green chiles, Thai chiles, jalapeños, poblanos, Anaheims, and more.

Sweet spices—Cinnamon, cardamom, nutmeg, allspice, and clove (can be used for desserts or mixed with savory spices in Middle Eastern, Moroccan, or Indian cuisine).

Store dried herbs and spices in a cool, dry location (e.g., not above the stove) and replace unused portions once or twice a year. Keep in mind that some spices are so strong that they may take over a dish. With rosemary, tarragon, smoked paprika, or chipotle peppers, a little goes a long way.

Keep Healthy Snack Foods Front and Center

Fresh nontropical fruits, raw vegetables (like carrots, celery, and bell peppers), roasted nuts and nut butters, hummus, cheese, and very dark chocolate are some of the easy items to keep on hand. Among the many snack recipes in the book, you can whip up a batch of crepes (page 197) or wraps (page 198), Socca Pinwheels (page 273), quesadillas (page 199), or Socca Crackers (page 202) anytime.

At the request of our Facebook community, we created Mint Chocolate Power Balls (page 279)—a mouth-watering and money-saving alternative to those nutritionally dubious snack bars. For other convenient grab-and-go options, try Chile Cheese Fritters (page 204), Quinoa Croquettes (page 232), or Grain-Free Pumpkin Spice Muffins (page 90).

Clean Out the Kitchen

Perform a complete kitchen cleanout as you begin your *Always Delicious* journey (see *Always Hungry?*, pages 134–138) and schedule cleanouts every three to six months. Mark them in your calendar now for a helpful reminder down the road. Regular cleanouts will not only rid the pantry of unsupportive foods that tend to creep back in, but also rekindle your energy and enthusiasm for the program. Every kitchen cleanout makes for a fresh start.

LET YOUR TOOLS DO THE WORK

Time efficiency in the kitchen means finding tools that make your life easier. Whether it's a food processor to chop vegetables or an immersion blender for soups and sauces, the right tools, appliances, and cookware provide years of return on investment. Here's a list of our favorites:

- **Food processor:** You don't need to spend a lot of money; most inexpensive models work just as well.
- **Immersion blender:** These often come with a small food processor and a whisk attachment. Using this tool, you can make any creamed soup in a flash, with quicker cleanup and less risk of splattering hot liquid than with a standing blender.
- **Blender:** Comes in handy for shakes, smoothies, sauces, and dips (you can forgo this one if you have an immersion blender).
- **Toaster oven:** Convenient for roasting nuts and reheating leftovers.
- **Vegetable spiralizer:** An optional but fun and inexpensive tool for making noodles or fun garnishes with zucchini, carrots, beets, and other vegetables.
- **Microplane zester or other fine grater:** This sharp little tool is perfect for grating ginger (see Chef Dawn's Tasty Tip, page 289).
- **Coffee grinder:** A separate grinder (in addition to the one you might use for coffee beans) for grinding spices, chia seeds, and flaxseeds will provide for the freshest ingredients.
- **Silicone spatulas:** These don't melt or stain like the rubber varieties.
- **Cast-iron skillet:** Naturally nonstick when properly "seasoned" (coated with a protective oil layer), this classic cookware evenly distributes heat, creating a nicely browned surface (see Chef Dawn's Tasty Tip, page 167).
- **Pressure cooker, slow cooker, or combination:** Modern pressure cookers, which can reduce cooking time by 50 percent or more, are virtually foolproof and require very little attention. Slow cookers allow you to start a meal in the morning and have it ready for dinner. Often these two appliances are combined into one convenient unit (such as the popular Instant Pot), saving time and money. On busy days, these appliances can be a saving grace.
- **Good-quality knife:** Keep your knives sharp, and learn how to use them properly (take a knife-skills class or find a video on the web).
- **Wooden cutting board:** Separate cutting boards for fruit, cheese, meats, and strong spices will keep your pears from tasting like garlic. When prepping oily foods, wipe the board with water before and after to prevent food oils from seeping into the cutting board. Although recommendations vary, wooden

cutting boards resist bacteria better than plastic, and they are easier on your knives.

- **Glass canning jars:** Use these jars to store everything from dried beans and grains to prepared sauces. Inexpensive and readily available, glass containers prolong the shelf life of dry foods and keep leftovers visible, increasing the likelihood that they will be eaten (remember, "out of sight, out of mind").

FRESH AND SEASONAL INGREDIENTS

Before rapid international transportation, most people naturally ate in rhythm with the seasons. Fresh berries simply weren't available during the winter in Boston, nor were apples in summer. Although today virtually any food can be purchased at any time of year, a tomato picked green and shipped halfway around the world can never compare with the vine-ripened variety. Often, fresh seasonal ingredients are available in abundance, at a lower price.

Using seasonal produce also instills a sense of adventure in the kitchen. Sign up for a Community Supported Agriculture (CSA) "crop share" to have weekly allotments of fresh produce either delivered to your home or available for pickup at the farm. Design your weekly meal plan around foods harvested at the peak of ripeness, potentially traveling from farm to table in just a day or two. You won't believe the difference in flavor from the standard industrial fare. Many grocers have begun carrying local produce as well. Plus, when buying local foods, you help stimulate your community's economy, while tending to reduce environmental impacts.

Make the Most of Every Ingredient

Once you have your fresh ingredients, make the most of them. Use green bags to extend the life of vegetables and fruits (for example, http://evertfresh.com). At the end of the week, make soups, casseroles, Summer Grilled or Roasted Vegetables (page 215), Herb Roasted Root Vegetables (page 214), or Pickles (pages 62 to 71) with leftover produce. You can even make soup stock with vegetable scraps like onion skins, celery tops, and parsley stems (store them in an airtight container in the refrigerator or in a bag in the freezer until ready to use).

Grow Your Own Kitchen Herbs

Many herbs are hearty and easy to grow, so you don't need any special gardening skills—a few pots on a well-lit windowsill will do. With a home herb garden, you just snip a little sprig for use in a recipe or as a garnish on soups and salads. Save money as you enjoy unsurpassed freshness. Some good options for a home garden include rosemary, thyme, basil, oregano, sage, cilantro, parsley, chives, dill, and mint.

Extend the Life of Your Herbs

Fresh herbs may have a short shelf life once harvested. If you can't maintain a garden, consider creative ways to preserve any leftover store-bought herbs. For example, basil can be made into Basil Walnut Pesto (page 297) and kept in the refrigerator for a week or two. Or freeze the pesto in ice cube trays, then store the cubes in a freezer-safe bag. These small portions can be added to soups or other recipes in the amounts needed. Ginger can be pureed and refrigerated, or peeled and frozen (see Chef Dawn's Tasty Tip, page 289). An elegant preservation method is to make herbed butters or infused olive oil.

Chef Dawn's Tasty Tip

The Essentials

A modern alternative to fresh herbs is food-grade essential oils. These natural extracts are relatively inexpensive, considering how little you use, and never go to waste. I keep a variety around for times when I don't have the right fresh ingredient. Add a small drop to entrées, sautéed vegetables, soups, or shakes for a time-saving blast of flavor. Lemon, ginger, dill, lemongrass, and orange are a few of my favorites.

MAKING THE SWAP: FOOD SUBSTITUTIONS

There are many reasons why people might have to modify their diet, including food allergies, medical indications (e.g., reduced sodium for high blood pressure), health preferences (sugar-, gluten-, or dairy-free), specific food aversions, and ethical preferences (vegetarian or vegan). If someone in the family has a severe allergy, that food might be excluded from the entire household. Whatever the reason, special diets present a special challenge for any chef.

Revisionist Recipes

All too often, special diets can feel restrictive, with an inevitable focus on the foods that *can't* be eaten—creating a desire for revised recipes made to taste the same with substituted ingredients. This revisionist approach may work well in certain circumstances, such as using chickpea flour instead of processed grains to make crepes, crackers, and piecrust (see chapter 7). Substituting peanuts with tree nuts makes perfect sense for someone with an allergy. However, many revisionist recipes frankly never stand up to the original, at least as we remember them, and may have nutritionally dubious results. Store-bought gluten-free baked goods usually contain highly processed starches with even higher glycemic load than the original versions, and imitation dairy may include a long list of artificial additives.

Another problem with the revisionist approach is a tendency to miss out on delicious new recipes that don't need to be altered at all. If you find yourself struggling to accommodate everyone in your family, choose from among the many options in *Always Delicious* designed for a wide range of special needs.

"I Just Don't Like That"

You or someone in your family might not like the flavor, texture, or even color of a food or recipe. That's okay! Simply choose another recipe or substitute a different ingredient for the one that doesn't appeal, using "like for like" to maintain macronutrient ratios (see the Equivalents Table, page 49, for guidance).

However, as we explored in chapter 2, virtually all food preferences (except for sugar) are "acquired tastes." When you retrain your fat cells with a diet that lowers insulin levels and calms chronic inflammation, you automatically retrain your taste buds, too. You'll naturally find yourself less attracted to the hyperprocessed, hypersweet stuff, and increasingly interested in new, more complex flavors. Give yourself some time as your body adjusts. Use symptom trackers to monitor hunger, cravings, energy level, and physical symptoms (download these forms at www.drdavidludwig.com). As your body responds to the *Always Delicious* way of eating, a whole new world of flavors may unfold.

My *Always Delicious* Story

Before *Always Hungry?*, I could never eat one cookie or just taste dessert. It was all or nothing. Carbs were everything, preferably crusty whole wheat bread and raisins—healthy cheats, I thought. I wanted to lose weight, but more important, I wanted to stop craving and thinking about food all the time.

AH has now been part of my life for fourteen months. Food in an *AH* balanced meal tastes unimaginably delicious. Bread no longer calls my name. A bag of raisins lasts a very long time. I savor the sweetness of berries, the richness of full-fat yogurt. I don't go looking for "something else" after dinner. In addition, I have more energy, improved mental clarity, and better quality time. This is invaluable.

Leslie N., age 75, Hillsdale, New Jersey

COMPOSE A MEAL EFFICIENTLY

Orchestrating a meal so that each dish comes out at the right time is one of the most challenging aspects of cooking for many people. However, with a little practice, it's not hard to become a true maestro. Try these tips:

- Prep Day: Prepare any time-consuming components that can be made in advance (see page 32).
- Read the recipe through before you start, and develop a mental timeline. Begin with steps that take the longest, using the intervals between productively. For example, if a recipe calls for 30 minutes of simmering, get that started first, then chop vegetables or do other tasks.
- Put a pot of water on the stove to boil, saving time in case you need hot water to add to soups, for blanching vegetables, etc.
- Chop as you go. Prechopped produce is convenient but expensive, and often not as fresh. Chopping all your vegetables beforehand typically takes extra time; it's more efficient to weave chopping into the inevitable downtimes during meal preparation. For example, if a recipe requires cooking onions for 3 to 5 minutes before adding other vegetables, chop the onion while the oil heats on low in the pan. Turn the heat up, add the onion, and chop the other vegetables as the onion cooks, pausing occasionally to stir.

- Let your tools do the work, like using a food processor for chopping. No need to wash the processor bowl between different vegetables.
- Distinguish between recipes that require precise timing (set a timer for these) and ones that don't. For example, sautéed onions or soups (and the sautéed vegetables that will be added to them) are often even more delicious with extra cooking time.
- Put dessert on to cook or to set in the refrigerator when you sit down for dinner, such as Chocolate-Dipped Fruit (page 313), Poached Pears (page 325), or even Apple Pie Parfait (page 319).
- Be adventuresome. If you don't have one ingredient, don't be afraid to experiment with something else instead. You might create a new masterpiece!

Chef Dawn's Tasty Tips

My Kitchen Rules

Years of training chefs, providing nutritional guidance, and cooking for my own family have taught me a lot about what works and what doesn't. In my kitchen, I have only a few rules:

1. Be gentle on yourself and others—not everyone is on the same path. Meet people where they are with love and compassion (including yourself). Model the behavior you want to see.
2. If it's not delicious, it's not worth it. A fundamental principle of the *Always Delicious* way of eating is "diet without deprivation." Find foods that you love instead of ones you just tolerate. Make your meals beautiful, be creative with ingredients and presentation, and have fun—all of which make great food taste even better!
3. Everything is a "learning opportunity." If a dish doesn't turn out right, or disaster strikes, remember Rule #1 and see what you can learn for the future. And remember, brilliant discoveries sometimes emerge by accident.
4. If you choose to eat something that you know doesn't support your health, do it mindfully and:
   a. Enjoy every bite.
   b. Leave shame, blame, and guilt at the doorstep.
   c. Start over in the next moment. Getting back on track is only one bite away.

My *Always Delicious* Story

I read *Always Hungry?* in February 2016, started my prep, and dived right into Phase I. I joined the fledgling Facebook community, and found a positive, supportive, loving group of people who became immediately important to me. My food cravings disappeared miraculously, but weight loss was slow at first.

Then in late August, my husband of forty-two years announced, out of the blue, that he was leaving—and a month later he did. *AH* was my salvation during this terrible time. Although my prep was derailed, I only had *AH* foods in my house and was totally comfortable with that. I was no longer attracted to the junk foods that previously comforted me in my sorrow. I didn't always have many choices at home, and ended up having lots of eggs and power shakes as I navigated being alone after a lifetime. Now, five months later, I still don't plan diverse menus like I'd like to, but am gentle to myself. I've been so aware through it all of how grateful I was for this plan and the Facebook community as my life crumbled and I began the hard work of rebuilding.

I'm not there yet. It really takes a long time. But I have an amazing pot of lentils in the slow cooker, fresh fruit ready for breakfast, and homemade almond butter chocolate chip cookies in the freezer as an occasional treat.

Speaking of healthy, I have lost 22 pounds and much of my over-sixties belly fat. Now that I'm putting myself out there more and even thinking about dating again, I love the way I look. A new hairstyle, some less frumpy clothes, and an attitude of trying new things and getting out of my comfort zone. Watch out world!

Nancy B., age 65, Houston, Texas

PLAN FOR AND USE LEFTOVERS CREATIVELY

To save time in the kitchen, learn to repurpose ingredients. Repurposing leftovers also saves money, and allows you to produce greater variety with less effort.

- Use leftover cooked vegetables from the day before as a base for a soup, sauce, or casserole. Precooked ingredients can add depth of flavor, which is why professional chefs build intricate recipes in a multistep process.
- Make extra portions of basic ingredients for use in other recipes. The same dish becomes boring by the third day. But you can keep things interesting with minor variations and additions. Serve soup chilled one night and hot

the next, perhaps garnished with toasted pumpkin seeds on one occasion and fresh herbs on another. Add beans for a heartier dish, or puree for a creamier texture. For any leftover soup, add cheese and a protein to create a casserole or use as the base for a gravy or cream sauce.

- Skip the prep step entirely with a strategic purchase. For example, a store-bought rotisserie chicken can be spiced up or down depending on the recipe. Make a chicken salad, a Buddha Bowl (pages 263 to 269), or a Socca Wrap (page 198) and serve with a sauce.

Like many kitchen skills, repurposing ingredients takes practice. Your dishes might not always work out, but experimenting with leftovers will build confidence. There's only one rule for leftovers—always add something fresh to keep meals lively and nutritionally varied. Skilled use of leftovers can transform cooking from a tedious chore to an outlet for creative expression.

OBSTACLES AND IF-THEN PLANNING

What gets in the way of achieving your diet-related health goals? For many people, the number one challenge is finding time to cook. As discussed in *Always Hungry?* (pages 130–131), we can use if-then planning to devise a list of quick, easy recipes for those extra-busy days. The key is to keep your kitchen stocked with the basics and know which choices to make when you need a quick meal. Here are some suggestions:

- **Quick-Cooking Beans:** Choose lentils when you want legumes but haven't soaked any in advance. Lentils take only 30 minutes to cook and require very little attention. Make them into a hot dish one day, a salad the next, and a soup after that.
- **Quick-Cooking Grains:** Quinoa, millet, and buckwheat take only 20 to 30 minutes to cook and can be used in a hot side dish, a soup, or a cold salad.
- **Stir-Fry:** Cut chicken thighs or tofu into small pieces or cubes and cook them on the stovetop in your favorite sauce. Toss in a few vegetables and serve over a bed of spinach, Cauliflower Couscous (page 211), or whole grains.

- **Sheet Pan Dinner:** Marinate or simply toss quick-cooking protein (tofu, shrimp, or small pieces of meat) with your favorite sauce and chopped vegetables. Spread the ingredients into a single layer on a baking sheet, and bake at 350°F until the protein is done for a no-fuss entrée.
- **Ready-to-Go Proteins:** Keep sardines (with skin and bones), canned salmon or tuna, canned chicken, smoked salmon, eggs, precooked and flavored tofu, or other quick proteins around as a base for emergency meals in minutes.
- **Buddha Bowls:** Turn a hodgepodge of leftovers into an impressive bowl topped with your favorite sauce. See page 263 for ideas.

Make your own list of obstacles to success, and plan for contingencies. With a bit of practice, you'll be able to adapt to almost anything life has to offer.

PRESENTATION AND FOOD APPEAL

We eat with our eyes first. Visually appealing food simply tastes better, and this principle has special importance when preparing to-go meals, presenting a new meal to your family, or serving food for parties. Opening a lunch container to find mush can be discouraging and make you head for the nearest vending machine. The extra few minutes needed for beautiful food presentation can mean the difference between your family devouring or rejecting an otherwise delicious meal.

On Prep Day, create colorful garnishes like scallions or carrot flowers (use specially designed vegetable cutters for this purpose), and store them covered with water in an airtight container to use throughout the week. Serve fun sauces, dips, and spreads in attractive small bowls to accommodate different taste preferences. Consider colors and textures as you prepare your recipes and meal plans. And involve your children as much as possible, for example arranging vegetables on a plate or combining ingredients for a special sauce. If they helped make it, they're more likely to eat it.

Invest in attractive food containers, especially those that can be used to serve and store food—which have the additional benefit of making cleanup easy. If someone in your family eats lunch away from home, find nonbreakable containers with sections to separate different foods. With lunches eaten, not returned, you'll maintain nutrition quality and save money.

My *Always Delicious* Story

As I was discussing mealtime "issues" with some other moms, I realized that *Always Hungry?* has given our family a special NSV—family breakfast and dinner! After starting the meal plan, I decided instead of two or three choices for the family (short-order cook that I was), we would all eat the same thing. We have been sharing hot breakfast together every morning ever since, and I feel like my children are now going to school with full bellies and full hearts—quite the contrast to our former hurried, stressful meals! We have also elevated our family dinners by using our good china and silverware every night. After all, this food is worthy of celebrating! The kids look forward to our "fancy" dinners, sit longer, try new things, talk more, and enjoy food I am proud to prepare and serve them!

Megan D., age 40, Dripping Springs, Texas

GETTING OUT OF COOKING RUTS

Many of us are creatures of habit, and tend to make the same familiar recipes over and over again. A repertoire of beloved recipes in rotation may save effort, but can also make for a food rut. As the quality of your diet improves, your palate likely will evolve. To keep things interesting and allow for continued growth, change something on a regular basis. Choose a few of these suggestions (or make up your own) and mark them on your calendar for automatic rut prevention.

- Make one recipe you've never tried from *Always Hungry?*, *Always Delicious*, or another cookbook or online source.
- Join a local CSA to receive a package of fresh produce each week or two. Then find creative ways to incorporate the changing seasonal items.
- Once a month, try one food you thought you didn't like, to see if your tastes have changed.
- If you eat meat at most meals, try a plant-based variation of any *Always Hungry?* or *Always Delicious* recipe.
- Invite a friend over to cook with you. Their food ruts might just inspire you, and vice versa.
- Explore an ethnic restaurant for new ideas about flavor combinations. Looking at menus online can provide inspiration even if you don't eat out.

- Choose a basic ingredient you enjoy, and challenge yourself to find new ways to use it.
- Mix your favorite herbs into softened butter or olive oil and serve as a garnish with plain proteins like steak, chicken, fish, tofu, or tempeh.
- Identify one entirely new ingredient each month and find out how to use it (go online for inspiration).
- Enroll in a culinary class to learn new techniques, or find some free cooking videos online.
- Do a reset by cooking the first 2 to 3 weeks' menus from *Always Hungry?*

Time Flies When You Are Having Fun

One of the best ways to sustain the practice of home cooking is to have fun! Put on your favorite music. Go ahead, play with your food. Arrange to cook with a friend. You could each make a double batch of three sauces to share, or do Prep Day together. If you have children, include them in the kitchen fun. This is an investment with returns for a lifetime.

GETTING STARTED WITH *ALWAYS DELICIOUS* RECIPES AND MEAL PLANS

Look through the Program Foods Summary for a quick review of the foods you'll eat on each of the three phases (for a more comprehensive list, see *Always Hungry?*, pages 110–117).

PROGRAM FOODS SUMMARY PHASE BY PHASE

	Phase 1	*Phase 2*	*Phase 3*
Grains (refer to Guide to Cooking Whole Grains, page 333)	No	Yes, 100% whole grains (intact-kernel), up to 3 servings per day	Yes, whole and processed grains as your body tolerates
Starchy Vegetables	No	Yes, except white potato	Yes, as tolerated

(continued)

	Phase 1	Phase 2	Phase 3
Legumes	Yes	Yes	Yes
Greens and other nonstarchy vegetables	Unlimited	Unlimited	Unlimited
Fruit	Yes, but avoid tropical, dried, and fruit juices	Yes, but avoid fruit juices	Yes, adjust as your body tolerates
High-Protein Foods	Yes, 4 to 6 ounces with every meal	Yes, 4 to 6 ounces with every meal	Yes, 4 to 6 ounces with every meal
Fats and High-Fat Foods	Yes, at every meal	Yes, at every meal (about 25% less than in Phase 1)	Yes, at every meal (about 25% less than in Phase 1)
Dairy and Nondairy Milks	Yes (no added sugar)	Yes	Yes
High-Carbohydrate Sweets and Snack Foods	No, except dark chocolate (at least 70% cacao) up to 1 ounce per day	No, except dark chocolate (at least 70% cacao) up to 1 ounce per day	Yes, as tolerated, up to 2 servings per day; avoid highly sweetened beverages
Sugar	No, except for the small amount in dark chocolate	Yes, up to 3 teaspoons of added sugar daily, preferable in the form of honey or maple syrup	Yes, up to 6 teaspoons of added sugar daily, preferable in the form of honey or maple syrup
Caffeinated Beverages (Feel free to add whole milk or cream in any phase.)	Yes, as desired, 2 or 3 servings daily, unsweetened	Yes, as desired, 2 or 3 servings daily. You may add 1 to 2 teaspoons honey, maple syrup, or sugar.	Yes, as tolerated. You may add 1 to 2 teaspoons honey, maple syrup, or sugar.
Diet Drinks and Artificial Sweeteners	Avoid	Avoid (occasional small amounts of natural stevia are okay)	Avoid (occasional small amounts of natural stevia are okay)
Alcohol	No (it's just 2 weeks!)	Yes, 1 to 2 drinks per day maximum as tolerated	Yes, 1 to 2 drinks per day maximum as tolerated

ALWAYS DELICIOUS RECIPES AND MEAL SUGGESTIONS

In the following chapters, you'll find Phase 1, 2, and 3 meal suggestions accompanying the main recipes. Pay special attention to the variations for ways to adapt them to your personal preferences and needs. Many recipes have vegetarian, vegan, dairy-free, egg-free, gluten-free, and spice options. In addition, some Phase 2 and 3 recipes have Phase 1 variations, and vice versa. Along the way, you'll also find Chef Dawn's Tasty Tips on specialty ingredients, tools, and preparations to make kitchen life a little easier.

The meal suggestions are intended to guide you in selecting what foods to serve with the recipes to make a complete meal. The Equivalents Table below offers suggestions on substituting "like for like" foods to maintain macronutrient ratios. Note that quantities shown are not suggested serving sizes, but instead the portion needed to equal the general macronutrient profile of the food being replaced. The table tells you, for example, how much chicken to substitute for beef to provide an equal amount of protein.

For additional guidance in meal design, see the Build-a-Meal tables for each phase in *Always Hungry?* or on our website at www.drdavidludwig.com. But remember, these are just suggestions. Ultimately, our goal is to dispense with counting numbers and rigid adherence to any plan, and instead listen to the wisdom of the body.

EQUIVALENTS TABLE

Meat or Soy	Equivalents
Lower fat/higher protein (0 to 6 g fat and 20 to 30 g protein)	• 4 ounces smoked salmon, turkey bacon, Canadian bacon, turkey breast, chicken breast or tenderloin, chicken or turkey sausage (unsweetened), pork tenderloin, or lamb tenderloin; • 3 or 4 slices Smoke-Dried Tomato Seitan (page 73); • 3½ ounces Basic Seitan (page 72); • 1 serving (approximately 22 grams protein) unflavored, unsweetened 100 percent whey or equivalent vegan protein powder

(continued)

Meat or Soy	Equivalents
Moderate fat/higher protein (6 to 10 g fat and 20 to 26 g protein)	• ½ cup Shredded Chicken (page 110); • 4 ounces cooked salmon or sardines (with skin, packed in oil); 1 large or 2 small chicken drumsticks; • 1 small lamb shank or a few lamb ribs; • 4 ounces ground turkey or buffalo; • 4 ounces beef loin or round, ground beef (90 to 95 percent lean), or boneless, skinless chicken thighs; • heaping ⅓ cup Crumbled Tempeh (page 192); • 5 to 6 ounces Baked Tofu (page 175); • 1 cup cottage cheese; • 1 cup shelled edamame
Higher fat/lower protein (10 to 24 g fat and 16 to 18 g protein)	• ¼ cup Shredded Beef (page 148); • 4 ounces cooked chicken thigh (bone-in, skin-on); • 3 ounces ground beef (85 percent lean) or beef chuck; • 6 ounces Panfried or Deep-Fried Tofu or 4 ounces Panfried or Deep-Fried Tempeh (pages 170 and 193); • 3 large eggs
Vegetarian proteins (10 to 13 g fat and 21 to 25 g protein) *Use to build vegetarian recipes or meals. These may need to be paired with supplemental proteins to create a balanced meal.*	• 6 ounces extra-firm tofu; • 4 ounces tempeh; • 1 cup cottage cheese; • 2 eggs plus 2 egg whites; • 1 cup Greek yogurt; • 3½ ounces Basic Seitan (page 72) (Note: Seitan has essentially no fat. Include an extra tablespoon of oil to the meal to make this vegetarian protein equivalent to the others in this category.) Peanuts, cheese, nuts, and seeds can be used as supplemental proteins, but they have more fat than other vegetarian proteins. Beans can also be used as supplemental protein; however, they are higher in carbohydrate.

Grains	Equivalents
Whole grain to accompany a meal	• ½ cup Cooked Quinoa (page 231), millet, barley, teff, or steel-cut oats; • Heaping ⅓ cup cooked brown rice, farro, or wheat berries; • ¾ cup cooked buckwheat (kasha)
Vegetables	**Equivalents**
Vegetables to accompany a meal	• Blanched or steamed nonstarchy vegetables (see Guide to Cooking Vegetables, page 329) with your favorite dressing or olive oil; • Sautéed vegetables; • Salad greens and chopped vegetables with your favorite dressing or olive oil; • Summer Grilled or Roasted Vegetables (page 215); • Nonstarchy vegetables in Herb Roasted Root Vegetables (page 214)
Fruits	**Equivalents**
Fruit with a meal	• 1 cup whole strawberries; • ½ cup blueberries; • ⅔ cup raspberries or blackberries; • 1 small peach or other stone fruit; • ½ medium apple; • ½ small pear; • 1 tangerine or ½ large orange

My *Always Delicious* Story

As a junior in college, I've watched my parents on the *Always Hungry?* program since the book came out and finally joined them when I was home for the holidays. I had spent the last seven years starving, frustrated, and sluggish while completing every diet fad I could find, beginning when I was just thirteen. It's been an incredibly long, painful journey with food, but I feel that I have finally found both security and freedom. Before, I ravenously craved sugary foods and had a diet extremely high in white starchy carbohydrates and nonfat, fake "diet" foods. Now my most common craving is berries, and I finish a meal or snack feeling calm and satisfied. I not only regained control of my relationship with food, but also noticed an incredible improvement in mental clarity and focus that has been directly reflected in my grade point average. This has been a true life-changer, and I can't imagine ever not eating this way.

Sophia A., age 20, Portland, Oregon

My *Always Delicious* Story

I started gaining weight after breaking four vertebrae in a snowboarding accident twelve years ago. I do not, nor have I ever, taken narcotic painkillers. Needless to say, I lived with a great deal of pain, and had basically given up hope for a physically active life. But I just now came in from a run. Yes…a run! And my energy levels are through the roof. I attribute my transformation to losing 100 pounds and the anti-inflammatory properties of *AH*. Okay, here's the data:

	Jan 2016 (pre AH)	May 2017
Weight, pounds	256	156
BMI	34.7	21.1
Waist, inches	48	30
Body Fat %	40+	14

As I started losing more and more weight, I was worried I would have excess skin around my belly. None at all, I mean none. I realize that is pure vanity, but that absolutely thrills me.

And here's a fun NSV. I recently needed new trousers, as again the ones I had were too big. (I've changed waist size so many times since *AH*, the Nordstrom's sales associates know me by name!) I tried on slim fit and to my shock, they fit!

Brian G., age 46, Charlotte, North Carolina

CHAPTER 4

Do It Yourself (DIY)

Why "do it yourself"? Once you begin changing your diet and reading nutrition labels, you'll start to notice everything that's been added to store-bought foods: hidden sugars and chemical additives galore. You'll also realize that constantly buying prepared foods is much harder on your wallet than preparing food at home.

We have found that our readers begin preparing their own food products for three main reasons: cost effectiveness, a desire for products not currently available, and an intention to replace currently available foods that use questionable or low-quality ingredients. Adding simple homemade items to your diet can help your budget as much as it does your health. At first glance, a can of beans seems like an inexpensive choice, but when you compare it to the price of dried beans, you'll realize you can save so much money by simply cooking the beans at home. The resulting dish is also tastier and more satisfying.

Gluten-free foods and vegetarian substitutes, such as seitan, vegan cheeses, and sour cream, are often only available with poor-quality, high-glycemic-index ingredients and additives. To get the full benefit from these products, they are best made at home so that you can be sure of what is and is not in your food.

With a little planning, doing it yourself can be quick and easy. You'll end up with a less-expensive, higher-quality food that tastes even better than store-bought. We'll show you how to make your own Greek yogurt, nut butters, bone broth, cold-brewed coffee, pickles, quick seitan, and beans, as well as some simple and inexpensive spa treatments.

DO-IT-YOURSELF GREEK YOGURT (ALL PHASES)

Making your own yogurt is simple and much less expensive than buying it. It also allows you to control the quality and ensure that you are getting the full-fat unsweetened version, which can be hard to find.

- 1 gallon whole milk
- ¼ cup plain full-fat Greek yogurt, to use as a starter

Step 1: Boil the milk.

Heat the milk in a large pot over medium heat until it starts to boil. Turn off the heat. (Note: In an effort to save time, we have occasionally skipped this step, but the resulting yogurt has a slightly slimy texture.)

Step 2: Pour the milk into jars.

Distribute the boiling milk evenly among four quart-size glass canning jars. (This serves the dual purpose of sanitizing the jars as you make the yogurt.)

Step 3: Cool the milk to 115°F.

Either let the jars cool naturally by setting them aside, or speed up the process by immersing the jars into a large pot or Dutch oven filled with ice water. Stir or whisk the milk inside the jars to cool. Measure the temperature using an instant-read thermometer (available at kitchen stores).

Step 4: Add the starter.

Once the milk has cooled to about 115°F, whisk 1 tablespoon of the Greek yogurt into each jar to start the fermentation process. Cover the jars loosely with their lids.

Step 5: Ferment the milk.

Place a large pot or Dutch oven on the counter and arrange the jars in it. (Use two pots if not all the jars fit.) Fill a kettle with hot tap water and pour the water into the pot around the outside of the jars to within 2 to 3 inches from the top of the jars.

Leave the pot on the counter for 8 to 10 hours. The hot tap water will slowly cool down, but will be enough to keep the yogurt at the right temperature for fermentation. (In colder climates, place the pot in the oven with the oven off.)

Remove the jars and strain (see step 6) or refrigerate until you have time. No transferring or dishwashing needed.

Step 6: Strain the yogurt.

Place a flour sack cloth, muslin cloth, or unbleached coffee filter inside a large mesh strainer or colander. Set the strainer over a large bowl. Pour the yogurt into the cloth or coffee filter and let it drain for an hour or two, stirring occasionally to redistribute the whey and facilitate drainage. Strain to the desired consistency; the more whey that drains, the thicker the yogurt will be.

Step 7: Store the yogurt.

Transfer the yogurt to clean containers or jars, or back to the original jar if you strained it immediately rather than refrigerating it; set the drained whey aside. Place the lids on the jars and store in the refrigerator for up to a few weeks.

Step 8: Store the whey.

Store the whey in clean jars (you should have 1½ to 2 quarts whey). Here are a few suggestions for using whey:

- Add a few tablespoons or more as a starter to the brine when making quick pickles.
- Use ½ to 1 cup as a hair conditioner after shampooing.
- Add ½ cup or more in place of water in soups or other recipes to add depth of flavor.

The flavor of the yogurt will be affected by:

- **Time**—The longer it ferments, the more sour the taste.
- **Type of Starter**—Different commercial and homemade yogurts have different strains of probiotics. Choose a yogurt starter with a taste profile that you like, and feel free to experiment.
- **Initial Heat**—Using unboiled milk will produce a less thickly set yogurt.

DO-IT-YOURSELF NUT AND SEED BUTTERS (ALL PHASES)

Why buy expensive nut butters when whole nuts cost less and automatically come sugar-free and without additives? Once you see how easy it is to make your own, you'll never go back to store-bought.

Step 1: Choose the nuts and any additions.

Keep in mind that however many nuts you begin with, you will end up with about half that amount in nut butter (i.e., 2 cups nuts = 1 cup nut butter). Make a simple single-nut butter or combine different types of nuts together. Combining stronger-tasting or drier nuts like almonds or hazelnuts with oily, neutral-tasting nuts like cashews creates a smoother, creamier product.

Get creative with additions as well. For example, include cocoa powder, unsweetened coconut flakes or coconut oil, spices, fresh or unsweetened dried fruit, citrus zest, or small amounts of honey or maple syrup.

Step 2: Roast the nuts, if necessary.

Oily nuts like macadamia, cashew, or Brazil nuts can be used raw. Pecans, walnuts, and seeds should be roasted to take full advantage of their flavors. Almonds, hazelnuts, and peanuts can be roasted or used raw—we prefer to lightly roast these to bring out their natural flavors.

Preheat the oven to 350°F.

Spread the nuts or seeds in a single layer on a baking sheet and roast until fragrant, 5 to 12 minutes. (Although buying preroasted nuts might save time, the taste of freshly roasted nuts is worth the little extra effort involved!) Seeds or lightly roasted nuts like almonds, hazelnuts, or peanuts will need only 5 to 8 minutes to become fragrant. Larger nuts like pecans, walnuts, or almonds will require 8 to 12 minutes. Let your nose be your guide. Once the nuts start to smell nutty, they're done. Take them out immediately, as perfectly roasted nuts become bitter quickly when overcooked.

Step 3: Process the nuts.

Place the nuts and any additions in a food processor. (If processing a small amount and including a watery ingredient like fresh fruit, put the nuts and additions in a jar and blend with an immersion blender, or use a high-powered blender.) Process the nuts, scraping the sides of the bowl regularly until the nuts reach the desired consistency. This process involves a few stages. Be patient. First the nuts will break down into coarse pieces. Then the pieces will begin to stick together. Finally the nuts will release their natural oils, becoming the creamy finished product!

Oily nuts like macadamia, cashews, and Brazil nuts will take less time to break down than drier nuts. Almonds and hazelnuts require the longest amount of time, 5 minutes or more. Walnuts and pecans will take an intermediate amount of time to break down into nut butter.

Step 4: Store the nut butter.

Transfer the nut butter to a glass jar with a lid. If you add fresh fruits as we did in the Pear Cinnamon Cashew Butter on page 58, the final product should be stored in the refrigerator. Otherwise, store the nut butter at room temperature for up to 1 month.

Some of our favorite combinations include Walnut Pecan Butter or Honey Peanut Butter. We've also put together a couple of specialty nut butter recipes for you to try.

Coconut Cardamom Macadamia Butter (All Phases)

"Luscious" is the only word for this nut butter. Great for any occasion; serve on apple slices or other fruit slices or with berries for a rich and delicious snack.

Preparation time: 5 minutes

Total time: 5 minutes

Makes about ¾ cup

- 1 cup macadamia nuts (5 ounces)
- ¼ cup unsweetened coconut flakes (¾ ounce)
- ¼ teaspoon ground cardamom
- ½ teaspoon pure vanilla extract

Place nuts and coconut in the food processor and process until smooth, 3 to 5 minutes. The nuts will go from a coarse meal to a fine meal to a creamy nut butter. Just keep processing until you get a smooth butter. Add cardamom and vanilla and pulse until fully incorporated.

Calories: 53 (Per 1 tablespoon)   Protein: 1 g
Carbohydrate: 2 g   Fat: 5 g

Variations

For Phases 2 and 3: Add 1 teaspoon honey.

Use other favorite spices in place of the cardamom or add other spices like cinnamon, nutmeg, or other sweet spices to enhance the flavor.

For a less expensive choice, use half macadamia nuts and half cashews.

Tip: This is best made at least a day ahead to allow flavors to mellow as they fully meld together.

Pear Cinnamon Cashew Butter (All Phases)

This nut butter acts as its own little snack package, like a bite-size PB&J. The lusciously creamy texture is sure to satisfy, and the sweetness of pears means you won't miss sugary jam. Use as a dip for fruit, a spread for muffins or pancakes, or just eat as is for the ultimate one-bite snack.

Preparation time: 5 minutes

Total time: 15 minutes

Makes about 2 cups

- 2 pears, cored and diced
- 2 tablespoons water
- 1 teaspoon ground cinnamon
- 1 teaspoon pure vanilla extract
- 1 cup cashews

Place the pears and water in a pot and bring to a boil over medium heat. Cover, reduce the heat to low, and simmer for 5 to 8 minutes, or until the pears are soft. Stir in the cinnamon, vanilla, and cashews. Puree directly in the pot with an immersion blender until smooth. It may take a few minutes for the mixture to become smooth—just keep blending until it has the consistency of nut butter.

Transfer to a jar and store in the refrigerator for up to a week or more.

Calories: 28 (Per 1 tablespoon)   Protein: 1 g
Carbohydrate: 3 g   Fat: 2 g

Variations

Use apples (cored) or other fruit of your choice in place of the pears.

DO-IT-YOURSELF BONE BROTH (ALL PHASES)

This deeply nourishing and delicious broth has recently become quite popular, even though the concept has been around since ancient times. When we first started making bone broth for our family, the many recipes, variations, and suggestions seemed overwhelming. After several rounds of trial and error, we landed on the simple, satisfying method described here. We'll also explore other options that can help you find a broth you love. You can use this broth in place of water in many of the recipes in this book.

Preparing and Making Some Decisions

Step 1: Choose the bones.

For rich broth with a thick texture, choose 2 to 5 pounds of bones, including a variety of marrow bones and especially joints like knuckle and neck bones, as they contribute extra collagen to the broth. (If you don't have joint bones, adding chicken feet to any broth will provide extra collagen.) The bones should have very little meat on them. Bones will vary in weight depending on the type you are using. Chicken bones, for example, will be lighter and require fewer pounds than beef bones. Buying bones from your grocer or butcher is usually inexpensive, or you can save leftover bones from home-cooked meals and freeze them in a freezer-safe zip-top bag until you have enough for making broth.

Step 2: Clean the bones and decide on a cooking method.

Wash the bones, making sure to wash your hands well between handling. Avoid cross-contaminating kitchen surfaces with raw meat. Go through the following list to decide how you will prep and cook your broth based on the result that you want.

To Roast or Not to Roast?

Roasting the bones will create a more flavorful broth, but some people prefer simplifying the recipe by skipping this step. Try it both ways. You may find that you like roasting a certain type of bones or using another type unroasted. If you use the roasting method, avoid overcooking, as charred meat contains compounds—including heterocyclic amines and polycyclic aromatic hydrocarbons—reported to be carcinogenic.

To Boil or Not to Boil?

Boiling will create a slightly faster but more cloudy broth with a less consistently subtle flavor; therefore, many recipes recommend gentle simmering, without letting the broth come to a full boil, for 24 to 48 hours. We find that pressure cooking makes an even quicker, convenient alternative, if you don't mind some cloudiness and a little more flavor. However, if you want a subtly flavored, clear broth, then choose the simmer method.

To Skim or Not to Skim?

When bringing the water to a simmer or a boil, a layer of foam may form on the surface. There is some debate as to the contents and impurities comprising the foam. If you want a clearer stock with a subtler flavor, skim off the foam.

Step 3: Consider adding herbs, vegetables, and seasonings if desired.

Depending on your preference for the final product, you may choose to add a few herbs or other ingredients. We prefer to keep it simple—most often the bones are sufficient, but if you are using this as a base for soup, a few large stalks of celery, a whole onion, and whole sprigs of parsley create a nice broth. Strain the broth and discard the vegetables or other solid additions when the broth is finished.

Other additions include:

Vinegar: Adding 1 to 2 tablespoons vinegar is an optional way to help extract minerals from the bones. However, the bones will break down even without the vinegar. Adding vinegar produces a more intense aroma in your home as the broth simmers.

Aromatic Herbs: For more flavor, you could add 1 or 2 bay leaves, a few whole garlic cloves, several sprigs of parsley or other fresh herbs, ½ to 1 teaspoon dried herbs, or whole black peppercorns.

Vegetables: Including vegetables can complicate a broth and cause the texture to become too thick, hard to strain, and/or less versatile in other recipes. You may also lose some of the delicious broth in the vegetable matter that remains after straining. If you do add vegetables, choose only large chunks of onion, leek, or celery and stay away from other root or cruciferous vegetables. Remember, you can always add these ingredients to the finished broth to make a vegetable soup.

Salt: Adding salt during cooking may limit your options for using the broth in other recipes. Taste the finished broth and season as needed.

Cooking the Broth

Step 1: Roast the bones (optional) and place the bones in a pot.

Preheat the oven to 400°F. Place the bones in a single layer in a roasting pan. Roast for about 30 minutes, or until the bones are well browned but not at all burned. Transfer the bones to a large stockpot, slow cooker, or pressure cooker. Add a bit of water to the roasting pan and use a wooden spoon to scrape up the browned bits on the bottom of the pan. Add the contents of the roasting pan to the stockpot.

Step 2: Add other optional ingredients and water.

If using vegetables, herbs, or seasonings, add them to the pot. Add water to cover the bones and vegetables, if using, by at least one inch.

Step 3: Cook the broth.

Simmer Method: Bring broth to a simmer over medium heat without letting the broth come to a boil. Reduce the heat to low, cover, and gently simmer for 24 to 48 hours, or until the bones crumble when crushed with light pressure. (Note, however, that some larger bones will not crumble even after having been fully cooked.) Chicken and turkey bones usually require 24 to 36 hours; larger bones like beef or lamb will require 48 hours or possibly more. Skimming any foam that accumulates on top will keep the foam from forming an insulating layer, facilitating a lower-temperature simmer.

Pressure Cooker: Bring the broth to a boil. Skim off the foam, if desired. Cover and bring to pressure. Pressure cook on high for 1½ to 2 hours for chicken or turkey; 2 to 3 hours for larger bones. Allow the pressure to release naturally.

Combination: Although pressure cooking is fast, simmering helps condense the broth. For a nice compromise with larger bones, pressure cook for 1 hour, then simmer for 24 hours.

Step 4: Strain the broth.

Strain the broth through a fine-mesh colander set over a clean pot or large bowl. Pick through and reserve any meat from the bones; discard the bones and any vegetables and/or herbs like bay leaves. The meat can be returned to the broth or used in soups and other recipes.

Step 5: Store the broth.

Refrigerator: Pour the hot broth, including the fat, immediately into glass canning jars. Place the lids on the jars and refrigerate, allowing the fat to form a protective top layer. Storing broth in this manner, an ancient technique, remains the easiest way to preserve freshness—the hot broth sterilizes the jar; the fat layer keeps moisture in and bacteria out. The broth under the fat layer will keep in the refrigerator for a month or more. Once you break the fat layer, use the broth within a few days.

Freezer: Let the broth cool, skim off the fat to use in other recipes, and pour the broth into a freezer-safe zip-top bag or in ice cube trays to freeze small portions. Once they are frozen, place the broth cubes into a freezer-safe zip-top bag and store in the freezer. It will keep for up to 6 months.

Step 6: Season the broth to use in your recipes.

You may not immediately know which recipes you'll be using the broth in, so it's best not to season it until ready to use. Taste the broth and season with salt, pepper, and/or herbs to taste. Use the broth in any of your favorite recipes or drink a simple cup of broth directly.

DO-IT-YOURSELF COLD-BREWED COFFEE CONCENTRATE (ALL PHASES)

For coffee shakes, it is nice to have a cold, concentrated brew that can be made ahead but doesn't get stale and bitter-tasting when stored. Our answer is DIY. Remember that this cold-brewed coffee is *concentrated*, with more caffeine per cup than your regular coffee or espresso. Either dilute it 50:50 with water, add cream to taste, or use it in a Creamy Vanilla Coffee Shake (page 84).

- 4 cups water
- ¼ pound coffee beans, coarsely ground (about 1½ cups whole beans or 1¼ cups ground)

Place the water and ground coffee in a large jar. Cover and steep in the refrigerator for 24 hours. Strain the coffee concentrate through a fine-mesh sieve lined with a coffee filter and discard the grounds (or let them dry and save them for your coffee scrub spa treatment; see page 78).

Transfer to a clean jar. Store the coffee concentrate in the refrigerator for up to 2 weeks, although the flavor is best within the first week. To serve as iced coffee, dilute the concentrate 50:50 with water or add cream to taste and pour over ice. Use the undiluted concentrate in your favorite recipes that call for coffee.

Tip: Experiment with different types of coffee, water temperatures, and steeping times to create your favorite concentrate. For a faster brew, start with warm water and steep for 8 to 10 hours on the counter, then store in the refrigerator.

DO-IT-YOURSELF PICKLES (ALL PHASES)

With recent research findings on the importance of the "gut microbiome" (the microbes living in our digestive tract), probiotics have been restored to their rightful place in a healthful diet. However, commercial preparations of these "good bacteria" can also come with an expensive price tag. What did our ancestors do before those little refrigerated probiotic capsules? They fermented their foods. Virtually all traditional cultures—around the world and throughout history—have relied on fermented foods to aid digestion and promote overall health. Fermentation was also revered for its ability to preserve foods that could be scarce through the winter and improve nutritional value. Fortunately, this lost art is making a comeback.

The basic concept of pickling is that, under the right condition (typically with salt), the growth of mold and other harmful microorganisms can be inhibited until probiotic bacteria produce enough lactic acid to act as an effective preservative. In the process, wonderful tastes and healthful nutrients are created.

Refer to any of a number of recent popular books on the topic (such as *Wild Fermentation: The Flavor, Nutrition, and Craft of Live-Culture Foods* by Sandor Ellix Katz) for additional guidance and safety measures on fermentation.

Enjoy a tablespoon or two of pickles or other fermented foods with every meal. Your entire digestive tract (including your taste buds) will thank you. Here are a few guidelines and recipes to get you started.

A Primer on Pickling

In this chapter, we consider three types of pickling: long fermentation lasting several weeks (such as Sauerkraut, page 65), short fermentation lasting several days (such as Easy Pickled Cabbage or Carrots, page 66) or nonfermented pickles (such as Quick Ume-Pickled Onions, page 69).

For long and short fermentation, an anaerobic (oxygen-free) environment is required. After a day or two, tiny bubbles will form as the vegetables begin to ferment. Some sources suggest burping the pickling jar lids by loosening them every day or so, to release these gasses (primarily carbon dioxide). However, a water-sealed fermentation lid provides for optimal control of the environment, and is essential for long fermentations.

Our favorite fermentation lid is an airlock lid that fits atop mason jars, allowing fermentation gasses to escape while preventing oxygen from getting in. Alternatively, you can find crocks designed with a water seal around the lid. Both systems can be found online and in specialty kitchen stores. (Note: Nonfermented pickles are made with higher concentrations of salt or vinegar and do not require special equipment.) Especially for smaller-batch ferments, we recommend clear glass jars so you're able to ensure that the vegetables stay packed beneath the level of the liquid, and also to see the tiny bubbles that let you know the fermentation process is working. Wedge a cabbage leaf over the pickled vegetables to hold them under the brine or purchase glass weights that fit into a mason jar to hold the vegetables down.

Use a variety of vegetables, herbs, and spices with any of the following solutions to make salt-based pickles. For best results, we recommend sea salt and filtered water. Regular iodized salt may have anticaking agents and other additives that can disrupt fermentation. Kosher salt is typically additive-free and can be substituted for sea salt. The chlorine in tap or unfiltered water may interfere with fermentation, so use filtered water.

Salt: Some pickles, like sauerkraut, are made by massaging a vegetable with salt, allowing the vegetable to create its own brine as the salt leaches water from the vegetable. This method works best for sturdy, higher-water-content vegetables like cabbage. Use 1½ to 2 teaspoons sea salt per pound of cabbage or other vegetable. This method can also be used to wilt vegetables for a couple of hours before rinsing and adding them to a salt brine (e.g., with watery vegetables like the napa cabbage used in making kimchi).

Salt Brine: Combine 1½ to 2 teaspoons sea salt and 1 cup water in a small saucepan. Heat to fully dissolve the salt. Let cool, then pour over vegetables in a clean canning jar to pickle.

Salt Brine with Vinegar or Liquid Whey: Vinegar or liquid whey from processing Greek Yogurt (see page 54) may also be added as a flavoring and fermentation starter in salt-brine pickles. Add anywhere from 1 tablespoon to ⅓ cup of your favorite vinegar or 2 tablespoons to ½ cup liquid whey per 1 cup water, or to taste. You may also choose to use a lower sodium concentration to pickle vegetables. In this case, you'll need to include the vinegar or liquid whey to inhibit the growth of harmful microorganisms and, in the case of whey, to enhance fermentation.

Soy Sauce: Add ¼ to ⅓ cup soy sauce, depending on the sodium content of the soy sauce and personal preference, to 1 cup water. Sodium content above 1,000 mg per tablespoon will typically require ¼ cup soy sauce, while lower-sodium brands will require up to ⅓ cup.

Umeboshi vinegar: Although it is labeled "vinegar," this product is not truly a vinegar but the pickling brine from the ume plum pickling process. (Note: Umeboshi, one of Chef Dawn's favorite ingredients, can add depth of flavor to salads, vegetables, soups, casseroles, and more. You can find this versatile condiment in whole plum, paste, or vinegar online, at natural foods stores, and in Japanese markets.) For pickling, add ¼ to ⅓ cup umeboshi vinegar, depending on the sodium content, to 1 cup water. Sodium content above 1,000 mg per tablespoon will typically require ¼ cup vinegar, while lower-sodium brands will require up to ⅓ cup.

Sauerkraut (All Phases)

This traditional fermented food is a fantastic source of probiotics and has recently become popular. Although inexpensive to make, sauerkraut can be very expensive to buy, so DIY will really pay off. Choose red or green cabbage and, if desired, add a few small carrots or other hearty root vegetables (shred them before adding). Then add herbs or spices, fresh ginger slices, or other flavorings to create interesting taste profiles. Once you have the basic principles of fermentation, getting creative with ingredients is fun.

- 2 small to medium heads cabbage (about 3 pounds), shredded, plus 1 or 2 whole leaves
- 1½ tablespoons sea salt
- 2 bay leaves, or 1 tablespoon caraway seeds, or to taste (optional)

Place the shredded cabbage into a large bowl. Sprinkle with the salt. Rub the salt into the cabbage, massaging with your hands until the cabbage wilts and releases its juices to form a liquid brine, 10 to 15 minutes with large batches. This may be easier to do with the cabbage and salt evenly divided into two or three smaller batches. At first it may feel like the cabbage is too dry to release enough liquid, but keep pressing and massaging firmly until the cabbage is wet and has released its liquid.

Place one ceramic crock or two quart-size glass canning jars in the sink and fill with boiling water to sterilize. Empty the jars and tightly pack the cabbage and liquid inside, adding a cup or so at a time and pressing until each layer is tightly packed and the liquid begins to rise above the cabbage. Fill the jars to 1 to 2 inches from the top of the jar. Wedge a clean cabbage leaf over the top of the shredded cabbage and tuck it around the edges to hold the shredded cabbage beneath the liquid. The liquid should remain above the top cabbage leaf. If there is not enough liquid, pour salted water (2 teaspoons sea salt dissolved in 1 cup warm filtered water) over the top until the liquid covers the cabbage by about 1 inch.

Cover with a fermentation lid (see A Primer on Pickling, page 63) and set on the counter. Let ferment for a minimum of 10 to 14 days, or up to a couple months, depending on the indoor temperature and the desired flavor. Check the taste after a couple of weeks, using clean utensils, to decide how long you prefer the sauerkraut to pickle. Vegetables will pickle faster in warmer climates. Check to make sure the cabbage stays packed beneath the level of the liquid and add salted water as needed. Skim off any foam that accumulates on the water when you check or taste the sauerkraut. Otherwise, leave the sauerkraut alone for the duration.

When the sauerkraut has fermented to your liking, divide it into smaller portions, if desired. Seal with a regular lid, and refrigerate. The cabbage will continue to slowly pickle in the refrigerator. It will keep longer in the refrigerator than most other pickles, up to 6 months.

Calories: 1 (Per 1 tablespoon)   Protein: 0 g
Carbohydrate: 0 g   Fat: 0 g

Easy Pickled Cabbage or Carrots (All Phases)

Many people consider freshly pickled vegetables more appealing, brighter, and easier to digest than raw vegetables. Use these short-fermentation pickles as a lively topping on salads, in wraps, or as a small vegetable side with each meal. A serving size ranges from a couple of tablespoons to ⅓ cup. Although we call for cabbage or carrots in this recipe, almost any vegetable or combination of vegetables can be used. You may also add garlic, herbs, and/or spices to add flavor variety.

- 1 cup filtered water
- 1½ to 2 teaspoons sea salt
- 4 cups packed shredded cabbage or carrots, or a mixture
- 1 cabbage leaf, rinsed
- A few slices of beet, for color (optional—especially nice to enhance the color of red cabbage)

Warm the water (no need to boil). Stir in the sea salt until it dissolves completely. Set aside to cool (use this time to cut the vegetables). The brine can be made ahead of time and stored in a sealed glass jar on the counter to use when ready to pickle.

Place a quart-size wide-mouthed glass canning jar in the sink and fill with boiling water to sterilize. Empty the jar and tightly pack the vegetable(s) inside to within 1 to 2 inches from the top of the jar.

Pour the brine over the vegetables to within 1 inch from the top. Wedge the clean cabbage leaf over the top of the vegetable(s) and tuck it around the edges to hold them down beneath the liquid.

Set on the counter and cover with a fermentation lid (see A Primer on Pickling, page 63). (Alternatively, use a standard lid and loosen it a bit each day for the first few days, then every other day, to allow gasses to escape.) Let pickle for 3 to 5 days, depending on the indoor temperature. Check the taste after a couple of days, using clean utensils. Vegetables will pickle faster in warmer climates. Make sure the vegetable(s) stay packed beneath the level of the liquid, and add salted water (2 teaspoons sea salt dissolved in 1 cup warm filtered water) as needed.

When the vegetable(s) have pickled to your liking, seal the jar with a regular lid and refrigerate. They will continue to slowly pickle in the refrigerator. The pickles will keep for about 1 month. Taste for saltiness before serving and, if desired, rinse gently to remove excess salt. (See photo insert page 15.)

Calories: 1 (Per 1 tablespoon)   Protein: 0 g
Carbohydrate: 0 g   Fat: 0 g

Middle Eastern Pickled Turnips (All Phases)

Pickled turnips are often found in traditional Middle Eastern cuisine. The natural pungent quality of turnips is enhanced in the pickling process to create a distinctly flavorful pickle. Often, a few slices of beet are added to produce a pink color.

- 2 cups filtered water
- 1 to 1¼ tablespoons sea salt
- 3 tablespoons distilled white vinegar or vinegar of your choice, or more to taste
- 2 medium turnips, cut into ½-inch-thick matchsticks
- ½ small beet, diced
- 1 clove garlic
- 1 bay leaf
- 1 cabbage leaf, rinsed

Warm the water (no need to boil). Stir in the sea salt until it dissolves completely. Set aside to cool (use this time to cut the vegetables). Add the vinegar just before using. The brine can be made ahead of time and stored in a sealed glass jar on the counter to use when ready to pickle.

Place a quart-size glass canning jar in the sink and fill it with boiling water to sterilize. Empty the jar and tightly pack the vegetables, garlic, and bay leaf inside to within 1 to 2 inches from the top of the jar, making sure the beets are mixed throughout the jar.

Pour the brine over the vegetables to within 1 inch from the top of the jar. Wedge the clean cabbage leaf over the top of the vegetables and tuck it around the edges to hold the vegetables beneath the liquid.

Set on the counter and cover with a fermentation lid (see A Primer on Pickling, page 63). (Alternatively, use a standard lid and loosen it a bit each day for the first few days, then every other day, to allow gasses to escape.) Let pickle for 3 to 5 days, depending on the indoor temperature. Check the taste after a couple of days, using clean utensils.

Vegetables will pickle faster in warmer climates. Make sure the vegetables stay packed beneath the level of the liquid and add salted water (2 teaspoons sea salt dissolved in 1 cup warm filtered water) as needed.

When the vegetables are pickled to your liking, seal the jar with a regular lid and refrigerate. Vegetables will continue to slowly pickle in the refrigerator. They will keep for about 1 month. Taste for saltiness before serving and, if desired, rinse gently to remove excess salt. (See photo insert page 15.)

Calories: 1 (Per 1 tablespoon)   Protein: 0 g
Carbohydrate: 0 g   Fat: 0 g

Spicy Pickled Vegetables (Escabeche) (All Phases)

These spicy pickles are reminiscent of the Mediterranean and Latin American culinary technique known as escabeche. This recipe leaves out the sugar. Traditionally, the larger vegetables would be lightly cooked before pickling, but we prefer to use a quick fermentation method and leave the vegetables a bit crisp instead.

- 2 cups filtered water
- 1 to 1¼ tablespoons sea salt
- 2 tablespoons apple cider vinegar
- 1 jalapeño or a few small hot chiles, or to taste, sliced
- 1 large carrot, cut into ¼-inch-thick rounds or diagonal slices
- 1 to 2 cups chopped cauliflower or small cauliflower florets
- 3 small stalks celery (use only small inner stalks from the heart), cut into 1-inch-long sticks
- 1 bay leaf
- 1 cabbage leaf, rinsed

Warm the water (no need to boil). Stir in the sea salt until it dissolves completely. Set aside to cool (use this time to cut the vegetables). Add the vinegar just before using. The brine can be made ahead of time and stored in a sealed glass jar on the counter to use when ready to pickle.

Set a quart-size canning jar in the sink and fill it with boiling water to sterilize. Empty the jar and tightly pack the vegetables and bay leaf inside to within 1 to 2 inches from the top of the jar. Pour the brine over the vegetables to fill the jar to within 1 inch from the top. Wedge the cabbage leaf over the top of the vegetables and tuck it around the edges to hold the vegetables beneath the liquid.

Set on the counter and cover with a fermentation lid (see A Primer on Pickling, page 63). (Alternatively, use a standard lid and loosen it a bit each day for the first few days, then every other day, to allow gasses to escape.) Let pickle for 3 to 5 days, depending on the indoor temperature. Check the taste after a couple of days, using clean utensils. Vegetables will pickle faster in warmer climates. Make sure the vegetables stay packed beneath the level of the liquid and add salted water (2 teaspoons sea salt dissolved in 1 cup warm filtered water) as needed.

When the vegetables are pickled to your liking, seal the jar with a regular lid and refrigerate. Vegetables will continue to slowly pickle in the refrigerator. They will keep for about 1 month. Taste for saltiness before serving and, if desired, rinse gently to remove excess salt. (See photo insert page 15.)

Calories: 1 (Per 1 tablespoon)   Protein: 0 g
Carbohydrate: 0 g   Fat: 0 g

Variation

Add 1 to 2 tablespoons liquid whey from making Greek Yogurt (page 54) to the salt water.

Quick Ume-Pickled Onions (All Phases)

Inspired by Rosa Vera, one of our original culinary students who is now an experienced chef, this pickled onion recipe remains one of our all-time favorites. While not a fermentation, these delicious preserved onions are easy to use in salads, as side dishes, or as toppings on recipes like The Perfect Cucumber-Tomato Salad (page 261), Texas Caviar (page 262), or any of the Buddha Bowls (pages 263 to 269). They also make a great nightshade-free salsa when tossed with cucumbers and avocados.

- 2 cups filtered water
- 2 medium red onions, halved and sliced into ⅛-inch-thick half-moons
- ¼ cup umeboshi vinegar (see page 64)
- 2 tablespoons unseasoned rice vinegar or vinegar of your choice
- ½ teaspoon coarsely ground black pepper
- ½ teaspoon dried oregano
- 2 cloves garlic, halved
- 1 (½-inch) piece fresh ginger, peeled and cut into thin rounds
- 1 cabbage leaf, rinsed

Bring the water to a boil in a small saucepan. Add the onion and cook for 1 minute. Drain the onion in a fine-mesh sieve set over a bowl; set aside the cooking liquid. Transfer the onion to a quart-size glass jar or other glass container with a lid.

In the same saucepan (no need to wash it), combine the umeboshi vinegar, rice vinegar, pepper, oregano, garlic, and ginger. Bring to a boil. Remove immediately from the heat.

Pour the hot vinegar mixture over the onion in the jar. Add the reserved onion cooking liquid to fill the jar to within 1 inch from the rim. Discard remaining cooking liquid. Wedge the cabbage leaf over the top of the onions and tuck it around the edges to hold the onion beneath the liquid.

Set on the counter and cover with a lid. Let pickle for 8 to 24 hours. Check the taste after a few hours, using clean utensils. Vegetables will pickle faster in warmer climates. Make sure the onion stays packed beneath the liquid and add salted water (2 teaspoons sea salt dissolved in 1 cup warm filtered water) as needed.

When the onion is pickled to your liking, seal the jar and refrigerate. The onion will continue to slowly pickle in the refrigerator. It will keep for about 1 month.

Calories: 2 (Per 1 tablespoon)   Protein: 0 g
Carbohydrate: 0 g   Fat: 0 g

Miso Pickles (All Phases)

Pickling vegetables in miso is easy because there is nothing to mix. The miso is its own premade pickling medium. From lighter white miso to the hearty barley or brown rice varieties, any will do here. This type of pickling is best with heartier vegetables that have a lower water content like carrot slices or broccoli stalks (an efficient way to use leftover broccoli stalks that might otherwise go to waste). Add garlic cloves for a special treat.

- 1 to 2 cups miso paste, or more as needed
- 2 broccoli stalks
- 2 cloves garlic, thinly sliced (optional)

Spread the miso into a shallow glass container, 1 to 2 inches deep.

Cut or peel off the tough outer layer of the broccoli stalks. Cut the stalk into ¼-inch-thick rounds.

Press the broccoli rounds into the miso, standing them on their sides and creating rows spaced as close together as possible without touching. The miso should cover the sides of the broccoli. Intersperse slim wedges of garlic (if using) among the rounds, again making sure the garlic is covered with miso on the sides. Smooth the top to create a miso layer over the vegetables.

Set on the countertop and cover with a lid or a thin towel tightly stretched and held in place with a rubber band so it won't touch the miso. This should keep the miso from drying out. Let pickle for 4 to 7 days.

Refrigerate, covered, for up to 6 months. The pickled broccoli and garlic can remain in the miso until ready to eat and will continue to slowly pickle in the refrigerator. Pull out a few at a time and rinse before serving with a meal. Once all the vegetables have been eaten, the miso remaining in the container can be used in soups, sauces, or other recipes (keep in mind that the garlic will flavor the miso).

Calories: 1 (Per 1 tablespoon)   Protein: 0 g
Carbohydrate: 0 g   Fat: 0 g

DO-IT-YOURSELF SEITAN (ALL PHASES)

Seitan starts as a simple dough made from whole wheat flour and water. The dough is then rested to allow gluten (protein) strands to form, then the starch and bran are washed out, leaving only the thick, meaty protein. The protein can be used as is or dried and ground into a substance called vital wheat gluten, which is available in grocery stores and online. Bakers often add a bit of vital wheat gluten to bread dough to improve the elasticity in the structure of the bread as it rises.

Everyone with celiac disease, an autoimmune disorder, must completely avoid gluten-containing grains (chiefly wheat, rye, and barley). In addition, some others avoid gluten out of concern for inflammatory reactions, and for this reason, we offer gluten-free alternatives for our recipes. However, gluten can provide a concentrated protein alternative for vegetarians and especially vegans—and Smoke-Dried Tomato Seitan is an especially tasty example!

Basic Seitan (All Phases)

Use this basic recipe to create a vegan meat substitute to use in any recipe. The soy sauce and ginger mellow to create the perfect umami flavor in the hearty vegetarian protein.

Preparation time: 10 minutes

Total time: 1¼ hours

Makes 4 servings (about 3½ ounces)

- 3 to 4 cups water
- 1 cup vital wheat gluten
- ¼ teaspoon garlic powder
- ½ teaspoon onion powder
- 1 to 2 tablespoons soy sauce or ½ teaspoon salt
- 1 (2-inch) piece fresh ginger, peeled and cut into thin slices

Heat water in a kettle over medium heat.

Combine the vital wheat gluten, garlic powder, and onion powder in a large bowl. Measure ¾ cup of the warm water, and slowly pour it over the gluten, quickly stirring to form a ball of dough. Knead for 1 to 2 minutes in the bowl to form a cohesive and elastic ball and to incorporate any remaining dry flour. Stretch to form a 1-inch-thick rectangle. Cut the dough into thin strips or cubes depending on the shape you prefer for your recipes, separating each slice as you cut it to prevent them from sticking together. The pieces will expand as they cook.

Add soy sauce, ginger, and the remaining water to a large, deep skillet or slow cooker pot. Bring to a simmer, turn the heat to low, and add the pieces of dough in a single layer or only slightly overlapping. Cover and simmer the dough in the broth for 1 hour, adding water as needed just to cover the pieces of dough, or turn the slow cooker to low and cook for up to 10 hours.

Remove the seitan from the broth to use in recipes. Retain the broth for storing leftover seitan. Store in an airtight container covered with the cooking broth for up to 2 weeks.

Tip: Since seitan is essentially fat-free, add additional oil or other fat to the meal when substituting for other meats.

Calories: 120
Carbohydrate: 4 g

Protein: 23 g
Fat: 0 g

Smoke-Dried Tomato Seitan (All Phases)

Calling this roast a "meat substitute" doesn't do justice to the rich, warm flavor of this fragrant loaf. Crumble it over salads or nibble a few slices alongside eggs for breakfast.

Preparation time: 10 minutes

Total time: 1¼ hours

Makes 12 servings

- 1 cup vital wheat gluten
- ¼ cup chickpea flour (see Tip, page 91)
- 2 tablespoons tahini
- 5 sun-dried tomatoes (no salt added), chopped
- ¾ cup warm water
- 1 teaspoon smoked paprika
- 1 tablespoon miso paste (heartier dark misos like red or barley miso work best)
- ¼ teaspoon garlic powder, or 1 clove garlic
- 1 tablespoon nutritional yeast (optional)
- 2 to 3 teaspoons soy sauce
- 2 tablespoons Sugar-Free Worcestershire Sauce (page 284)
- ½ teaspoon ground black pepper

Preheat the oven to 350°F.

Place the vital wheat gluten and chickpea flour in a large bowl. Add the tahini and mix with a spatula or with clean hands until completely combined. Set aside.

In a blender, combine the tomatoes, water, paprika, miso, garlic, nutritional yeast (if using), soy sauce, Worcestershire, and pepper. Blend until smooth. (Alternatively, combine the ingredients in a wide-mouthed mason jar and blend using an immersion blender.)

Add the tomato mixture to the bowl with the vital wheat gluten. Stir until the liquid has been completely absorbed. Knead by hand until soft and well combined.

Form the dough into a 2-inch-thick rectangle. Cover tightly with parchment paper, sealing the top and sides to completely surround the seitan. Wrap the edges under the bottom. Cover the parchment with foil to completely seal the package. Bake directly on an oven rack for 1 to 1¼ hours.

Remove from the heat and set aside to cool. Once cool enough to handle, unwrap the seitan and store it in an airtight container in the refrigerator. The seitan is better the next day, after flavors have fully developed. Cut the loaf into 12 equal slices. Use immediately or refrigerate for up to a week or more. Reheat in a cast-iron skillet or toaster oven before serving. (See photo insert page 8.)

Calories: 70	Protein: 9 g
Carbohydrate: 4 g	Fat: 2 g

Variations

Mushroom Seitan: Substitute ½ ounce dried porcini mushrooms for the sun-dried tomatoes.

Substitute other spices or form the package into other shapes before baking, like link sausage shapes, to create other meat substitutes.

DO-IT-YOURSELF BEANS (ALL PHASES)

Cooking dried beans yourself is one of the easiest ways to cut costs in your food budget. In addition to being cost-effective, this method also creates tastier recipes. While discarding the liquid from canned beans is generally recommended, you can use the cooking liquid from homemade beans to enhance the flavor and texture of your dish. Quicker-cooking beans or locally sourced, freshly dried beans can be prepared in a pot on the stove. The best way to cook all other beans is to use a pressure cooker or slow cooker.

- **Quicker-Cooking Beans:** lentils, mung beans, adzuki beans, lima beans, black-eyed peas, fava beans (use small beans to avoid having to peel them), navy beans, and split peas
- **Medium-Cooking Beans:** pinto, black (turtle), great northern, cannellini, red beans
- **Long-Cooking Beans:** chickpeas (garbanzo beans), kidney beans, and soybeans

Step 1: Sort and wash the beans.

Put the beans in a colander or sieve. Pick through the beans and remove any grit or stones. Rinse well. Beans generally triple in size when cooked, so use 1 cup dried beans to yield about 3 cups cooked.

Step 2: Soak, if necessary.

Quicker-cooking beans do not need to be soaked. If you are pressure cooking, medium- and long-cooking beans can also be prepared without soaking, however, both do best with at least a 4- to 6-hour soak. For many people, soaking makes all beans more digestible. Try them both ways to see which you prefer.

Long Soak:

Place the rinsed beans in a large pot and add enough water to cover by 3 to 4 inches. Keep in mind that the beans will triple in size and absorb much of the water. Set aside on the counter to soak for 8 hours or up to overnight.

Quick Soak:

Place the rinsed beans in a large pot or bowl and pour over enough hot or boiling water to cover by 3 to 4 inches. Set aside on the counter to soak for 1 hour.

Step 3: Add water.

If you haven't soaked the beans, put them in a pot and add water to cover by about 3 inches (or more for larger beans). If you have soaked the beans, drain them, discarding the soaking water, return them to the pot, and add fresh water to cover by about 2 inches (use more water if you are making a soup or a recipe that will require extra cooking liquid).

Step 4: Cook the beans.

Bring the water to a boil, uncovered. If desired, add a 1-inch piece of kombu (kelp) seaweed for more depth of flavor (see Chef Dawn's Tasty Tip, page 104). Skim off any foam that rises to the surface.

Add ¾ to 1 teaspoon salt per pound of dried beans (2 to 2½ cups); more salt can be added to taste later (if you are using the beans in a recipe that already contains a significant amount of salt, postpone this step and add the salt at step 5).

For Quicker-Cooking Beans:

General Stovetop Cooking: Reduce the heat to medium-low. Cover and simmer for 30 minutes to 2 hours, or until the beans are soft. Older dried beans will take longer to cook, and unfortunately it is hard to determine this by looking at them.

- **Split peas:** Pressure cook on high for 25 minutes to create a creamy soup consistency.
- **Dried fava beans:** Pressure cook on high for 20 minutes.
- **Lentils and mung beans:** Simmer, covered, for 30 minutes, or until tender.
- **Adzuki beans, baby lima beans, navy beans, and black-eyed peas:** Simmer, covered, for 30 minutes to 2 hours, or until the beans are tender. Alternatively, pressure cook them on high for 15 minutes, then simmer until tender.

For Medium- or Long-Cooking Beans

- **Pressure Cooker:** Pressure cook on high for 25 to 30 minutes, or according to the manufacturer's instructions.
- **Slow Cooker:** Bring to a boil in a saucepan, stovetop-safe slow cooker insert, or using the slow cooker's sauté setting, if it has one. Transfer to the slow cooker or return the insert to the slow cooker, if necessary. Cover and cook on medium for 6 to 8 hours, or according to the manufacturer's instructions.
- **Stovetop:** Bring to a boil, reduce the heat to low, cover, and simmer for 2 to 8 hours, until the beans are tender.

Step 5: Season the beans and use in recipes.

Herbs or spices can be added in the beginning for shorter stovetop cooking. However, seasonings tend to lose their flavor with pressure cooking or slow cooking and are best added at the end.

Taste and add or adjust the salt, considering how beans will be used (e.g., whether a recipe also calls for salt).

Step 6: Store the beans.

Let the beans cool in their cooking liquid. Transfer the beans and cooking liquid to a jar or other container with a tight-fitting lid. Freshly cooked beans will keep in the refrigerator for up to 1 week. The cooking liquid can be used to enhance the flavor and texture of many dishes.

The recipes in this book will indicate if you measure the beans with the cooking liquid or instead use them drained and rinsed. To serve the beans on their own, put the beans and their liquid in a saucepan and bring to a simmer, uncovered. Cook for about 30 minutes, or until the liquid has reduced to the desired texture. This method enhances the flavor and creates a rich, thick consistency. The liquid will further thicken as it cools.

Note on using canned beans: If using canned beans in a recipe that calls for cooking liquid, always drain and rinse the beans, then add fresh water to the desired level. Canned beans with water added may need to be cooked longer to create a creamy texture.

DO-IT-YOURSELF SELF-CARE

Self-care is an essential part of the *Always Delicious* program. Better sleep and stress relief importantly contribute to a healthy body that doesn't hoard calories. These simple DIY self-care treatments are not only quick and easy, but also won't put a dent in your budget.

Chef Dawn's Tasty Tip

Forget the Spa

One of my greatest sources of satisfaction on this journey has been watching readers in our community let go of the "no pain, no gain" mentality as they shift their relationship with food and physical activity, and move toward more self-care. It's liberating to realize that instead of whipping your body into shape, you can love and nourish it to lasting health.

In this spirit, we've included some simple, inexpensive DIY spa treatments as a practical alternative to the fancy spas. With just a few common items in your kitchen, you can enjoy hours of soothing relaxation in the comfort of your own home. And they don't take a lot of time. A maximum of enjoyment for a minimum of effort and cost.

Relaxing Foot Soak (All Phases)

This bedtime ritual relaxes the body with minimum effort and cost. Using salt is optional; try it with and without to see which best supports you.

- Large bath towel
- Large plastic tub that will fit your feet immersed in water
- 3 to 6 quarts hot water
- ½ cup sea salt or Epsom salt (optional)
- 3 to 5 drops lavender or geranium essential oil
- Cream or lotion (optional)

Find a place that has enough room for you to comfortably sit with the plastic tub in front of you.

Place the bath towel, folded in half, on the floor in front of your seat.

Fill the plastic tub with hot water from the bathtub or sink, leaving enough room for your feet to be immersed without spilling the water, usually about halfway up the side of the tub. Add sea salt (if using). Center the tub of water on the towel, leaving room to blot your feet dry on either side of the tub.

Add a few drops of essential oil to the water.

Immerse your feet in the hot water and soak for about 15 minutes as you relax and gently breathe in the aroma of the essential oil.

Remove your feet from the water and blot them dry on the edges of the towel. If desired, finish with a quick rub using your favorite cream or lotion.

Coffee Scrub (All Phases)

Skin is the largest organ in the body. Revive and exfoliate it with a Coffee Scrub. Although there are expensive commercial products with fancy moisturizers and caffeine extracts touting detoxifying properties, this simple and inexpensive home scrub is all you need. Coffee Scrubs a few times per week will leave your skin feeling soft and smooth as the natural oils in the coffee beans do their magic. Used coffee grounds work great for this scrub. Spread the grounds onto a plate to completely dry (to avoid mold), then store in a clean, dry pint jar. Once the jar is filled, keep it in your bathroom for use in the shower. Experiment with different grinds to see which you like best. A fine espresso grind will feel different from a typical brewed coffee grind. If you don't drink coffee, check with your local coffee shop. Many coffee shops will happily give you some used grounds at no cost.

- ½ to ¾ cup dry coffee grounds (fresh or used)

Shower as normal. Place a small mound of coffee grounds, about 1 tablespoon, in the palm of your hand, then spread the grounds over each part of your body, gently rubbing the grounds over your skin to exfoliate. Repeat until your body is completely scrubbed, using about 1 tablespoon of the grounds at a time. Avoid scrubbing your face unless you are gently using a fine espresso grind. Rinse.

Body Rub (All Phases)

Another great way to stimulate and soothe your body without spending a dime is a Body Rub. The hot water opens your pores as the cotton wicks out dirt and toxins and gently exfoliates the skin.

- Cotton washcloth

Fill the bathroom sink with hot tap water and plug the drain. Place the cloth in the hot water and wring it out. Using just the weight of your hand, gently rub the hot cloth over your dry skin, one body part at a time. Dip the cloth back into the water and repeat until your whole body has been rubbed. Pay special attention to the body parts with lymph glands, including the armpits and groin. As you do this treatment, tension melts away and your body relaxes. Experiment with using this technique daily for two weeks, especially before bed, and see how you feel.

Tip: This works well after a warm shower when your pores are open and your muscles are warm. For best results, dry your body with a towel first so that the wet washcloth effectively wicks toxins from the skin, rather than just absorbing excess water.

Egg Yolk Face Mask (All Phases)

Who knew how luxurious having egg on your face could be? This simple DIY spa treatment is a useful tool for repurposing any leftover yolks in your refrigerator. This moisturizing mask will leave your skin feeling soft and smooth for only pennies per treatment. Use it a few times per week, or whenever you have an extra yolk.

- 1 egg yolk

Wash and dry your face. Gently spread the yolk over your face and neck, avoiding your eyes. Allow the mask to dry completely, 5 to 10 minutes. Place a hot, wet washcloth over your face to soften the mask, then gently rub to remove the yolk. Rinse with warm water until all egg has been removed.

Follow your regular moisturizing regimen after removing the mask.

My *Always Delicious* Story

Always Hungry? has given me permission to let go of the "calories in, calories out" model that fooled me into an unhealthy relationship with food my entire adult life. As a thirty-year-old mother to two young children, I didn't want to accept my body or lack of energy as a side effect of motherhood. I had tried exercise fads, counting calories, point systems, and juice cleanses, but they left me more ravenous and tired than ever. *Always Hungry?* has given me so many valuable tools with so many amazing results. First comes improved sleep, lasting energy, clear skin, mental clarity, and finally an easily maintained body I love, who some say shows no physical proof it has carried children!

Pamela B., age 31, Martha's Vineyard, Massachusetts

CHAPTER 5

Breakfasts

Chef Dawn's Tasty Tip

Nutritious, Delicious, *and* Expeditious!

In working with our readers over the past two years, I've learned that many people face a common challenge at breakfast—not enough time! Often, they skip breakfast entirely and are left feeling hungry and drained long before lunch. To solve this problem once and for all, we've designed many grab-and-go recipes for complete meals on the run. Most can be made in advance, so all you need to do in the morning is open your fridge!

Cherry Chocolate Power Shake (Phases 2 and 3, with Phase 1 Variation)

The rich, classic combination of cherries and chocolate is sure to please your taste buds as this nutrient-balanced meal helps you power through to lunch.

Preparation time: 5 minutes

Total time: 5 minutes

Makes 1 serving

- ½ cup unsweetened frozen dark cherries
- ¼ ripe banana
- ¾ cup whole milk or unsweetened soy milk
- ⅓ cup cashews
- 1 serving unsweetened, unflavored 100% whey protein powder (check the package nutritional info—1 serving should yield 22 g protein)
- 1 tablespoon unsweetened cocoa powder, or more to taste
- ¼ teaspoon pure vanilla extract

Place all the ingredients in a high-speed blender or a wide-mouthed glass jar or cup that will fit an immersion blender without splashing. Blend until creamy.

Calories: 522
Carbohydrate: 43 g (32%)
Protein: 36 g (27%)
Fat: 24 g (41%)

Variations

For a less filling shake, use ½ serving protein powder *or* use unsweetened almond milk in place of whole milk or soy milk to reduce the density but still keep the ratios in the Phase 2 range.

For Phase 1: Omit the banana and add 1 tablespoon heavy cream or canned coconut milk.

Calories: 546
Carbohydrate: 37 g (27%)
Protein: 36 g (26%)
Fat: 30 g (47%)

For Phase 3: Use 1 whole banana and reduce the protein powder to ½ serving.

Calories: 545
Carbohydrate: 62 g (44%)
Protein: 26 g (18%)
Fat: 24 g (38%)

Berry Vanilla Coconut Shake (with Ice Cream Dessert Variation) (All Phases)

Many of our readers have asked for dairy-free and vegan versions of our shakes. This one fits the bill. The creamy coconut and naturally sweet berries pair perfectly for a satisfying morning meal. Add a bit of ice and it converts into a soft-serve dessert!

Preparation time: 5 minutes

Total time: 5 minutes

Makes 1 serving (2 to 4 servings for dessert variation)

- ¼ cup unsweetened canned coconut milk
- ¾ cup frozen berries (cherries, blueberries, or strawberries)
- 1 serving unsweetened, unflavored 100% whey protein powder or vegan protein powder (check the package nutritional info—1 serving should yield 22 g protein)
- 1 teaspoon pure vanilla extract
- 1½ tablespoons unsweetened almond butter
- ⅓ cup whole milk or unsweetened soy milk

Place all the ingredients in a high-speed blender or a wide-mouthed mason jar or cup that will fit an immersion blender without splashing. Blend until creamy.

Calories: 493
Carbohydrate: 30 g (25%)
Protein: 32 g (25%)
Fat: 29 g (50%)

Variations

For Dessert: Add about ⅓ cup ice cubes (or enough to reach desired consistency) before blending, then divide among two to four bowls. Serve as a soft-serve ice cream substitute.

For Phases 2 and 3: Substitute ½ cup frozen berries and 1 frozen banana for the ¾ cup berries. Reduce the almond butter to 1 tablespoon.

Calories: 528
Carbohydrate: 50 g (38%)
Protein: 31 g (22%)
Fat: 25 g (40%)

Creamy Vanilla Coffee Shake (Phases 2 and 3)

Skip the expensive coffee house drinks! This is the only espresso beverage you'll ever need. It's so smooth and creamy, you'd never guess it was a balanced meal. The base makes a great starter for any number of favorite coffee flavors, including luscious chocolate mocha. Rather than feeling the crash of a typical sugary coffee drink, this one will leave you energized all morning.

Preparation time: 5 minutes

Total time: 5 minutes

Makes 1 serving

- 2 shots of espresso, ⅓ cup Cold-Brewed Coffee Concentrate (page 62), or 1 serving instant espresso powder
- ½ cup whole milk or unsweetened soy milk
- ⅓ cup cashews
- 2 large or 4 small dates (about 1 ounce), pitted
- 1 teaspoon pure vanilla extract
- 1 serving unsweetened, unflavored 100% whey protein powder (check the package nutritional info—1 serving should yield 22 g protein)
- ⅓ cup ice cubes

Place the coffee, milk, cashews, dates, and vanilla in a high-speed blender or a wide-mouthed glass mason jar or cup that will fit an immersion blender without splashing. Blend until the dates and cashews are well pulverized and smooth. Add the protein powder and ice. Blend until smooth.

Tips: To make the cashews easier to blend to a smooth consistency, soak them in water overnight, then drain.

If you use hot coffee, the dates can be soaked in the coffee for a few minutes to soften them, or they can be soaked overnight in the milk.

Even with the ice, this shake is meant to be a frothy, room-temperature or slightly chilled drink rather than an iced or frozen drink.

Calories: 491
Carbohydrate: 41 g (35%)
Protein: 33 g (26%)
Fat: 22 g (39%)

Variations

Add 1 tablespoon unsweetened cocoa powder for a mocha flavor.

Add 1 teaspoon MCT (medium-chain triglyceride) oil (typically derived from coconut oil) or coconut oil for a higher-fat option.

Shakshuka (All Phases)

One of the most popular recipes from *Always Hungry?* was the Ranchero Sauce. We created a Middle Eastern version of that sauce and topped it with eggs—irresistible! Although shakshuka is often served for breakfast, the chickpeas make it work as a quick lunch or dinner entrée as well.

Preparation time: 10 minutes

Total time: 30 minutes

Makes 4 servings

- 1 large clove garlic
- 1 medium onion, cut into large chunks
- 1 red or yellow bell pepper, cut into large chunks
- 1 jalapeño, poblano, Anaheim, or other fresh mild to medium chile, seeded and cut into large chunks
- 2 tablespoons extra-virgin olive oil
- ¾ teaspoon salt, plus more if needed
- ¼ teaspoon ground black pepper, plus more if needed
- 1 to 2 teaspoons paprika
- ¼ teaspoon smoked paprika (optional)
- Dash of cayenne pepper, or to taste (optional)
- 1¼ cups diced fresh tomatoes, or 1 (14.5-ounce) can diced tomatoes
- 1½ cups cooked chickpeas (see Do-It-Yourself Beans, page 74), or 1 (14.5-ounce can) chickpeas, drained and rinsed
- 8 eggs
- 1 avocado, sliced, for garnish
- ¼ cup chopped fresh cilantro, for garnish

Place the garlic, onion, pepper, and chile in a food processor and process until finely minced, or mince them with a knife.

Heat the olive oil in a large, deep skillet over medium heat. Add the minced vegetables, salt, black pepper, paprika, and smoked paprika and cayenne (if using). Cook, stirring, until the vegetables begin to soften, about 5 minutes.

Add the tomatoes. Bring to a boil, then reduce the heat to low and simmer for about 10 minutes. Taste and adjust the seasonings.

Stir in the chickpeas and simmer for 5 minutes more. (This sauce can also be made ahead of time, stored in the refrigerator for 1 week or in the freezer for up to 6 months, and reheated before adding the eggs.)

Crack the eggs over the top of the sauce one at a time, spacing them evenly in the pan. Sprinkle lightly with additional salt and pepper, if desired. Cover the skillet and simmer, or place in the oven and bake at 350°F, until the eggs reach the desired consistency. Traditionally, the eggs are served with soft yolks, about 5 minutes on the stovetop or in the oven.

Scoop 2 eggs with sauce onto a plate for each person. Garnish with a few slices of avocado and the cilantro.

Calories: 389
Carbohydrate: 29 g

Protein: 19 g
Fat: 23 g

Phase 1 Meal: Serve with ⅓ cup plain whole-milk Greek yogurt or 4% cottage cheese.

Calories: 486; Carbohydrate: 27%; Protein: 24%; Fat: 49%

Phase 2 Meal: Omit the avocado. Serve with ¾ cup berries and 2 slices cooked turkey bacon (about 2 ounces) or equivalent vegetarian protein (see Equivalents Table, page 49).

Calories: 483; Carbohydrate: 36%; Protein: 26%; Fat: 38%

Phase 3 Meal: Serve with a slice of crusty artisan sourdough bread (1 to 2 ounces).

Calories: 503; Carbohydrate: 41%; Protein: 18%; Fat: 41%

Red Pepper Ring Omelets (Phases 2 and 3, with Phase 1 Variation)

These omelets are simple to make and almost too pretty to eat. Make them ahead and even pop them on top of half a Rosemary Biscuit (page 203) with a bit of turkey bacon or equivalent vegetarian protein (see Equivalents Table, page 49) for a perfect morning meal on the run.

Preparation time: 5 minutes

Total time: 20 minutes

Makes 1 serving

- ½ large red bell pepper
- 1 egg
- 1 egg white
- ⅓ cup Cooked Quinoa (page 231)
- 1 ounce baby spinach or arugula, chopped (about ½ cup packed)
- ⅛ teaspoon salt
- ⅛ teaspoon ground black pepper
- 1 teaspoon neutral-tasting oil, such as high-oleic safflower or avocado oil
- ½ ounce cheese, such as mozzarella, provolone, or cheddar, shredded

Cut the pepper crosswise into two rings 1 to 1½ inches thick. Remove and discard the seeds.

Whisk the egg, egg white, quinoa, spinach, salt, and black pepper together in a bowl.

Heat the oil in a medium ovenproof skillet, such as a cast-iron skillet, over medium heat. Place the red pepper rings into the skillet cut-side down. Cook for a minute on each side.

Slowly pour the egg mixture into the red pepper rings, evenly distributing it between the two, so that the bottom seals and the egg mixture fills the rings. Reduce the heat to low. Cover and cook for 3 to 5 minutes to allow the eggs to cook on the bottom.

Uncover and transfer the pan to the oven. Broil for 2 to 3 minutes, or until the eggs are done on top. Sprinkle evenly with the cheese and broil until the cheese melts, 1 to 2 minutes. Serve immediately.

Calories: 257
Carbohydrate: 21 g
Protein: 17 g
Fat: 12 g

Variations

For Phase 1: Use 2 whole eggs, increase the cheese to 1½ ounces, and omit the quinoa.

Calories: 278   Protein: 20 g
Carbohydrate: 9 g   Fat: 18 g

Phase 1 Meal: Use the Phase 1 Variation. Serve with 1 cup berries and ½ cup plain whole-milk Greek yogurt.

Calories: 528; Carbohydrate: 26%; Protein: 27%; Fat: 47%

Phase 2 Meal: Serve with 1 cup berries and ½ cup plain whole-milk Greek yogurt.

Calories: 507; Carbohydrate: 37%; Protein: 25%; Fat: 38%

Phase 3 Meal: In place of the quinoa, fry ⅔ cup shredded white potatoes in 1 teaspoon olive oil until soft, about 5 minutes and divide them between the red pepper rings before adding the egg mixture. Serve with 1 cup berries and ¼ cup plain whole-milk Greek yogurt.

Calories: 502; Carbohydrate: 41%; Protein: 20%; Fat: 39%

Breakfast Biscuit Stacks (All Phases)

A warm biscuit with soft fried eggs and crunchy bacon will leave anyone nostalgic for diners with checkerboard tablecloths, but these special breakfast stacks would also be right at home in your favorite upscale brunch spot. The rosemary in the biscuit combined with the basil in the stack make for a perfect, savory bite.

Preparation time: 5 minutes

Total time: 15 minutes

Makes 1 serving

- 1 teaspoon olive oil
- 2 eggs
- 1 Rosemary Biscuit (page 203)
- 1 ounce smoked salmon, Canadian bacon, or cooked turkey bacon, or 1 slice Smoke-Dried Tomato Seitan (page 73) or other vegetarian protein (see Equivalents Table, page 49)
- 3 fresh basil leaves, chopped
- 2 large slices tomato
- 1 ounce mozzarella cheese, sliced or shredded

Preheat the broiler.

Heat the oil in a medium ovenproof skillet over medium heat. Crack the eggs gently into the skillet and fry to the desired doneness. Remove from the pan and set aside on a plate.

Cut the biscuit in half, put the halves cut-side up in the skillet, and top each half evenly with the salmon, basil, tomato, eggs, and mozzarella.

Place under the broiler for a few minutes, or until the cheese has melted. Serve immediately.

Calories: 489	Protein: 32 g
Carbohydrate: 20 g	Fat: 31 g

Variations

For Phase 2: Substitute 1 Red Pepper Ring Omelet (page 87) for the fried eggs and mozzarella.

Calories: 481	Protein: 30 g
Carbohydrate: 39 g	Fat: 23 g

Phase 1 Meal: Serve with 1 cup strawberries.

Calories: 535; Carbohydrate: 23%; Protein: 24%; Fat: 53%

Phase 2 Meal: Use the Phase 2 Variation. Serve with ½ cup berries.

Calories: 504; Carbohydrate: 35%; Protein: 24%; Fat: 41%

Phase 3 Meal: Use the Phase 2 Variation. Substitute a couple of slices of crusty artisan sourdough bread for the Rosemary Biscuit, and spread ¼ avocado on each slice.

Calories: 550; Carbohydrate: 41%; Protein: 21%; Fat: 38%

Grain-Free Pumpkin Spice Muffins (Phases 2 and 3)

A quick breakfast or the perfect grab-and-go snack for classroom celebrations, office potlucks, or any occasion that calls for allergen-free treats. Your friends don't even have to know these muffins are healthy! They've been taste-tested by hundreds of kids and adults alike, with rave reviews.

Preparation time: 10 minutes

Total time: 40 minutes

Makes 6 servings (6 large muffins)

- Olive oil spray (optional)
- ¾ cup chickpea flour (see Tip)
- ¼ cup coconut flour or almond flour
- ¼ teaspoon baking soda
- 1 teaspoon baking powder
- ⅓ cup neutral-tasting oil, such as high-oleic safflower or avocado oil (use ¼ cup if using almond flour)
- 1 egg, beaten, or 1 tablespoon chia or flaxseeds, ground and mixed into ¼ cup water
- ½ cup packed steamed winter squash, such as kabocha, butternut, buttercup, etc., or sweet potato
- ½ cup whole milk or unsweetened soy milk
- ¼ teaspoon pure vanilla extract
- 3 tablespoons honey or pure maple syrup
- ¾ teaspoon ground cinnamon
- ¼ teaspoon ground ginger
- ⅛ teaspoon ground cardamom
- ⅛ teaspoon ground cloves
- ⅛ teaspoon freshly grated nutmeg
- ¼ teaspoon salt

Preheat the oven to 350°F. Line six wells of a large muffin tin with paper liners or coat with olive oil spray.

Combine the chickpea flour, coconut flour, baking soda, and baking powder in a large bowl.

In a separate medium bowl, combine the oil, egg, squash, milk, vanilla, honey, spices, and salt. Blend with an immersion blender until smooth.

Add the wet ingredients to the dry ingredients and stir, whisk, or blend until smooth. (Because the batter is gluten-free, it's okay to use the immersion blender to get the lumps out.) Divide the batter evenly among the prepared muffin cups.

Bake for 25 to 30 minutes. Remove the muffins from the tin and let cool on a wire rack for at least 15 to 20 minutes before serving. Cool completely and store in an airtight container for a couple of days on the counter, up to 10 days in the refrigerator, or up to 3 months in the freezer. (See photo insert page 3.)

Tips: This recipe makes 6 large muffins. Depending on the size of your muffin tins, use any excess batter to make a few pancakes or to make 7 or 8 smaller muffins.

Chickpea flour is also known as garbanzo bean flour, gram flour, or besan and may be labeled that way at your grocery store. You could also use garbanzo–fava bean flour, if you prefer.

Calories: 245
Carbohydrate: 20 g

Protein: 5 g
Fat: 17 g

Variations

To make pancakes: For each pancake, pour a scant ¼ cup of the batter onto a hot skillet brushed with oil. Cook until golden brown and the edges appear done and lift easily, then flip and brown on the second side. *Makes about 12 medium pancakes.*

For Apple Cinnamon Muffins: Substitute 2 medium apples, cored, chopped, and cooked with 2 tablespoons water, then pureed for the squash, and 1 teaspoon ground cinnamon with 1 teaspoon pure vanilla extract in place of all the other spices.

For Banana Nut Muffins: Substitute 2 ripe bananas, mashed, for the squash and ½ teaspoon ground cinnamon with 1 teaspoon pure vanilla extract in place of all the other spices. Add ¼ cup chopped walnuts.

Phase 1 Meal: None (contains honey and starchy vegetables).

Phase 2 Meal: Serve with 3 slices cooked turkey bacon or equivalent vegetarian protein (see Equivalents Table, page 49), ¼ cup plain whole-milk Greek yogurt, and 1 cup blueberries.

Calories: 496; Carbohydrate: 34%; Protein: 23%; Fat: 43%

Phase 3 Meal: Use the pancake variation. Serve each person 2 pancakes, each drizzled with 1 teaspoon pure maple syrup. Serve with 3 slices cooked turkey bacon or equivalent vegetarian protein (see Equivalents Table, page 49) and 1 cup blueberries.

Calories: 469; Carbohydrate: 40%; Protein: 20%; Fat: 40%

Chef Dawn's Tasty Tip

Egg Substitutes

Looking to master egg-free cooking? First, determine the function of the egg in the recipe.

Main ingredient: For recipes like quiches, scrambles, or egg salads, tofu is the best egg substitute. Consider various types of tofu, depending on the texture you want to produce. Silken tofu has a similar texture to boiled egg white. Crumbled firm tofu works well as an egg salad substitute. For scrambled eggs, use firm or extra-firm tofu, crumble, and panfry in oil with spices. You can also use firm or extra-firm tofu, pureed in a food processor, for baking into a quiche.

Binding structure or rising agent: Although tofu will work in muffins, cakes, and meat or veggie patties, I prefer to use flax- or chia seeds as binding or rising agents. To make a simple egg substitute, combine 1 tablespoon ground chia or flaxseeds with ¼ cup water. Let it rest for a few minutes to form an eggy consistency. Choose chia rather than flaxseeds in baking unless you are using strong spices to mask the distinct flavor of flax. These substitutes work especially well in gluten-free baking that requires more structure to hold the final product together. (Grind chia and flaxseeds fresh with a coffee or spice grinder, since the pre-ground meal tends to go rancid fairly quickly.) For other types of binders, as in meatballs or latkes, chickpea flour makes an effective egg substitute.

Emulsifier: In mayonnaise or other sauces that use egg as an emulsifier, milk, soy milk, or a bit of silken tofu make good substitutes.

Keep in mind that tofu is quite bland and will need more salt and other seasonings than an egg would.

Spinach Feta Quiche (All Phases)

This is the quickest quiche recipe you've ever encountered. It takes just a few minutes to whip up a batch of bite-size quiches that you can eat on the run, and a little fruit and yogurt completes the meal. A quick staple breakfast for your hectic mornings. You can even leave off the crust and make little mini egg muffins.

Preparation time: 10 minutes

Total time: 30 minutes

Makes 4 to 6 servings (12 muffin-size or one 9- or 10-inch quiche)

- 1 recipe Grain-Free Piecrust dough (page 206)
- 8 ounces frozen chopped spinach
- 8 eggs
- ¼ teaspoon salt, or to taste
- ¼ teaspoon ground black pepper, or to taste
- 4 ounces feta cheese

Preheat the oven to 350°F.

Roll out the pie dough between two pieces of parchment paper to fit either one 9-inch pie plate or one 10-inch quiche pan, or roll it into a thick log, then cut 12 equal pieces to roll individually to line 12 wells of a muffin tin. Press the dough into the pie plate, pan, or wells and prick the bottom with a fork. (No need to oil the pan if using a nonstick plate, pan, or wells.) Prebake the crust for about 5 minutes while assembling the filling.

Rinse the frozen spinach in a colander to thaw it a bit. Leave to drain, and squeeze out the excess water before using.

Beat the eggs, salt, and pepper in a large bowl. Crumble the feta into the eggs, and mix in the spinach.

Pour the mixture into the prebaked crust or spoon about ⅓ cup of the mixture into each prebaked muffin crust.

Bake for 20 minutes, or until the egg is completely set. Cool mini quiches for 5 minutes before removing from the tins by sliding a thin spatula or knife around the edges to loosen each mini crust.

Serve 2 to 3 mini quiches per person or cut the quiche into 4 to 6 slices. Cool completely, then cover and store in the refrigerator for up to a week or in the freezer for up to 3 months. Quiches may be served at room temperature or warm, reheated in the oven or toaster oven.

Calories: 329	Protein: 17 g
Carbohydrate: 17 g	Fat: 21 g

Variations

For Phase 2: Add 1½ cups Cooked Quinoa (page 231) to the egg mixture before pouring and baking.

Calories: 385	Protein: 19 g
Carbohydrate: 27 g	Fat: 22 g

Phase 1 Meal: Serve with ½ cup blueberries and ½ cup plain whole-milk Greek yogurt, topped with 1 tablespoon cashews.

Calories: 535; Carbohydrate: 26%; Protein: 23%; Fat: 51%

Phase 2 Meal: Use the Phase 2 Variation. Serve with ¾ cup blueberries and ⅓ cup plain whole-milk Greek yogurt.

Calories: 530; Carbohydrate: 35%; Protein: 21%; Fat: 44%

Phase 3 Meal: Use the Phase 3 Variation for the Grain-Free Piecrust (page 206). Serve with ¾ cup blueberries and 2 tablespoons plain whole-milk Greek yogurt.

Calories: 525; Carbohydrate: 40%; Protein: 17%; Fat: 43%

Bacon-Cheddar Quiche (All Phases)

The classic combination of bacon and cheese in these minis will keep even your quiche-skeptic family members happy. Make them in muffin tins, with or without the crust, for a quick grab-and-go breakfast or a nutritious snack any time of the day.

Preparation time: 10 minutes

Total time: 30 minutes

Makes 4 to 6 servings (12 muffin-size or one 9- or 10-inch quiche)

- 1 recipe Grain-Free Piecrust dough (page 206)
- 4 eggs
- 4 egg whites
- ⅛ teaspoon salt, or to taste
- ¼ teaspoon ground black pepper, or to taste
- 3 ounces cheddar cheese, shredded
- 2 ounces cooked bacon (about 2¾ ounces uncooked), crumbled

Preheat the oven to 350°F.

Roll out the pie dough between two pieces of parchment paper to fit either one 9-inch pie plate or one 10-inch quiche pan, or roll it into a thick log, then cut 12 equal pieces to roll individually to line 12 wells of a muffin tin. Press the dough into the pie plate, pan, or wells and prick the bottom with a fork. (No need to oil the pan if using a nonstick plate, pan, or wells.) Prebake the crust for about 5 minutes while assembling the filling.

Beat the eggs, egg whites, salt, and pepper in a medium bowl, then mix in the cheese and bacon.

Pour the egg mixture into the prebaked crust or spoon about ⅓ cup of the mixture into each prebaked muffin crust.

Bake for 20 minutes, or until the egg is completely set. Cool for 5 minutes and, if serving immediately, slice the whole quiche or remove mini quiches from the tins by sliding a thin spatula or knife around the edges to loosen. To serve later, remove from tins, cover, and store in the refrigerator up to 1 week or in the freezer up to 3 months.

Serve 2 to 3 mini quiches per person. Quiches may be served at room temperature or warm, reheated in the oven or toaster oven.

Calories: 338
Carbohydrate: 15 g
Protein: 19 g
Fat: 22 g

Variations

For Phase 2: Substitute turkey bacon or equivalent vegetarian protein (see Equivalents Table, page 49) for the bacon, and add 1½ cups Cooked Quinoa (page 231) to the egg mixture before pouring and baking.

Calories: 380
Carbohydrate: 25 g
Protein: 20 g
Fat: 22 g

Phase 1 Meal: Serve with ½ cup blueberries and ½ cup plain whole-milk Greek yogurt.

Calories: 504; Carbohydrate: 24%; Protein: 24%; Fat: 52%

Phase 2 Meal: Use the Phase 2 Variation. Serve with ¾ cup blueberries and ¼ cup plain whole-milk Greek yogurt.

Calories: 505; Carbohydrate: 34%; Protein: 21%; Fat: 45%

Phase 3 Meal: Use the Phase 3 Variation for Grain-Free Piecrust (page 206) and the Phase 2 Variation for the Quiche. Serve with ¼ cup blueberries.

Calories: 503; Carbohydrate: 39%; Protein: 18%; Fat: 43%

Apple Spice Pancakes (All Phases)

These fluffy pancakes are designed for celebratory birthday brunches, or just regular mornings around the house. Freeze them for a quick weekday breakfast. The sweet apples and cinnamon bring a warm, familiar flavor that will satisfy even the pickiest eaters.

Preparation time: 5 minutes

Total time: 30 minutes

Makes 4 servings (about eight 5-inch pancakes)

- 2 medium apples, cored and diced *OR APPLE SAUCE* *(makes ½ cup)* *2/3*
- ¼ cup water
- ¾ cup chickpea flour (see Tip, page 91)
- ¼ cup almond flour
- ¾ teaspoon baking soda
- 1 teaspoon ground cinnamon
- ⅛ teaspoon salt
- 1 egg, beaten, or 1 tablespoon chia or flaxseeds, finely ground and mixed with ¼ cup water
- ¼ cup whole milk or unsweetened soy milk
- 2 tablespoons neutral-tasting oil, such as high-oleic safflower or avocado oil, plus more for frying
- ½ teaspoon pure vanilla extract
- ⅛ teaspoon white wine vinegar

Place the apples and water in a saucepan with a lid. Bring to a boil. Cover, reduce the heat to low, and simmer for 5 to 10 minutes, or until apples are soft. Place in a wide-mouthed glass jar or cup that will fit an immersion blender without splashing. Blend until smooth. Set aside. This can be made ahead and stored in the refrigerator for up to 2 weeks.

Combine the chickpea flour, almond flour, baking soda, cinnamon, and salt in a large bowl. (This step can be done ahead of time. Store the dry pancake mix in a jar or other airtight container in a cool, dark place and use it when you need it.)

In a separate medium bowl, combine the egg, milk, oil, vanilla, vinegar, and half the pureed apples, about ⅓ cup.

Add the wet ingredients to the dry ingredients. Stir until well combined.

Heat a cast-iron skillet or nonstick griddle over medium heat. Brush the pan with oil.

Pour the batter onto the hot skillet in 5-inch rounds, using about ¼ cup batter per pancake. Cook until bubbles appear throughout and the edges begin to lift easily from the skillet, 2 to 3 minutes. The bottom should be lightly browned. Turn and cook on the other side until golden brown. Transfer the cooked pancakes to a plate and cover with a towel to keep warm, or keep warm in a low oven until ready to serve. Repeat with the remaining batter.

Serve each pancake topped with a heaping tablespoon of the remaining pureed apples. Store cooled, leftover pancakes in an airtight container for up to a week in the refrigerator, or up to 3 months in the freezer.

Tip: Using unpeeled apples ensures a more balanced applesauce appropriate on occasion for all phases.

Calories: 276
Carbohydrate: 26 g
Protein: 8 g
Fat: 17 g

Variations

Banana or Pumpkin Spice (Phases 2 and 3): Substitute a ripe banana or ⅓ cup packed, cooked sweet potato, winter squash, or pumpkin for the apples and water. Use all of it in the batter instead of reserving half for the topping. Add pumpkin pie spice to taste.

Add sweet spices like ground cardamom or freshly grated nutmeg.

Phase 1 Meal: Serve each portion with 3 (1-ounce) slices cooked turkey bacon or equivalent vegetarian protein (see Equivalents Table, page 49), and Pear Cinnamon Cashew Butter (page 58) and 2 tablespoons plain whole-milk Greek yogurt to top the pancakes.

Calories: 468; Carbohydrate: 27%; Protein: 25%; Fat: 48%

Phase 2 Meal: Serve each portion with 3 (1-ounce) slices cooked turkey bacon or equivalent vegetarian protein (see Equivalents Table, page 49), ¾ cup blueberries, and 1 tablespoon Pear Cinnamon Cashew Butter (page 58).

Calories: 473; Carbohydrate: 36%; Protein 22%; Fat 42%

Phase 3 Meal: Serve each portion with 2 (1-ounce) slices cooked turkey bacon or equivalent vegetarian protein (see Equivalents Table, page 49), ¼ cup blueberries, 1 tablespoon pure maple syrup, and 1 tablespoon Pear Cinnamon Cashew Butter (page 58).

Calories: 475; Carbohydrate: 41%; Protein: 17%; Fat 42%

Sweet Breakfast Crepe (All Phases)

Creamy Greek yogurt and rich fruit compote all rolled together in a delicious breakfast crepe. This recipe shows you how to take two leftover foods, or even desserts, and combine them to make a quick and simple meal.

Preparation time: 5 minutes

Total time: 5 minutes

Makes 4 servings (6 crepes)

Socca Crepes

- 1 cup chickpea flour (see Tip, page 91)
- 1 cup sparkling water
- 1 tablespoon extra-virgin olive oil
- 1 egg
- ¼ teaspoon salt

Cooking and Filling

- Neutral-tasting oil, such as high-oleic safflower or avocado oil, for frying
- ¾ recipe (6 servings) Apple Pie Parfait (page 319)

Make the crepes: Place all the crepe ingredients in a wide-mouthed glass jar or cup that will fit an immersion blender without splashing. Blend until smooth. Use right away so that the sparkling water brings a lighter texture to the crepe.

Cook and fill the crepes: Heat a 10- to 12-inch cast-iron skillet over medium-high heat. Brush ¼ to ½ teaspoon of the oil onto the hot skillet and adjust the heat as necessary—the pan should be hot, but the oil should not smoke.

Pour about ⅓ cup of the batter onto the hot oiled skillet, tilting the pan in a circular motion as you pour so the batter coats the surface evenly.

Cook until the edges brown and lift easily from the skillet, about 3 minutes. Turn and cook on the second side for 2 to 3 minutes. Remove from the heat and use immediately or refrigerate and reheat to soften before using.

Spread 1 serving of the parfait, including Greek yogurt, inside each crepe. Serve 1½ crepes per person.

Tip: If you make the entire Apple Pie Parfait recipe, you will have 2 servings of parfait left over to serve with another meal.

Calories: 408   Protein: 20 g
Carbohydrate: 46 g   Fat: 17 g

Phase 1 Meal: Use the Phase 1 Variation for the Apple Pie Parfait. Serve with 2 (1-ounce) slices cooked turkey bacon or equivalent vegetarian protein (see Equivalents Table, page 49).

Calories: 464; Carbohydrate: 25%; Protein: 28%; Fat: 47%

Phase 2 Meal: Serve with 2 (1-ounce) slices cooked turkey bacon or equivalent vegetarian protein (see Equivalents Table, page 49).

Calories: 478; Carbohydrate: 37%; Protein: 26%; Fat: 37%

Phase 3 Meal: Substitute buckwheat flour for half the chickpea flour. Add a drizzle of pure maple syrup (about 1 teaspoon). Serve with 1 (1-ounce) slice cooked turkey bacon or equivalent vegetarian protein (see Equivalents Table, page 49).

Calories: 460; Carbohydrate: 43%; Protein: 22%; Fat: 35%

Spinach Mushroom Crepes (All Phases)

A classic combination for the perfect savory breakfast. Make the filling ahead for a delicious breakfast in minutes.

Preparation time: 5 minutes

Total time: 30 minutes

Makes 4 servings (6 crepes)

- 1 recipe Socca Crepes (page 197)
- 1 tablespoon olive oil
- 2 cloves garlic, minced or pressed
- 1 pound baby bella/cremini mushrooms, sliced
- ⅛ teaspoon salt
- 1 pound baby spinach (about 8 cups packed)
- 6 ounces cheese, such as mozzarella or cheddar, shredded

Reheat the crepes, if necessary.

Heat the olive oil in a large skillet over medium heat. Add the garlic, mushrooms, and salt. Cook, uncovered, stirring occasionally, until the mushrooms are soft and all liquid they release has absorbed, 10 to 15 minutes.

Add the spinach and cook until wilted.

Working with one at a time, place the cooked crepes flat in a large cast-iron or nonstick skillet. Spread one-sixth of the spinach-mushroom mixture inside the crepe and top with 1 ounce of the cheese. Fold over or roll each side over the middle to close the crepe. Heat the filled crepe over medium heat, gently turning over once, until the cheese melts.

Remove from the heat and repeat with the remaining crepes. Keep the filled crepes warm in a 200°F oven until ready to serve. Serve 1½ crepes per person, warm from the oven or skillet.

Calories: 350	Protein: 23 g
Carbohydrate: 25 g	Fat: 18 g

Variations

For Phase 3: Substitute buckwheat flour for half the chickpea flour.

Phase 1 Meal: Serve with a few slices of avocado, 1 (1-ounce) slice cooked turkey bacon or equivalent vegetarian protein (see Equivalents Table, page 49), and ¼ cup berries topped with 1 tablespoon Cardamom Whipped Cream (page 324).

Calories: 479; Carbohydrate: 25%; Protein: 25%; Fat: 50%

Phase 2 Meal: Serve with 1 (1-ounce) slice cooked turkey bacon or equivalent vegetarian protein (see Equivalents Table, page 49) and 1 cup blueberries.

Calories: 469; Carbohydrate: 38%; Protein: 25%; Fat: 37%

Phase 3 Meal: Use the Phase 3 Variation. Serve with 1 cup blueberries tossed with a drizzle of pure maple syrup and 1 heaping tablespoon Cardamom Whipped Cream (page 324).

Calories: 489; Carbohydrate: 41%; Protein: 19%; Fat: 40%

Make-Your-Own Whole-Grain Porridge (Phases 2 and 3)

A whole-grain porridge is a comforting way to break the overnight fast. A variety of different whole grains, add-ins, and toppings can be used to create delicious savory or sweet concoctions for your morning routine. Try a few to find the ones you like best, then mix and match for new treats. You might be surprised to find how satisfying savory breakfasts can be. For a morning time-saver, cook the porridge the night before, then just reheat for breakfast.

Preparation time: 2 to 5 minutes

Total time: 20 to 30 minutes

Makes 4 servings

Phase 2 Base Porridge 1

- 1½ cups cooked brown rice, wheat berries, millet, or quinoa (or any combination of leftover cooked whole grains)
- 3 cups water, milk, or broth
- Pinch of salt

Phase 2 Base Porridge 2

- ½ cup cooked brown rice, millet, farro, barley, or quinoa (or any combination of leftover cooked whole grains)
- ⅓ cup uncooked steel-cut oats, amaranth, teff, or other quick-cooking whole grain
- 3 cups water, milk, or broth
- Pinch of salt

Phase 2 Base Porridge 3

- 1 cup uncooked steel-cut oats, amaranth, teff, or other quick-cooking whole grain
- 3 cups water, milk, or broth
- Pinch of salt

Place the grains, water, salt, and any add-ins (see list on page 102), if using, in a pot with a lid. Bring to a boil, uncovered. Stir well, reduce the heat to low, cover, and simmer for about 20 minutes, or until the water has been absorbed and the porridge is smooth and creamy. Stir once or twice while cooking to ensure that the water is distributed throughout for even absorption.

Serve plain or with toppings (see list on page 102) to complete the meal.

Add-ins:

Sweet:

- Dried fruit (apricots, raisins, currants, apples, figs, etc.), chopped
- Fresh or frozen fruit (apples, pears, berries, etc.), chopped
- Root vegetables (onion, carrot, turnip, rutabaga, parsnip, fennel, etc.), diced small
- Raw nuts or seeds (pecans, walnuts, cashews, sunflower seeds, pumpkin seeds, sesame seeds, etc.), chopped
- Coconut oil

Savory:

- Cooked protein (chicken, beef, bacon, lamb, sardines, tofu, tempeh), diced
- Cooked or canned beans, drained and rinsed
- Root vegetables (carrot, turnip, rutabaga, parsnip, onion, fennel, etc.), chopped
- Raw nuts or seeds (pecans, walnuts, cashews, sunflower seeds, pumpkin seeds, sesame seeds, etc.), chopped
- Herbs, spices, garlic
- Fresh Salsa (page 302)
- Coconut oil
- Egg (cracked on top halfway through cooking)

Toppings:

- Fresh or dried fruit (apples, pears, berries, etc.), chopped
- Roasted nuts or seeds (pecans, walnuts, cashews, sunflower seeds, pumpkin seeds, sesame seeds, etc.), chopped
- Flax- or chia seeds, whole or ground
- Cheese, shredded
- Avocado, sliced
- Hard-boiled egg, sliced
- Fresh Salsa (page 302)
- Spicy Pickled Vegetables (page 68) or kimchi
- Fresh herbs (parsley, cilantro, scallions, or dried herbs like oregano, basil, or others)
- Scallion-Miso Condiment (see page 105)
- Oils or fats (coconut oil, extra-virgin olive oil, or flax oil)
- Plain whole-milk Greek yogurt

If you choose a version without protein, serve it with an egg; turkey bacon or equivalent vegetarian protein (see Equivalents Table, page 49); cottage cheese; plain whole-milk Greek yogurt; or other higher-protein side to complete the meal.

Creamy Coconut Teff (Phases 2 and 3)

Teff is a nutty-flavored whole grain that pairs well with creamy coconut. Add a touch of dried or fresh fruit, and you have a lusciously sweet breakfast porridge. If you know you'll be in a hurry, make this ahead and set it like polenta for quick breakfast squares.

Preparation time: 5 minutes

Total time: 25 minutes

Makes 4 servings

- 4 cups water
- ⅛ teaspoon salt
- 1 cup uncooked teff
- ½ cup dried fruit, such as figs, prunes, raisins, etc., chopped
- 3 tablespoons coconut oil
- ⅓ cup walnuts or other nuts of your choice, lightly toasted

Bring the water to a boil in a medium saucepan. Stir in the salt, teff, dried fruit, and coconut oil. Cook over medium heat, stirring frequently with a whisk, until the liquid has been absorbed, 15 to 30 minutes.

Serve warm, topped with toasted nuts.

Tip: Teff will set like polenta when it cools. If you are not eating it right away, either scoop it into decorative mounds with an ice cream scoop or spread it into an 8 x 4-inch loaf pan and let cool to set. Reheat it in the oven or toaster oven at 350°F for 10 to 15 minutes for an easy grab-and-go breakfast option, or add ¼ to ½ cup milk to reheat to a creamy consistency.

Calories: 381
Carbohydrate: 50 g

Protein: 8 g
Fat: 18 g

Variations

Omit the dried fruit and serve as a sweet or savory breakfast porridge.

Phase 2 or 3 Meal: Serve with 3½ ounces smoked salmon, cooked turkey bacon, or equivalent vegetarian protein (see Equivalents Table, page 49).

Calories: 497; Carbohydrate: 39%; Protein: 22%; Fat: 39%

Phase 2 or 3 Meal Variation: Use the variation without dried fruit. Serve with ½ cup strawberries and ⅔ cup cottage cheese.

Calories: 516; Carbohydrate: 36%; Protein: 21%; Fat: 43%

Chef Dawn's Tasty Tip

The Original Flavor Enhancer

The taste sensation known as *umami*—described as savory richness—was originally identified in kombu, a type of kelp. The sensation of umami is produced by a newly identified class of taste receptors specific for glutamate, an amino acid found in the food additive MSG. Before the chemical version of MSG was commercially available, the Japanese obtained this rich flavor naturally from kombu broth. We often add a 1-inch piece of kombu to grain or bean dishes to achieve a subtle depth of flavor. Kombu, as with most sea vegetables, also provides vital trace minerals (such as iodine) and is traditionally believed to improve the digestibility of beans.

Brown Rice Congee (Phases 2 and 3)

Congee, also known as *jook*, is a staple savory breakfast food in many Asian countries. Although traditionally made with white rice, the brown rice version makes a deliciously creamy dish. Shiitake, kombu, and beans provide a lavish umami flavor in this little porridge, while the ginger and salty miso condiment top it off for a big win. The recipe requires some planning the night before, but if you haven't explored savory for breakfast, this one could be a game-changer!

Preparation time: 25 minutes

Total time: 8 hours (slow cooker)

Makes 4 servings

- 5½ cups water
- 1 (½- to 1-inch) piece fresh ginger, peeled and thinly sliced
- 2 to 3 tablespoons extra-virgin olive oil (1 tablespoon with tofu option)
- 1 stalk celery, cut into ½-inch pieces
- 2 fresh or 1 dried shiitake mushrooms, cut into small pieces
- 1 pound boneless, skinless chicken thighs, diced, or 1¼ pounds extra-firm tofu, pressed with an absorbent towel and crumbled
- ½ teaspoon salt, or to taste
- ⅔ cup uncooked short-grain brown rice
- ⅓ cup dried adzuki or mung beans, or ⅔ cup cooked (see Do-It-Yourself Beans, page 74) or drained and rinsed canned beans
- 1 (1-inch) piece kombu or kelp seaweed (optional)
- 1 small rutabaga or other root vegetable (8 ounces)
- 1½ cups large chunks cabbage

Scallion-Miso Condiment

- 2 tablespoons toasted sesame oil
- 16 scallions or 2 small leeks, thinly sliced on an angle
- ¼ cup miso paste (see Tip)
- ½ cup sesame seeds, toasted, for garnish

Bring 5 cups of the water to a boil in a large saucepan.

Place the ginger in a wide-mouthed glass jar or cup that will fit an immersion blender without splashing. Add the remaining ½ cup water. Blend until smooth. Set aside in the refrigerator.

Heat olive oil in a slow cooker on the sauté setting or in a large Dutch oven or stovetop-safe slow cooker insert over medium heat. Add the celery, mushrooms, chicken, and salt. Cook, stirring, for 5 to 8 minutes, or until the vegetables soften and release their juices and the chicken begins to brown slightly.

Add the rice, beans, kombu (if using), rutabaga, cabbage, and the boiling water to the slow cooker or pot and bring to a boil. Transfer the mixture to the slow cooker or return the insert to the slow cooker, if necessary, cover, and cook on low overnight or for about 8 hours. (If you'd rather skip the slow cooker, simmer on low heat in the Dutch oven for 4 to 5 hours, or until all water has been absorbed and the porridge is creamy.)

Make the scallion-miso condiment: Heat the sesame oil in a small skillet over medium-high heat. Add the scallions and cook, stirring, until soft and slightly caramelized, about 2 minutes. Reduce the heat to low. Pile the scallions in the middle of the pan. Put the miso on top and cover with a lid. Leave on low heat for 5 minutes, until the miso begins to soften. Uncover and stir the scallions and miso together. Refrigerate until ready to serve.

Once the congee is done, stir the reserved ginger puree into the hot congee. Serve garnished with the sesame seeds and scallion-miso condiment.

Tip: This congee is lightly salted but served with a salty condiment that allows it to reach its full flavor. Experiment with different types of miso from the hearty dark miso to the mellow light miso to find the one you love for this condiment. Adjust the seasonings to taste.

Calories: 573   Protein: 35 g (24%)
Carbohydrate: 50 g (34%) Fat: 28 g (42%)

Variations

Add 1 (½-inch) piece fresh turmeric, peeled and thinly sliced, or ¼ teaspoon ground turmeric to the jar with the ginger, blend, and set aside.

On-the-Go Breakfast Parfait (All Phases)

This delicious meal in a jar is a satisfying, self-contained masterpiece. Make it the night before for an easy, out-the-door breakfast so you'll never leave home hungry again. Swap out the nutmeg for your favorite spices, or alter the fruit to tailor this dish to your preferences.

Preparation time: 5 minutes

Total time: 10 minutes

Makes 1 serving

- ¼ cup half-and-half
- 1 tablespoon chia seeds, ground (see Tip)
- ½ teaspoon pure vanilla extract
- ¼ teaspoon freshly grated nutmeg, ground cinnamon, or ground cardamom
- 1 teaspoon lemon zest (optional)
- ¾ cup 4% whole-milk cottage cheese

Fruit Sauce

- ¾ cup fresh or frozen berries
- 1 tablespoon water
- 3 tablespoons chopped cashews, peanuts, or other nuts of your choice, for garnish

Heat the half-and-half in a small saucepan, stirring frequently, until the edges begin to bubble. Pour into a medium bowl and set the saucepan aside to use for the fruit sauce—no need to wash it.

Stir the chia seeds, vanilla, nutmeg, lemon zest, and cottage cheese into the warm half-and-half. Set aside.

Make the fruit sauce: Place the berries and water into the saucepan used to heat the half-and-half. Bring to a boil. Reduce the heat to low, cover, and simmer until the berries are soft. Mash lightly with a spatula.

Assemble the parfait: Spoon 3 to 4 tablespoons of the cottage cheese mixture into the bottom of a pint-size jar. Pour about 2 tablespoons of the warm berries on top, then layer 1 tablespoon of nuts on top of the berries. Repeat this layering, ending with berries and nuts.

Serve warm, or put the lid on the jar and refrigerate for a quick breakfast-on-the-run when you need it. (See photo insert page 2.)

Tip: Use a coffee grinder or spice mill to grind the chia seeds. This step can be skipped and the chia seeds used whole, but their texture and digestibility are improved when they are ground.

Calories: 529
Carbohydrate: 36 g (27%)
Protein: 31 g (23%)
Fat: 30 g (50%)

Variations

For a spiced apple or pear parfait, substitute an apple or ½ pear, cored, and use apple pie or pumpkin pie spices (cinnamon, ginger, nutmeg, and clove) in place of the berries and nutmeg.

For Phases 2 and 3: Substitute whole milk for the half-and-half. Add 1 tablespoon pure maple syrup or honey to the Fruit Sauce.

Calories: 539
Carbohydrate: 50 g (37%)
Protein: 31 g (23%)
Fat: 25 g (40%)

Chia Seed Pudding (All Phases)

This creamy pudding is so delicious it can double as dessert! Serve the full portion for a complete breakfast, or one-third portion for a rich and satisfying after-dinner treat.

Preparation time: 5 minutes plus resting time

Total time: 1 hour

Makes 4 servings (3 cups)

- 1 cup whole milk or unsweetened soy milk
- 1 (14.5-ounce) can unsweetened coconut milk
- 1/3 cup chia seeds
- 1 teaspoon pure vanilla extract
- 3 servings unsweetened, unflavored 100% whey protein powder (check the package nutritional info—1 serving should yield 22 g protein)
- 4 cups berries, quartered

Heat the milk and coconut milk in a saucepan over medium heat, stirring occasionally, until it is creamy and starts to bubble at the edges.

Grind the chia seeds in a coffee grinder or spice mill and stir them into the hot milk mixture. Add the vanilla, stir, and remove from the heat. Transfer to a bowl and set aside to cool for about 1 hour, or set the bowl in a larger bowl of ice water to cool.

Make sure the pudding is cool, then stir in the protein powder until well combined.

Divide the pudding evenly among four jars. Top with the berries and serve, or place the lids on the jars and store in the refrigerator.

Calories: 447
Carbohydrate: 30 g (26%)

Protein: 26 g (21%)
Fat: 29 g (53%)

Variations

Serve one-third of each portion as a dessert, with or without the protein powder.

Dairy-free version: Vegetarian protein powders don't work well in this recipe. Omit the whey powder and use 1 cup coconut milk and 1½ cups unsweetened soy milk. Serve it with 3 ounces of a lower-fat, higher-protein side like turkey bacon or equivalent vegetarian protein (see Equivalents Table, page 49).

For Phases 2 and 3: Reduce the coconut milk to 1 cup and increase the whole milk to 1¼ cups. Cook ⅓ cup dried fruit of your choice with the coconut milk in addition to the berries in the recipe.

Calories: 444
Carbohydrate: 41 g (34%)

Protein: 26 g (22%)
Fat: 23 g (44%)

My *Always Delicious* Story

Thirty years ago, at age twenty-one, I read *Fit or Fat* and committed myself to avoiding fat. The book said fat had 9 calories per gram, while sugar had 4. Clearly fat was the enemy—eat fat, get fat. I ate pasta, fruit, SnackWell's, the crust of the pizza to avoid the cheese, the pretzels instead of the hummus. I wouldn't touch anything with oil, and I'd panic if fat passed my lips unintentionally. As my struggles with weight continued, I restricted calories more and more, I took my own food to social events, and I logged my calories and walked around with a persistent dull headache. And I exercised *a lot*. My entire adult life has been fraught with confusion and shame as to why I was fat.

Enter *Always Hungry?* What a paradigm shift. I read it with intermittent gasps and tears of frustration from years of self-loathing and energy wasted. I have gratitude for my liberation mixed with mourning for the things I might have accomplished physically, mentally, and emotionally had I been twenty-one when I read this book.

Kathleen N., age 51, Running Springs, California

CHAPTER 6

Entrées

CHICKEN

Shredded Chicken (All Phases)

Use this shredded chicken as a starting point for your favorite recipes. Add it to salads, casseroles, wraps, and stir-fries, or just serve it on its own. Switch up the spices to create different flavor profiles. This is also a fantastic base recipe to freeze in individually portioned zip-top bags for a quick protein when you haven't planned ahead. It is generally lower in fat, making it a great dinner choice when you're planning to serve one of our higher-fat desserts.

Preparation time: 5 minutes

Total time: 30 minutes

Makes 6 servings (about 3 cups)

- 2 teaspoons extra-virgin olive oil
- 1 large clove garlic, minced or pressed
- 1½ tablespoons All-Purpose Seasoned Salt (page 283), or ½ teaspoon salt
- 1¾ pounds boneless, skinless chicken thighs
- ½ cup water, unsalted chicken broth, or Bone Broth (page 58)
- 2 teaspoons Sugar-Free Worcestershire Sauce (page 284)

Heat the olive oil in a skillet over medium heat. Add the garlic, seasoned salt, and chicken and cook, turning to lightly brown the chicken on both sides, about 2 minutes per side. Add the water and Worcestershire. Bring to a boil.

Reduce the heat to low. Cover and simmer for about 20 minutes, turning the chicken a few times, until it is fully cooked and no longer pink in the middle.

Shred the chicken in the pot, using two forks and pulling along the grain to create thin strands. Heat the shredded chicken, uncovered, stirring frequently, until the liquid and spices have been absorbed, 3 to 5 minutes. Serve immediately or cool and store in the refrigerator for 3 to 4 days or in the freezer for up to 6 months.

Calories: 172
Carbohydrate: 1 g

Protein: 27 g
Fat: 6 g

Phase 1 Meal: Serve with 1 cup Cuban Black Bean Soup (page 253) garnished with ¼ avocado and 1 heaping tablespoon sour cream, and Zucchini with Garlic and Greens (page 212). **For Dessert:** ½ cup strawberries topped with 2 to 3 tablespoons heavy cream.

Calories: 632; Carbohydrate: 25%; Protein: 25% Fat 50%

Phase 2 or 3 Meal: Serve with ¾ cup Mexican Rice (page 227) drizzled with 1 teaspoon olive oil, and Zucchini with Garlic and Greens (page 212). **For Dessert:** 1 Coconut BonBon (page 316) or Orange Chocolate Pudding (page 317).

Calories: 665; Carbohydrate: 36%; Protein: 21%; Fat: 43%

Creamy Dijon Chicken and Mushrooms (All Phases)

Rich and satisfying, the sauce is really the star here. Using a lower-fat protein like chicken tenderloins leaves room for all the fat in the sauce. At the same time, the sauce keeps those lower-fat meats from tasting too dry. This is a great casserole to make ahead and freeze for those days when you just don't have time to cook.

Preparation time: 10 minutes

Total time: 45 minutes

Makes 6 servings

- 1½ pounds chicken tenderloins (or sliced pork tenderloins)
- 1 teaspoon salt
- ¼ teaspoon ground black pepper
- 2½ tablespoons extra-virgin olive oil
- 3 or 4 cloves garlic, minced
- 1 pound sliced baby bella/cremini mushrooms
- 2 tablespoons Dijon mustard
- Leaves from 5 large sprigs thyme or tarragon, or ½ teaspoon dried thyme or tarragon
- ⅓ cup dry white wine, unsalted chicken stock, Bone Broth (page 58), or water
- ½ cup heavy cream
- 1½ cups whole milk or unsweetened soy milk
- 1 (8-ounce) bag fresh baby spinach (about 4 cups packed)

Sprinkle the tenderloins with ½ teaspoon of the salt and ⅛ teaspoon of the pepper.

Heat the olive oil in a very large skillet over medium heat. Add the chicken and cook, turning, to brown on all sides. Remove from the pan and set aside on a plate.

Raise the heat to medium-high and add the garlic, mushrooms, and the remaining ½ teaspoon salt and ⅛ teaspoon pepper to the pan. Cook, stirring, until the mushrooms have softened and the liquid they release has reduced, 8 to 10 minutes.

Stir in the mustard, then add the thyme and wine, stirring to scrape up the browned bits in the pan. Cook for a few minutes more.

Return the chicken and any juices that have collected on the plate to the pan. Reduce the heat to medium and stir in the cream and milk.

Simmer for 10 to 15 minutes, until the sauce has thickened and the tenderloins are cooked through.

Stir in the spinach leaves. Cover and cook until the spinach is just wilted but still bright in color and not overcooked.

Serve immediately or cool and store in the refrigerator for 3 to 4 days or in the freezer for up to 6 months.

Calories: 311   Protein: 31 g
Carbohydrate: 9 g   Fat: 17 g

Variations

Add 1 tablespoon butter and reduce the olive oil to 1¾ tablespoons.

Dairy-free version: Increase the olive oil to ⅓ cup, add 3 tablespoons chickpea flour with the mushrooms, and substitute 2 cups unsweetened soy milk for the cream and the whole milk.

Fish version: Substitute 2 pounds white-fleshed fish like cod, hake, or haddock for the chicken.

Phase 1 Meal: Serve with Cauliflower Couscous (page 211) and a side of salad greens and chopped raw vegetables tossed with 1 to 2 teaspoons Creamy Sun-Dried Tomato Dressing (page 287). **For Dessert:** 1 Chocolate Truffle (page 314) and 1 cup strawberries topped with 2 tablespoons Cardamom Whipped Cream (page 324).

Calories: 610; Carbohydrate: 26%; Protein: 25%; Fat: 49%

Phase 2 Meal: Serve with ½ cup cooked brown rice and 1 cup steamed broccoli with a drizzle of olive oil. **For Dessert:** 4 Chocolate-Dipped Strawberries (page 313).

Calories: 637; Carbohydrate: 36%; Protein: 24%; Fat: 40%

Phase 3 Meal: Use the Phase 2 Meal, but substitute 1 cup cooked white potatoes for the brown rice.

Calories: 611; Carbohydrate: 37%; Protein: 24%; Fat: 39%

Fried Fish Fillets or Chicken Fingers (All Phases)

Chickpea flour works perfectly for frying and breading your favorite proteins. If you want an even crispier version, try using Chickpea Bread Crumbs (page 196) as we do in Chicken Parmesan (page 126).

Preparation time: 5 minutes

Total time: 35 minutes

Makes 4 servings

Coating

- 1 cup chickpea flour (see Tip, page 91)
- ¼ teaspoon garlic powder
- ½ to 1 teaspoon salt
- ¼ teaspoon ground black pepper

Protein

- 1 cup neutral-tasting oil with a high smoke point, such as high-oleic safflower or avocado oil
- 2 pounds fish fillets (leave small, thin fillets whole and cut thicker fillets into 2-inch-wide strips), or 1¼ pounds boneless, skinless chicken thighs, cut into 1-inch-wide strips
- Salt and ground black pepper

Preheat the oven to 200°F.

Make the coating: Combine the chickpea flour, garlic powder, salt, and pepper in a shallow dish or pie plate.

Coat and fry the protein: Heat the oil in a large cast-iron skillet over medium heat. (The oil should be ¼ to ⅓ inch deep in the skillet and hot enough to sizzle when the protein is added, about 350°F.)

If using fish, rinse it and pat dry. If using chicken, do not rinse, just handle carefully by patting it dry with paper towels to avoid cross contaminating any surface with liquid from the raw chicken.

Season the fish or chicken lightly with salt and pepper. (Remember that there is salt in the coating as well.)

Dredge the fish or chicken in the coating to completely cover, shaking off any excess, and gently place in the hot oil in a single layer. Work in batches as necessary to avoid crowding the pan. Cook, uncovered, until the coating is browned and crispy, about 5 minutes, then turn and cook on the other side for 5 to 8 minutes, or until the protein is fully cooked.

Remove from the pan and drain on a plate lined with paper towels or a bamboo sushi mat. Transfer to a baking sheet and keep warm in the oven until ready to serve.

Skim any bits of flour from the oil with a mesh strainer or spoon, add oil as needed, and reheat it. If the oil isn't hot enough, the batter will be soggy instead of crispy, so let the oil come back to temperature between batches and avoid crowding. Repeat to fry the remaining fish or chicken.

Serve warm.

Calories: 404   Protein: 32 g
Carbohydrate: 10 g   Fat: 26 g

Variations

For a thicker, crispier coating, dredge the fish or chicken in chickpea flour, then dip in a beaten egg, then dredge in the flour again before frying.

Vegetarian version: See Crispy Tofu Fries (page 173).

Higher-protein, lower-fat version: Substitute chicken tenderloins for thighs. This option works well when serving with higher-fat sides, higher-fat desserts, or larger portions of dipping sauces.

Phase 1 Meal: Serve with 1 to 2 tablespoons Lemon Aioli (page 298) for dipping, a bowl (2 cups) of Minestrone Soup (page 248), and ½ small cucumber, sliced and seasoned with salt and lemon juice. **For Dessert:** A few strawberries.

Calories: 701; Carbohydrate: 25%; Protein: 24%; Fat: 51%

Phase 2 Meal: Serve with Millet Mashed Fauxtatoes (page 236) and ½ small cucumber, sliced and seasoned with salt and lemon juice. **For Dessert:** 1 medium apple, cored, sliced, and dipped in 2 tablespoons plain whole-milk Greek yogurt mixed with 1 teaspoon honey.

Calories: 690; Carbohydrate: 35%; Protein: 22%; Fat: 43%

Phase 3 Meal: Serve with 1 cup boiled potatoes seasoned with salt, pepper, and 1 teaspoon olive oil, and ½ small cucumber, sliced and seasoned with salt and lemon juice. **For Dessert:** 1 cup diced mango.

Calories: 690; Carbohydrate: 39%; Protein: 21%; Fat: 40%

Chef Dawn's Tasty Tip

Worth Your Salt

Knowing how much salt to use and "seasoning to taste" can be a maddening task when reading recipes that aren't specific. How can you salt meat loaf or chicken "to taste" before cooking, when you can't taste it until done? To make matters more complicated, commercial marinades, sauces, or soup stocks contain widely varying amounts of salt. So here are guidelines to get you started. For boneless raw meat, chicken, or fish, start with about ½ teaspoon salt per pound, then taste and add more salt if needed before serving. For beans, add ¾ to 1 teaspoon salt per pound (2½ cups) dried beans or per 5 cups cooked beans. For soups, start with about 1 teaspoon salt, or 2 to 3 tablespoons soy sauce per quart of water or unsalted broth. Soups with beans or meat will need more salt if the ingredients weren't seasoned before adding them to the soup. For vegetarian proteins like tofu or tempeh, start with about 1 teaspoon salt per pound.

Add proportionately less salt if using a commercial ingredient that already contains salt like broths or canned beans (look at the Nutrition Facts Label). Taste and season with salt at the end of cooking to balance the other flavors. For example, creamy or spicier dishes lend themselves to a bit more salt.

NOTE: 1 teaspoon salt = 6 grams salt = 2.3 grams sodium

On-a-Budget Marinated Chicken (All Phases)

The secret is in the sauce. Use any of our sauces or marinades to quickly and easily turn inexpensive chicken into restaurant-quality masterpieces. This is a definite go-to for busy nights when you haven't planned ahead. For a complete meal, add vegetables and beans or grains.

Preparation time: 10 minutes plus overnight marinating

Total time: 1 hour

Makes 4 servings

- 2½ to 2¾ pounds skin-on chicken drumsticks
- ½ cup Lemon Thyme Marinade (page 296), or any of your favorite marinades or sauces from pages 284 to 306
- Salt, depending on the saltiness of the sauce
- Fresh parsley, cilantro, or scallions, chopped, for garnish

Arrange the chicken in a 9 x 13-inch baking dish in a single layer. Pull back the skin from the large side of the chicken and pour or rub half the marinade or sauce over the top, making sure to get the marinade under the skin. Put the skin back in place and pour or rub the rest of the marinade or sauce over the top.

These can be baked right away. To create a more flavorful dish, cover the dish with plastic wrap, or place the chicken and marinade in a zip-top bag, making sure that the chicken is covered in the marinade. Place in the refrigerator to marinate for at least 1 hour and up to overnight.

When ready to bake, preheat the oven to 350°F.

If marinating in a zip-top bag, transfer the chicken and marinade to a baking dish.

Bake for about 45 minutes, or until the chicken is done and no longer pink in the center, basting every 15 to 20 minutes by spooning marinade from the bottom of the pan over the top of each piece of chicken and adding water as needed to prevent burning.

Garnish with parsley and serve hot.

Calories: 356   Protein: 36 g
Carbohydrate: 1 g   Fat: 24 g

Variations

Toss large chunks of onion and/or other root vegetables or dried fruit with a bit of the marinade and arrange in the baking dish around the chicken before cooking.

Slow cooker version: Place chicken in a slow cooker with the marinade, cover, and cook on medium for 4 to 5 hours or on low for about 8 hours, or according to the manufacturer's instructions. For crispier skin, once the drumsticks are done, place in the oven under the broiler for a few minutes, turning until the skin reaches desired crispiness. The time needed under the broiler will depend on the sauce used.

Higher-protein, lower-fat version: Substitute 2 pounds boneless, skinless chicken thighs for the drumsticks. This option works well when serving higher-fat sides, dipping sauces, or desserts.

Vegetarian version: See Marinated Baked Tofu (page 175).

Substitute ½ cup Fresh Turmeric Garlic Marinade (page 295), Chimichurri (pages 300 and 301), Basil Walnut Pesto (page 297), Miso-Sake Marinade from Drunken Marinated Shrimp Kebabs (page 144), Lime Cilantro Pesto (page 298), Greek Dressing (page 285), or 1 cup Spicy Asian Marinade (page 294), or Enchilada Sauce from the Quinoa Enchilada Casserole (page 183) for the Lemon Thyme Marinade.

Chicken Potpie (with Tofu Variation) (All Phases)

Our chickpea crust transforms this old favorite into a homey meal that everyone can enjoy. Simple chicken combined with a luscious filling creates a savory, homestyle dish that you can feel good about feeding to your family.

Preparation time: 20 minutes

Total time: 45 minutes to 1 hour

Makes 6 servings

- 3 tablespoons extra-virgin olive oil
- 1 large onion, diced
- 2 stalks celery, diced
- 1 large carrot, diced
- 1 or 2 cloves garlic, minced
- ½ teaspoon dried thyme
- 1 to 1½ teaspoons salt, or to taste
- ½ teaspoon ground black pepper
- 1¾ pounds boneless, skinless chicken thighs, diced
- ⅓ cup chickpea flour (see Tip, page 91)
- 1½ cups unsalted chicken broth, Bone Broth (page 58), or water
- ½ cup half-and-half
- 1 recipe Grain-Free Piecrust dough (page 206)

Preheat the oven to 375°F.

Heat the olive oil in a large skillet over medium heat. Add the onion, celery, carrot, garlic, thyme, salt, and pepper. Cook, stirring, until the onion is translucent, 3 to 5 minutes. Add the chicken and cook for 8 to 10 minutes more.

Add the chickpea flour and cook, stirring, for 5 minutes to lightly brown the flour.

Combine the broth and half-and-half in a measuring cup, pour over the vegetable mixture, and cook, stirring, until thickened, 5 to 10 minutes.

Evenly distribute the filling among six large ramekins or pour it into one 9-inch pie plate.

Roll out the pie dough and cut it into 6 rounds to fit over the ramekins, or into a large round to fit over the top of the pie plate. Place the crust over the filling, covering the edges of the ramekins or pie plate. Decoratively flute or crimp the edges of the dough to seal it, and cut a few small vents in the middle to allow steam to escape.

Bake for 20 to 40 minutes (smaller ramekins will cook more quickly), or until the filling is bubbling and the crust is golden brown.

Calories: 457
Carbohydrate: 22 g

Protein: 35 g
Fat: 25 g

Variations

Vegetarian version: Substitute 2 pounds extra-firm tofu, drained, pressed with an absorbent towel, and crumbled, for the chicken. Reduce the oil to 1 tablespoon. Use vegetable stock or water in place of chicken stock, and increase the salt to 2 teaspoons, or to taste; or substitute 1½ recipes Basic Seitan (page 72), minced, for the chicken. Increase the oil to 5 tablespoons, and omit the salt.

Dairy-free version: Use ½ cup unsweetened soy milk in place of the half-and-half and increase the olive oil to ¼ cup.

For Phase 3: Reduce the chicken to 1½ pounds and reduce the salt to 1 to 1¼ teaspoons.

Double-crust version: Use 2 Grain-Free Piecrusts (one for the bottom and one for the top). These can even be made into 6 individual grab-and-go, complete-meal mini pies as we describe in Meat Pies (page 155).

Calories: 630
Carbohydrate: 36 g

Protein: 40 g
Fat: 36 g

Phase 1 Meal: Serve with 1 cup Minestrone Soup (page 248) drizzled with ½ teaspoon olive oil and a side of salad greens and chopped raw vegetables tossed with 1 to 2 teaspoons Greek Dressing (page 285). **For Dessert:** ½ cup strawberries topped with 1 heaping tablespoon Cardamom Whipped Cream (page 324).

Calories: 687; Carbohydrate: 27%; Protein: 24%; Fat: 49%

Phase 1 Meal (Double-Crust Variation): Serve with sliced tomatoes and cucumbers seasoned with salt and lemon juice and a drizzle of olive oil. **For Dessert:** A few strawberries.

Calories: 686; Carbohydrate: 25%; Protein: 24%; Fat: 51%

Phase 2 Meal: Serve with a bowl (2 cups) of Creamy Millet Vegetable Soup (page 255) and sliced tomatoes and cucumbers seasoned with salt and lemon juice. **For Dessert:** 1 cup strawberries.

Calories: 676; Carbohydrate: 36%; Protein: 24%; Fat: 40%

Phase 3 Meal: Use the Phase 3 Variation. Serve with a bowl (2 cups) of Creamy Millet Vegetable Soup (page 255) and sliced tomatoes and cucumbers seasoned with salt and lemon juice. **For Dessert:** ¾ cup diced mango.

Calories: 682; Carbohydrate: 40%; Protein: 21%; Fat: 39%

Citrus Teriyaki Chicken Stir-Fry (Phases 2 and 3, with Phase 1 Variation)

This is a go-to recipe when you want something fresh, quick, and delicious. Make the sauce on Prep Day and use precut vegetables to make this meal in a flash. It's also delicious in a lettuce wrap the next day.

Preparation time: 10 minutes

Total time: 30 minutes

Makes 4 servings

- 1¼ pounds boneless, skinless chicken thighs, cut into 1-inch cubes
- ¾ cup Citrus Teriyaki Sauce (page 293)
- 1 tablespoon neutral-tasting oil, like untoasted sesame, avocado, or high-oleic safflower
- 4 ounces fresh shiitake, baby bella/cremini, or white button mushrooms, sliced (about 2 cups)
- 1 head broccoli, cut into small florets, stalk peeled and cut into small pieces
- 2 medium carrots, cut into matchsticks or coarsely shredded (about 1 cup)
- 2 cups shredded cabbage
- 8 ounces snow peas or snap peas (15 to 20 pods)
- Salt or soy sauce
- 3 cups packed fresh spinach (about 6 ounces)
- Scallions, sliced, for garnish

Place the chicken and teriyaki sauce in a shallow pan or in a zip-top bag, stirring or shaking the sealed bag to make sure the sauce covers all sides of the chicken. Place in the refrigerator to marinate for at least 1 hour and up to overnight (or cook the chicken in the sauce immediately, if you have less time).

Heat the oil in a large skillet over medium heat. Add the chicken and sauce. Cook, stirring, for 5 minutes, or until chicken begins to brown.

Add the mushrooms. Cook, stirring, until the chicken is no longer pink in the middle and the mushrooms are softened, 5 to 7 minutes.

Stir in the broccoli, carrots, cabbage, and snow peas. Reduce the heat to medium-low, cover, and simmer, stirring a few times, until the vegetables are tender but still bright in color, 2 to 3 minutes. Taste and adjust the seasonings with salt or soy sauce as needed.

Spread the spinach on a serving tray or divide among individual bowls. Spoon the hot chicken and vegetables on top of the spinach, leaving any excess liquid in the skillet. The spinach should begin to wilt under the heat of the chicken.

Bring the liquid in the skillet to a boil, reduce the heat to medium-low, and simmer, uncovered, until the sauce thickens, 3 to 5 minutes. Pour the thickened sauce over the stir-fry.

Garnish with scallions. Serve immediately, while the vegetables are still bright in color.

Tip: Since we are not using cornstarch to thicken the sauce, you will need to cook it down a bit to thicken it. Although it will not have the same volume of liquid, the reduced sauce will add all the flavor you need to the final product.

Calories: 307
Carbohydrate: 23 g

Protein: 34 g
Fat: 9 g

Variations

Add or substitute other vegetables of your choice.

Shrimp version: Substitute 16 to 20 ounces peeled and deveined shrimp for the chicken.

Whole-grain version: Add the spinach and 1⅓ cups cooked brown rice or Cooked Quinoa (page 231) when you add the vegetables, then sauté them together. The grain will absorb the sauce and you may not need to reduce it at the end.

Vegan version: Substitute 1¾ pounds extra-firm tofu, drained, pressed with an absorbent towel, and cut into bite-size pieces, for the chicken, reduce the oil to 1 teaspoon, and season with additional salt or soy sauce; or substitute 1 recipe Basic Seitan (page 72) for the chicken and increase oil to 2 to 3 tablespoons.

Calories: 324
Carbohydrate: 17 g

Protein: 33 g
Fat: 13 g

Phase 1 Meal: Substitute Spicy Asian Marinade (page 294; without honey) for the Citrus Teriyaki Sauce.

Phase 2 Meal (Grain-Free): Serve with Cauliflower Couscous (page 211) drizzled with 1 teaspoon olive oil, and a bowl (2 cups) of Miso Soup (page 258). **For Dessert:** ½ cup blueberries and 1 Coconut BonBon (page 316).

Calories: 688; Carbohydrate: 35%; Protein: 26%; Fat: 39%

Phase 2 Meal (Whole-Grain Version): Make the whole-grain version with brown rice or quinoa. Serve with a bowl (2 cups) of Miso Soup (page 258). **For Dessert:** 2 or 3 Almond Coconut Macaroons (page 312).

Calories: 683; Carbohydrate: 35%; Protein: 27%; Fat: 38%

Phase 3 Meal: Cook 1½ ounces dry udon or soba noodles per serving, and sauté them with a slightly smaller portion of stir-fry. **For Dessert:** ½ cup blueberries topped with 1 heaping tablespoon of Cardamom Whipped Cream (page 324) and sprinkled with ¼ cup Candied Nuts (page 324).

Calories: 669; Carbohydrate: 37%; Protein: 22%; Fat: 41%

Spicy Asian Stir-Fry (Phases 2 and 3, with Phase 1 Variation)

Slightly spicy with a touch of sweetness. This restaurant-quality stir-fry packs all the flavor of a takeout meal without the refined sugars and additives. Feel free to experiment with different proteins, vegetables, and spices as you create your own version of the perfect stir-fry.

Preparation time: 15 minutes plus overnight marinating

Total time: 30 minutes

Makes 4 servings

- 1¼ pounds boneless, skinless chicken thighs, cut into bite-size pieces
- 1 recipe Spicy Asian Marinade (page 294)
- 1 teaspoon toasted sesame oil or a neutral-tasting oil, such as avocado or high-oleic safflower oil
- 2 medium carrots, cut into matchsticks or coarsely shredded (about 1 cup)
- 2 cups shredded cabbage, chopped bok choy, or napa cabbage
- 1 head broccoli, cut into small florets, stalk peeled and cut into small pieces
- 1 medium zucchini, cut into ½-inch-thick half-moons
- Soy sauce
- 3 cups packed fresh spinach (about 6 ounces)

Place the chicken and marinade into a shallow pan or in a zip-top bag, stirring or shaking the sealed bag to make sure the sauce covers all sides of the chicken. Place in the refrigerator to marinate for at least 1 hour and up to overnight.

Heat the sesame oil in a large skillet over medium heat. Add the chicken and marinade. Cook, stirring, until the chicken is no longer pink in the middle, about 10 minutes.

Stir in the carrots, cabbage, broccoli, and zucchini. Cover and simmer, stirring regularly, until the vegetables are tender-crisp and still bright in color and the chicken is completely cooked throughout, 1 to 3 minutes. Season with soy sauce.

Serve over a bed of spinach.

Calories: 296   Protein: 34 g
Carbohydrate: 20 g   Fat: 10 g

Variations

Vegan version: Substitute 1¾ pounds extra-firm tofu, drained, pressed with an absorbent towel, and cut into bite-size pieces, for the chicken, but keep in mind that the tofu will absorb more marinade and make the final dish have a more subtle flavor. We recommend increasing spiciness by doubling the ginger and chile in the marinade, and increasing soy sauce to taste.

Phase 1 Meal: Use the Spicy Asian Marinade (page 294; without honey). Drizzle each serving with 1 to 2 teaspoons toasted sesame oil. Serve over Cauliflower Couscous (page 211), and with a bowl (2 cups) of Miso Soup (page 258; omit the tofu if using chicken for the stir-fry). **For Dessert:** Fruity Coconut Ice Pops (page 310; without honey).

Calories: 564; Carbohydrate: 24%; Protein: 28%; Fat: 49%

Phase 2 Meal: Use the Spicy Asian Marinade (page 294; with or without the honey). Serve over ½ cup cooked brown rice, and with a bowl (2 cups) of Miso Soup (page 258; omit the tofu if using chicken for the stir-fry). **For Dessert:** Fruity Coconut Ice Pops (page 310; with the honey).

Calories: 586; Carbohydrate: 36%; Protein: 27%; Fat: 37%

Phase 3 Meal: Serve slightly smaller portions of the stir-fry with the Spicy Asian Marinade (page 294; with honey). Serve each portion over ¾ to 1 cup cooked soba noodles. **For Dessert:** 2 or 3 mini Almond Coconut Macaroons (page 312).

Calories: 574; Carbohydrate: 37%; Protein: 24%; Fat: 39%

Green Chile Chicken or Beef Enchilada Casserole (All Phases)

Who can resist the smoky flavor of green chiles? A premade casserole is always a time-saver, and this one is best made ahead so the flavors have time to fully meld. Make a big batch on Prep Day and refrigerate or freeze individual portions for quick and delicious meals.

Preparation time: 10 minutes

Total time: 1 to 1¼ hours

Makes 6 to 8 servings

- 3 tablespoons extra-virgin olive oil
- 2 cloves garlic
- 1¾ pounds boneless, skinless chicken thighs, cut into small chunks
- ½ teaspoon salt
- ¼ teaspoon ground black pepper
- 1 large onion, diced
- 1 medium leek, cut into thin rounds and rinsed well
- 4 cups packed spinach (about 8 ounces)
- 1 recipe Green Chile Cream Sauce (page 305)
- 1 large zucchini, thinly sliced on an angle

Preheat the oven to 375°F.

Heat the olive oil and garlic in a large skillet over medium heat. Add the chicken, salt, and pepper. Cook, stirring, until the chicken is browned on all sides, about 5 minutes.

Add the onion and leek. Cook, stirring, until the onion is translucent, about 5 minutes.

Add the spinach, cover, and cook until the spinach is just wilted, 1 minute or less. Remove from the heat.

In a casserole pan, layer 1 cup of the chile cream sauce, one layer of zucchini slices, and then one-third of the chicken mixture. Repeat, using about 2 cups of the sauce on subsequent layers, until all the chicken and zucchini have been used. Top with the remaining sauce.

Bake until the casserole is bubbling throughout, 30 to 40 minutes. Serve immediately or cool and store in the refrigerator for 3 to 4 days or in the freezer for up to 6 months.

Based on 6 servings   Carbohydrate: 27 g   Fat: 23 g
Calories: 456   Protein: 36 g

Variations

Dairy-free version: Use the dairy-free variation of the Creamy Green Chile Sauce (page 188).

Ground beef version: Substitute 1½ pounds ground or shredded beef (90% lean) for the chicken, and reduce the oil from 3 tablespoons to 1 tablespoon.

Vegetarian version: See Creamy Green Chile Casserole (page 187); or substitute 1½ recipes Basic Seitan (page 72), minced, for the chicken, omit the salt, and increase the olive oil to 5 tablespoons.

For Phase 3: Add two layers of corn tortillas (about 12 tortillas) and increase the servings to 8 per casserole.

Phase 1 Meal: Serve with a side of salad greens and chopped raw vegetables tossed with 1 to 2 teaspoons Greek Dressing (page 285). **For Dessert:** ½ cup raspberries with 1 tablespoon heavy cream, whipped if desired. **If using the beef version:** Serve with plain whole-milk Greek yogurt instead of cream for the dessert.

Calories: 601; Carbohydrate: 26%; Protein: 25%; Fat: 49%

Phase 2 Meal: Serve the casserole in smaller portions, each with ⅓ cup cooked brown basmati rice tossed with 2 tablespoons chopped fresh cilantro, ½ teaspoon olive oil, a squeeze of lime juice, and the same salad as for the Phase 1 Meal. **For Dessert:** ½ cup raspberries with 3 tablespoons plain whole-milk Greek yogurt mixed with ½ teaspoon honey.

Calories: 597; Carbohydrate: 36%; Protein: 23%; Fat: 41%

Phase 3 Meal: Use the Phase 3 Variation. Serve with the same salad as for the Phase 1 Meal. **For Dessert:** 1 cup berries and ½ ounce dark chocolate (at least 70% cacao).

Calories: 625; Carbohydrate: 38%; Protein: 20%; Fat: 42%

Chicken Parmesan (All Phases)

Our chickpea bread crumbs make this breaded chicken perfectly crisp and golden without the processed carbohydrate of bread. Pair with tasty marinara and gooey melted cheese for a winning combination. While this dish is typically done with chicken breasts, the fattier thighs are even more luscious and satisfying, and often less expensive.

Preparation time: 15 minutes

Total time: 45 minutes

Makes 6 servings

- 1½ pounds boneless, skinless chicken thighs
- ½ cup chickpea flour (see Tip, page 91)
- 1 cup Chickpea Bread Crumbs (page 196)
- ¾ cup grated Parmesan cheese
- ¼ teaspoon salt
- ¼ teaspoon garlic powder
- ¼ teaspoon ground black pepper
- 2 eggs, or 2 tablespoons ground chia or flaxseeds mixed with ½ cup water
- ½ cup neutral-tasting oil, such as high-oleic safflower or avocado oil
- 1½ cups prepared marinara sauce (no added sugar)
- 4 ounces mozzarella or provolone cheese, sliced or grated (about 1 cup)

Preheat the oven to 350°F.

Chicken thighs are often thin and even enough to make this recipe without pounding them; however, if they are thick or uneven, place them between two sheets of plastic wrap or in an unsealed zip-top bag. Pound with a kitchen mallet or any heavy object (a can of vegetables or a rolling pin will work if you don't have a conventional meat mallet) to ¼- to ½-inch thickness. Set aside.

Spread the chickpea flour in a shallow dish. In a separate shallow dish or pie plate, mix the chickpea bread crumbs, Parmesan, salt, garlic powder, and pepper. In a third separate shallow bowl, beat the eggs.

Heat the oil in a large cast-iron or other heavy skillet over medium heat.

Dredge the chicken in the chickpea flour, shaking off any excess, then dip in the eggs to cover both sides, letting any excess drip off, and finally dredge in the Parmesan–bread crumb mixture to cover on both sides. Gently place the chicken in the hot oil, working in batches as needed to avoid crowding the pan. Cook until browned on each side, about 5 minutes, turning once the edges begin to look golden brown. Transfer to a baking pan and repeat with the remaining chicken.

Arrange the cooked chicken in a single layer in the baking pan. Top each piece with a generous spoon of marinara sauce and a slice of mozzarella. Bake for 10 to 15 minutes, or until warm throughout and the cheese is bubbling and melted. If desired, switch the oven to broil and broil for a minute or more to lightly brown the cheese topping.

Calories: 548   Protein: 38 g
Carbohydrate: 21 g   Fat: 35 g

Variations

Vegetarian version: Omit the salt, and substitute 1½ recipes Basic Seitan (page 72) for the chicken—form and cook the seitan into 6 thin, flat chicken-thigh shapes and use salt instead of soy sauce to season the cooking broth.

For Phase 2: Reduce the Parmesan to ½ cup and the mozzarella to 2 ounces (about ½ cup shredded).

Calories: 505   Protein: 35 g
Carbohydrate: 21 g   Fat: 32 g

Phase 1 Meal: Serve with a side of salad greens and chopped raw vegetables tossed with 1 to 2 teaspoons Creamy Peppercorn Vinaigrette (page 286). **For Dessert:** ¾ cup blueberries.

Calories: 668; Carbohydrate: 24%; Protein: 24%; Fat: 52%

Phase 2 Meal: Use the Phase 2 Variation. Serve with Fresh Quinoa Salad with Pomegranates (page 262). **For Dessert:** 1 small pear, cored, raw or cooked.

Calories: 680; Carbohydrate: 34%; Protein: 22%; Fat: 44%

Phase 3 Meal: Use the Phase 2 Variation. Serve a smaller portion of chicken for each person along with ½ cup cooked pasta lightly tossed with ¼ cup prepared marinara (no salt added). **For Dessert:** 1 small pear, cored, raw or cooked.

Calories: 661; Carbohydrate: 38%; Protein: 21%; Fat: 42%

Easy Dijon Chicken or Salmon (All Phases)

Quick, easy, and delicious. This dish is the perfect go-to dinner when you only have a few minutes and you need a protein that tastes like you went to a lot of effort.

Preparation time: 5 minutes

Total time: 30 to 50 minutes

Makes 4 servings

- 1 teaspoon olive oil (1 tablespoon for salmon)
- ½ teaspoon salt
- ¼ teaspoon ground black pepper
- 2 tablespoons Dijon or spicy brown mustard
- ½ to 1 teaspoon dried thyme, rosemary, tarragon, or other herbs of your choice (optional)
- 2 pounds bone-in, skin-on chicken thighs, or 1½ pounds skin-on salmon fillets

Preheat the oven to 350°F.

Combine the olive oil, salt, pepper, mustard, and herbs (if using) in a small bowl.

Rub the mustard mixture over the chicken and under the chicken skin or on both sides of the salmon until completely covered. Cook immediately, or for a more flavorful dish, cover and set aside in the refrigerator to marinate for at least 1 hour; salmon should marinate for no longer than 3 hours, while chicken is better marinated overnight.

Place the chicken or salmon skin-side up in a 9-inch square baking dish or medium baking sheet. Bake the chicken for 45 minutes or the salmon for about 15 minutes, or until cooked through. For chicken, if there are juices in the pan, use them to occasionally baste while cooking by spooning the juices in the baking dish over the chicken.

If desired, turn the oven to broil, and broil for 1 to 2 minutes at the end of the cooking time for crispier skin.

Serve.

Tip: If using salmon, include a higher-fat dessert with your meal.

Calories: 307 (Chicken)	Protein: 29 g
Carbohydrate: 0 g	Fat: 21 g

Calories: 272 (Salmon)	Protein: 34 g
Carbohydrate: 0 g	Fat: 14 g

Variations

Grill instead of baking.

Use 1¾ pounds thick white-fleshed fish fillets or tuna fillets in place of the chicken or salmon. Increase the oil to 3 tablespoons to accommodate the lower fat content of the protein or serve with higher-fat sides. Bake for 15 to 25 minutes (depending on the thickness of the fish), until fish is opaque throughout. **Tip:** Tuna steaks can be pan-seared or grilled until done instead of baked.

Sheet Pan Meal: Prep Herb Roasted Root Vegetables (page 214) and spread on the baking sheet to cook with the chicken, or do the same with Summer Grilled or Roasted Vegetables (page 215) and the salmon.

Phase 1 Meal (Chicken): Use the Sheet Pan Meal with Herb Roasted Root Vegetables (page 214). Serve with a side of salad greens and chopped raw vegetables tossed with 1 to 2 teaspoons Creamy Peppercorn Vinaigrette (page 286). **For Dessert:** 1 cup blueberries topped with 1 tablespoon heavy cream.

Calories: 604; Carbohydrate: 27%; Protein: 22%; Fat: 51%

Phase 1 Meal (Salmon): Use the Sheet Pan Meal with Summer Grilled or Roasted Vegetables (page 215). Serve with ½ small cucumber, sliced and seasoned with salt and lemon juice. **For Dessert:** 1 cup blueberries and 1 Chocolate Truffle (page 314).

Calories: 614; Carbohydrate: 27%; Protein: 26%; Fat: 47%

Phase 2 Meal (Salmon or Chicken): Serve with a bowl (2 cups) of Creamy Millet Vegetable Soup (page 255) and Sautéed Bok Choy and Shiitake (page 213). **For Dessert:** 1 cup blueberries topped with 1 tablespoon heavy cream. If using chicken, omit the cream to accommodate the higher fat content of the chicken.

Calories: 622; Carbohydrate: 35%; Protein: 27%; Fat: 38%

Phase 2 or 3 Meal (Chicken or Salmon): Serve with Brown Rice Mushroom Risotto (page 229; without Parmesan), and ½ small cucumber, sliced and seasoned with salt and lemon juice. If using salmon, substitute a side of salad greens and chopped raw vegetables tossed with 1 to 2 teaspoons Greek Dressing (page 285) for the cucumber, to accommodate the lower fat content of the salmon. **For Dessert:** 1 Poached Pear with Dried Plums (page 325).

Calories: 659; Carbohydrate: 38%; Protein: 22%; Fat: 40%

Phase 3 Meal: Serve a slightly smaller portion of chicken or salmon with Cornbread (page 205), drizzled with 1 teaspoon olive oil or butter, and Perfect Cucumber-Tomato Salad (page 261). If using salmon, substitute a side of salad greens and chopped raw vegetables tossed with 1 to 2 teaspoons Greek Dressing (page 285) for the Cucumber Salad, or add more olive oil or butter to the cornbread in order to accommodate the lower fat content of the salmon. **For Dessert:** 1 Poached Pear with Dried Plums (page 325).

Calories: 663; Carbohydrate: 40%; Protein: 20%; Fat: 40%

No-Fuss Coq au Vin (All Phases)

This traditional French recipe was the perfect way for a peasant to turn a tough old rooster into an extravagantly flavorful meal with whatever ingredients were available. If you can find one, use a stewing hen, a much less expensive but very flavorful older chicken. Although the dish can be prepared on the stovetop, the slow cooker makes it even more tender. Start in the morning and have the whole house smell delicious by dinnertime.

Preparation time: 25 to 30 minutes

Total time: 5 to 8 hours (slow cooker)

Makes 4 to 6 servings

- 1 tablespoon olive oil
- 1 (3-pound) chicken (a stewing chicken or whole fryer), bone-in, skin-on, cut into large pieces
- 1 to 1¼ teaspoons salt
- ½ teaspoon ground black pepper
- ¼ cup cognac or Armagnac (optional)
- 1 large onion, cut into large chunks, or about 25 pearl onions, peeled
- 2 large cloves garlic, minced or pressed
- 8 to 10 ounces baby bella/cremini mushrooms, quartered
- ½ teaspoon dried thyme
- 1 bay leaf
- 1 tablespoon tomato paste
- 1½ cups dry red wine
- ½ cup unsalted chicken broth, Bone Broth (page 58), or water
- 2 large carrots, cut into large chunks
- ¼ cup chickpea flour (see Tip, page 91)

- ¼ teaspoon garlic powder
- ½ cup chopped fresh parsley, for garnish

Heat the olive oil in a large Dutch oven or stovetop-safe slow cooker insert over medium heat or in a slow cooker on the sauté setting. Lightly season the chicken pieces with about ½ teaspoon of the salt and ¼ teaspoon of the pepper.

Working in batches so as not to crowd the pan, brown the chicken on all sides, a few minutes on each side. Remove the chicken from the skillet and set aside on a plate.

Add cognac (if using) or ¼ cup of the broth to the skillet and scrape up any browned bits on the bottom of the pan. Add the onion, garlic, mushrooms, thyme, bay leaf, and remaining salt and pepper to the skillet. Cook, stirring, until the onion softens and the mushrooms begin to release their juices, about 5 minutes.

Stir in the tomato paste and pour in the wine and broth. Return the chicken pieces and any juices that have collected on the plate to the pan, pressing the chicken down into the broth. Arrange the carrots on top of and around the pieces of chicken. Bring to a boil.

Transfer to a slow cooker or return the insert to the slow cooker, if necessary, cover, and cook on high for about 5 hours or on low for 8 to 9 hours, or according to the manufacturer's instructions for poultry. (Alternatively, reduce the heat under the Dutch oven to low and simmer, covered, for about 3 hours, or until the chicken is tender.)

When the chicken is done, arrange the chicken and vegetables on a serving platter. Or, if you like the chicken skin a bit crispy, preheat the broiler, place the chicken on a broiler pan, and broil for 3 to 5 minutes, or until crispy to your liking.

Using a measuring cup, remove 1 cup of liquid from the slow cooker or Dutch oven. Add the chickpea flour and garlic powder and whisk or use an immersion blender to blend until all lumps are gone. Pour the chickpea flour mixture back into the pot (or pour it into a saucepan and then add the liquid remaining in the slow cooker). Taste and season with salt and pepper as needed. Bring to a boil, whisking as it heats. Cook until the liquid has slightly thickened, easily coats a spoon, and drips off versus pouring off in a steady stream, 5 to 10 minutes.

Pour the thickened gravy on top of the chicken and vegetables. Garnish with parsley and serve.

Tip: To serve 8 to 10 people or to have more leftovers, add an additional 1 to 1½ pounds of boneless, skinless chicken thighs without increasing the sauce. Add these when you return the chicken pieces to the pot with the vegetable mixture. The additional chicken thighs don't require browning at the beginning or broiling at the end.

Based on 4 servings	Carbohydrate: 20 g	Fat: 18 g
Calories: 406	Protein: 40 g	

Variations

Bacon version: Reduce the olive oil to 1 teaspoon. Heat the oil and add 2 ounces lardons, thick-cut bacon, or 2 teaspoons fat reserved from making Bone Broth (see page 58). Cook until the fat has rendered, then remove the lardons or bacon (if you used them), and use the fat for browning the chicken. Return the lardons or bacon to the pan when you return the chicken.

Quick-and-easy version: Although it won't create the depth of flavor that browning and sautéing will, you can skip those steps and still have a delicious dish. Place all the ingredients except the chickpea flour, garlic powder, and parsley into a slow cooker pot with a sauté setting or in a Dutch oven, or stovetop-safe slow cooker insert on the stovetop. Bring to a boil. Transfer to the slow cooker, if necessary. Cover and cook on high for 5 to 6 hours or low for 8 to 9 hours, or according to the manufacturer's instructions for poultry. Follow the directions in the recipe for adding the chickpea flour and thickening the gravy.

Pressure cooker version: Follow the recipe directions but pressure cook for 20 minutes on high, or according to the manufacturer's instructions for poultry, instead of slow cooking. Allow the pressure to release naturally. Alternatively, pressure cook on low for 20 minutes, then simmer, covered, over low heat on the stovetop for an hour or more. Follow the directions in the recipe for adding the chickpea flour and thickening the gravy.

Phase 1 Meal: Serve with a side of salad greens and chopped raw vegetables tossed with 1 to 2 teaspoons Greek Dressing (page 285). **For Dessert:** ½ cup blueberries, 1 heaping tablespoon Cardamom Whipped Cream (page 324), and 1 Chocolate Truffle (page 314).

Calories: 658; Carbohydrate: 27%; Protein: 26%; Fat: 47%

Phase 2 Meal: Serve with Millet Mashed Fauxtatoes (page 236) and a side of salad greens and chopped raw vegetables tossed with 1 to 2 teaspoons Greek Dressing (page 285). **For Dessert:** 1 cup blueberries.

Calories: 684; Carbohydrate: 36%; Protein: 26%; Fat: 38%

Phase 3 Meal: Serve a smaller portion of Coq au Vin with ⅔ cup boiled and mashed potatoes topped with a pat of butter, and a side of salad greens and chopped raw vegetables tossed with 1 to 2 teaspoons Greek Dressing (page 285). **For Dessert:** ½ cup blueberries topped with 1 heaping tablespoon Cardamom Whipped Cream (page 324) with 1 teaspoon honey drizzled on top.

Calories: 687; Carbohydrate: 40%; Protein: 22%; Fat: 38%

Moroccan Chicken Stew with Apricots (Phases 2 and 3)

Rich warm spices and sweet dried fruit make this Moroccan stew an instant favorite. Once you've prepped the ingredients, it's only a matter of letting it cook. A slow cooker makes for even easier prep. Leave in the morning and come home to the sweet and savory aromas of dinner ready to eat.

Preparation time: 10 minutes plus overnight marinating

Total time: 1 to 1½ hours

Makes 4 servings

- 1 recipe Moroccan Sauce (page 292)
- 1½ pounds boneless, skinless chicken thighs, cut into 1-inch cubes or slices
- 1 to 2 tablespoons extra-virgin olive oil
- 1 medium onion, diced
- 2 medium carrots, cut into chunks (about 1 cup)
- 1 small sweet potato or ½ small winter squash (kabocha, butternut, buttercup, etc.; peeled), cut into 1-inch pieces (about 1½ cups)
- 6 dried apricots, whole or diced, or 4 fresh apricots, quartered and pitted
- ¼ cup water
- ¼ teaspoon salt

Place the sauce in a large zip-top bag, add the chicken, seal the bag, and massage to completely coat the chicken with the sauce. Place it in the refrigerator to marinate for at least 1 hour and up to overnight (or cook it immediately if you have less time).

Heat the olive oil in a Dutch oven or stovetop-safe slow cooker insert over medium heat, or in a slow cooker on the sauté setting. Add the onion and cook, stirring, until translucent, 3 to 5 minutes.

Stir in the chicken and sauce from the bag, carrots, sweet potatoes, apricots, water, and salt. Cook, stirring, for 5 to 7 minutes. Reduce the heat to low, or transfer the ingredients or the slow-cooker insert to the slow cooker. Cover and simmer for at least 30 minutes or up to 1½ hours on the stovetop (longer, slow cooking creates a more savory dish) or cook on low in a slow cooker for up to 8 hours or according to the manufacturer's instructions. If desired, remove the lid for the last 15 to 30 minutes to thicken the sauce.

Serve hot. (See photo insert page 7.)

Calories: 459
Carbohydrate: 22 g

Protein: 37 g
Fat: 26 g

Variations

Vegetarian version: Substitute 1½ pounds extra-firm tofu, drained, pressed with an absorbent towel, and crumbled, and increase the salt to taste, or 1 recipe Basic Seitan (page 72) plus 2 additional tablespoons olive oil, for the chicken.

Phase 2 Meal: Serve over Cauliflower Couscous (page 211) or ¼ cup Cooked Quinoa (page 231), with a side of salad greens and chopped raw vegetables tossed with 1 to 2 teaspoons Greek Dressing (page 285). **For Dessert:** 1 small apple, cored, sliced, and drizzled with ½ teaspoon honey and sprinkled with ground cinnamon and ground cardamom.

Calories: 658; Carbohydrate: 34%; Protein: 24%; Fat: 42%

Phase 3 Meal: Serve over ½ cup cooked regular or whole wheat couscous, with a side of salad greens and chopped raw vegetables tossed with 1 to 2 teaspoons Greek Dressing (page 285). **For Dessert:** ½ medium apple, cored and sliced, drizzled with ½ teaspoon honey and sprinkled with ground cinnamon and ground cardamom.

Calories: 669; Carbohydrate: 36%; Protein: 24%; Fat: 40%

Barbecue Baked Chicken (Phases 2 and 3, with Phase 1 Variation)

A classic dish you won't feel guilty eating, this irresistible meal is perfect for a summertime barbecue or a simple night in.

Preparation time: 10 minutes plus overnight marinating

Total time: 1 hour

Makes 4 servings

- 2 pounds bone-in, skin-on chicken thighs
- ¾ cup Barbecue Sauce (page 290)
- ¼ teaspoon salt
- ¼ cup water

Arrange the chicken in a baking dish in a single layer or in a zip-top bag. Add the sauce, making sure it completely covers the chicken. (For best results, pull back the skin and rub the sauce over the chicken, making sure to get the sauce under the skin. Put the skin back into place and coat the outside with the sauce as well.) Cover the dish with plastic wrap or seal the bag, and place it in the refrigerator to marinate for at least 1 hour or up to overnight (or cook it immediately if you have less time).

When ready to cook, preheat the oven to 350°F.

If the chicken was marinated in a bag, transfer it to a baking dish, arranging it in a single layer with the sauce completely covering it. Sprinkle the chicken with the salt, and stir the water into the sauce at the bottom of the dish to keep it from burning.

Bake for about 45 minutes, basting every 15 to 20 minutes by spooning sauce from the bottom of the pan over the top of each piece of chicken, until the chicken is cooked through and no longer pink in the center.

Serve. Or, if you like the chicken skin a bit crispy, preheat the broiler, place the chicken on a broiler pan, and broil for 3 to 5 minutes, or until crispy to your liking.

Calories: 328   Protein: 30 g
Carbohydrate: 7 g   Fat: 20 g

Variations

Add onions and root vegetables, cut into large chunks, to the baking dish before cooking.

Grilled version: Marinate the chicken pieces in the sauce, then place each piece on a hot, lightly oiled grill; set aside the excess sauce. Grill, turning and brushing with the excess sauce, until cooked throughout. Heat any leftover sauce in a small pot until boiling (this is essential, as it will kill any bacteria from the raw chicken), then reduce the heat to low and simmer for 3 to 5 minutes. Spoon the sauce over the grilled chicken before serving.

Vegetarian version: Substitute 1 recipe Basic Seitan (page 72) for the chicken. Omit the salt and add 1½ tablespoons oil with the sauce.

Phase 1 Meal: Substitute 1 recipe Moroccan Sauce (page 292) for the Barbecue Sauce. Serve with 1 cup Sicilian Fava Bean Soup (page 244), blanched or steamed kale or other greens tossed with 1 to 2 teaspoons Creamy Sun-Dried Tomato Dressing (page 287), and ½ cucumber, sliced and seasoned with salt and lemon juice. **For Dessert:** 1 cup blueberries.

Calories: 679; Carbohydrate: 26%; Protein: 22%; Fat: 52%

Phase 2 Meal: Serve with a bowl (2 cups) of Creamy Millet Vegetable Soup (page 255), Garlicky White Beans with Broccoli Rabe (page 221), ½ cucumber, sliced and seasoned with salt and lemon juice. **For Dessert:** ½ cup berries.

Calories: 684; Carbohydrate: 38%; Protein: 24%; Fat: 38%

Phase 3 Meal: Serve a smaller portion of the chicken with Cornbread (page 205), topped with a pat of butter, and 1 cup Minestrone Soup (page 248). **For Dessert:** 1 cup diced mango or other tropical fruit.

Calories: 679; Carbohydrate: 40%; Protein: 21%; Fat: 39%

SEAFOOD

Fish and Mushrooms in Tarragon Cream Sauce (All Phases)

The delicate flavor of tarragon adds an herby touch to brighten up this creamy sauce. Pairs well with fish or any of your favorite proteins. With a simple substitution, you can make a vegetarian or vegan alternative.

Preparation time: 5 minutes

Total time: 45 minutes

Makes 4 servings

- ¼ cup extra-virgin olive oil
- 1 clove garlic, minced
- 1 shallot, minced
- 1 pound baby bella/cremini mushrooms, quartered
- ¾ teaspoon salt
- ¼ teaspoon ground black pepper
- 1 teaspoon dried tarragon, or 1 tablespoon minced fresh tarragon
- 1 tablespoon Dijon mustard
- 1½ tablespoons chickpea flour (see Tip, page 91)
- ½ cup white wine
- 2 cups whole milk or unsweetened soy milk (Phases 2 and 3); half-and-half (Phase 1)
- 1¼ pounds white-fleshed fish, such as cod, haddock, or hake, cut into 2- to 3-ounce pieces
- 1 small bunch hearty greens, such as kale, collards, mustard greens, or other leafy greens, chopped (8 to 12 ounces)

Heat the olive oil in a very large skillet over medium-high heat. Add the garlic, shallot, mushrooms, salt, pepper, and dried tarragon (if using fresh tarragon, add later with the milk). Cook, stirring, until the mushrooms have softened and the liquid has reduced, 8 to 10 minutes.

Stir in the mustard and chickpea flour. Cook, stirring, for 2 to 3 minutes to allow the flour to cook slightly.

Add the wine and cook, stirring or whisking continuously to evenly distribute the flour into the sauce, for 1 to 2 minutes. Reduce the heat to medium. Stir in the milk and fresh tarragon (if using). Simmer, stirring regularly, for about 5 minutes, or until the sauce begins to thicken. Taste and adjust the seasonings.

Gently nestle the pieces of fish into the simmering sauce. Cover the skillet and cook until the fish is completely cooked and opaque throughout, 8 to 10 minutes or more, depending on the thickness of the fillets.

In a separate pot, bring 1 inch of water to a boil. Add the chopped greens and cover the pot with a tight-fitting lid to steam the greens. Cook for 2 to 3 minutes, or until the greens are tender but still bright in color.

Remove from the heat, drain, and arrange on a serving tray or on individual plates.

Serve the fish and sauce on a bed of cooked greens.

Tip: For most hearty greens, chop the stems either with the leaves, or separate the stems from leaves and thinly slice the stems. If the stems are too tough, they can be discarded, but stems are usually tasty and nutritious.

Calories: 390 (Cod)   Protein: 36 g
Carbohydrate: 19 g   Fat: 20 g

Variations

Substitute 1 pound boneless, skinless chicken tenderloins for the fish; or substitute 1¼ pounds boneless, skinless chicken thighs for the fish and reduce the olive oil to 2 to 3 tablespoons.

Vegetarian or vegan version: Substitute 1½ pounds extra-firm tofu, crumbled or cut into cubes, for the fish. Increase the salt to 1 teaspoon, and reduce the olive oil to 1 tablespoon. Add the tofu with the mushrooms at the beginning.

Phase 1 Meal: Use the Phase 1 version. Serve with a side of salad greens, chopped raw vegetables, and ¼ cup cooked or canned chickpeas tossed with 1 to 2 teaspoons of Creamy Peppercorn Vinaigrette (page 286). **For Dessert:** 2 Chocolate-Dipped Strawberries (page 313).

Calories: 645; Carbohydrate: 25%; Protein: 25%; Fat: 50%

Phase 2 Meal: Serve over ½ cup cooked brown rice, with a side of salad greens and chopped raw vegetables tossed with 1 to 2 teaspoons Creamy Peppercorn Vinaigrette (page 286). **For Dessert:** 2 Chocolate-Dipped Strawberries (page 313).

Calories: 628; Carbohydrate: 35%; Protein: 25%; Fat: 40%

Phase 3 Meal: Serve a slightly smaller portion over about 1 cup cooked pasta, with a side of salad greens and chopped raw vegetables tossed with 1 to 2 teaspoons Creamy Peppercorn Vinaigrette (page 286). **For Dessert:** 2 Chocolate-Dipped Strawberries and 2 Chocolate-Dipped Banana Slices (page 313).

Calories: 614; Carbohydrate: 40%; Protein: 22%; Fat: 38%

Parchment-Baked Fish (Fish en Papillote) (All Phases)

Cooking fish in parchment or, as the French say, *en papillote*, keeps the fish from drying out. The paper ensures that it's still hot at the table, while also providing an impressive, full-of-flair presentation. Get creative as you plan which flavors, colors, and textures will go together in each packet. Everyone can choose the ingredients to fill their own packet—an empowering experience for kids. Have fun as you experiment with this simple yet inspiring method of cooking.

Preparation time: 15 minutes

Total time: 30 minutes

Makes 4 servings

- 1½ to 2 pounds fish fillets
- ½ to 1 teaspoon salt, or to taste
- ¼ teaspoon ground black pepper, or to taste
- Flavorings: fresh or dried herbs or spices, citrus zest, thinly sliced lemon or other citrus, olives, chiles, capers, ginger, garlic, parsley, cilantro, scallions, nuts, seeds, etc.
- 1 cup thinly sliced vegetables, such as onion, zucchini, carrot, mushroom, fennel, bell pepper, asparagus, artichoke hearts, snap peas, green beans, arugula, etc.
- 4 to 6 teaspoons olive oil, butter, coconut oil, or other fat
- 3 to 4 teaspoons white wine, soy sauce, vinegar, broth, mirin, sake, or other liquid seasoning, or your favorite sauce like Chimichurri (pages 300 and 301), Gremolata (page 299), Lemon Thyme (page 296), Basil Walnut Pesto (page 297), etc.

Preheat the oven to 425°F. Cut four pieces of parchment paper measuring 12 to 14 inches on each side. Fold each in half. Cut each sheet into a large heart shape, using the fold as the center of the heart. Arrange the parchment on one or two baking sheets.

Place 6 to 8 ounces of fish onto one side of each heart. Evenly distribute the salt and pepper over the fish, using more or less to taste depending on the saltiness of the flavorings you plan to use. Layer the flavorings on top of each piece of fish. Place ¼ cup of the vegetables either on top of or surrounding the fish on each parchment heart. Drizzle each with 1 to 1½ teaspoons oil or other fat and ½ to 1 teaspoon liquid seasoning, if not using a premade sauce. Make sure not to fill the packet too full or add too much liquid.

Close the parchment into a half heart over the fillings. Seal the open edges of the parchment by starting at the top end of the fold (opposite from the bottom point of the heart). Make a small triangle fold on that edge to begin to seal the cut edge. Crease the edge so that it stays down. Moving around the open end of the half heart, make another triangle fold that overlaps the first fold a bit, creasing well to keep it sealed down. Keep folding overlapping creases around the open side of the parchment heart to create a well-sealed packet with no open holes, ending at the bottom point of the heart. Either fold that final edge under or twist it closed and fold it to seal the bottom end. A well-sealed packet will create a mini steam tent that will keep the fish moist and the flavors and aromas in. (See photo insert page 5.)

Arrange the packets next to one another on the baking sheet(s).

Bake for 10 to 20 minutes, depending on the thickness of the fish and the types of vegetables used. Thinner fillets of fish will only require 10 minutes of cooking; thicker cuts will need longer. If well sealed, the packets will gently puff up (if they don't puff, don't worry—the fish will still cook). For longer cooking times, the parchment may brown slightly on top.

Serve each packet on its own plate and let everyone open their own, being careful to avoid the hot steam that escapes.

If you use a less fatty fish such as cod, you will want to serve this with a fattier sauce, dessert, or side dish. If you use a fattier fish such as salmon, serve with any sides or desserts. See meal suggestions for guidance.

Tip: If using a sauce or dressing that includes oil, omit the additional drizzle of oil. Also omit additional liquids and other flavorings if using a premade sauce. Simply add the sauce and vegetables to each packet.

Variations

Some of our favorite fish and flavor combinations:

- Italian or Mediterranean: white-fleshed fish (hake, cod, flounder, sole, haddock, etc.) with fresh oregano or basil, garlic, Kalamata olives, zucchini, onion, red bell pepper, and olive oil
- Asian: white-fleshed fish (see above) or salmon with fresh ginger (see Chef Dawn's Tasty Tip on ginger, page 289), garlic, soy sauce, shiitake mushrooms, carrots, snap peas, and toasted sesame oil (optional drizzle of honey)
- Basic French: white-fleshed fish (see above) with a sprig of thyme or dill, garlic, lemon slices, olive oil or butter, and a splash of white wine
- Thai: white-fleshed fish (see above) or salmon with fresh ginger, garlic, cayenne pepper or minced fresh chiles, lime juice or thin slices, onion, carrot, snow peas, chopped cashews, and coconut oil
- Herbed: white-fleshed fish (see above) with Gremolata (page 299) and olive oil, Chimichurri (pages 300 and 301), Basil Walnut Pesto (page 297), or any other sauces or marinades

Based on Italian or Mediterranean combination, 7 ounces per serving	Calories: 244 Carbohydrate: 3 g Protein: 36 g	Fat: 8 g

Phase 1 Meal (white-fleshed fish): Serve with Cauliflower Couscous (page 211) drizzled with 2 teaspoons olive oil, and ½ cup Ful Mudammas (page 222). **For Dessert:** ½ cup blueberries topped with 2 tablespoons heavy cream. **If using salmon:** Reduce the olive oil to 1 teaspoon and the heavy cream to 1 tablespoon.

Calories: 630; Carbohydrate: 23%; Protein: 28%; Fat: 49%

Phase 2 Meal Option 1 (white-fleshed fish): Serve with Brown Rice Mushroom Risotto with Parmesan (page 229), and a side of salad greens and chopped raw vegetables tossed with 1 to 2 teaspoons Greek Dressing (page 285). **For Dessert:** 1 cup blueberries topped with 1 heaping tablespoon Cardamom Whipped Cream (page 324). **If using salmon:** Use 1½ pounds salmon (6 ounces per serving). Substitute ½ cucumber, sliced and seasoned with salt and lemon, for the salad, and omit the whipped cream for dessert.

Calories: 642; Carbohydrate: 34%; Protein: 27%; Fat: 39%

Phase 2 Meal Option 2 (white-fleshed fish): Serve with Brown Rice "Tater" Tots (page 228) and 2 tablespoons Lemon Aioli (page 298) for dipping. **For Dessert:** 1 cup blueberries.

Calories: 626; Carbohydrate: 32%; Protein: 25%; Fat: 43%

Phase 3 Meal (white-fleshed fish): Serve smaller portions of the fish. Serve with 1 cup boiled potatoes or sweet potatoes with a pat of butter. **For Dessert:** Pear Cranberry Pie (page 320) topped with 1 heaping tablespoon Cardamom Whipped Cream (page 324). **If using salmon:** Use 1¼ pounds salmon (5 ounces per serving). Substitute an extra-thick slice of crusty, sourdough bread (2½ to 3 ounces) for the potatoes and 1 Coconut BonBon (page 316) and ½ small mango, diced (about ½ cup), for the pie.

Phase 3 Meal (white-fleshed fish), Whole-Grain Option: Serve smaller portions of the fish. Serve with Brown Rice "Tater" Tots (page 228) with 2 tablespoons ketchup for dipping, and Jicama, Clementine, and Avocado Salad (page 260). **For Dessert:** 3 Chocolate-Dipped Strawberries (page 313).

Calories: 637; Carbohydrate: 40%; Protein: 21%; Fat: 39%

Teriyaki Salmon (with Chicken Kebab Variation) (Phases 2 and 3)

Enjoy this timeless Asian favorite without all the added sugar in most recipes.

Preparation time: 5 minutes

Total time: 25 minutes

Makes 4 to 6 servings

- 1½ pounds skin-on salmon fillets
- ¾ to 1 cup Citrus Teriyaki Sauce (page 293)
- ¼ cup chopped fresh cilantro or scallions

Preheat the oven to 350°F.

Arrange the salmon in a baking dish in a single layer or in a zip-top bag. Add the sauce, making sure it completely covers the salmon. Cover the dish with plastic wrap or seal the bag, and place it in the refrigerator to marinate for about 1 hour (or cook it immediately if you have less time).

If you used a zip-top bag, transfer the fish and sauce from the bag to a baking dish. The salmon should be skin-side up.

Bake for 15 to 20 minutes, basting occasionally by spooning the juices in the baking dish over the fish. For a crispy skin, broil for the last 5 minutes of cooking.

Serve warm, garnished with cilantro or scallions. (Or, if you like the salmon skin a bit crispy, preheat the broiler, place the salmon on a broiler pan, and broil for a few minutes, until crispy to your liking, then garnish and serve.) (See photo insert page 4.)

Based on 4 servings	Carbohydrate: 10 g	Fat: 11 g
Calories: 282	Protein: 35 g	

Variations

Teriyaki Chicken Kebabs: Substitute 1¾ pounds boneless, skinless chicken thighs for the fish. Cut the chicken into squares or strips and marinate overnight. After marinating, toss the meat with chunks of vegetables like zucchini, red pepper, onion, and mushrooms, and thread onto bamboo skewers that have been soaked in water. Grill over high heat on a lightly oiled grill or bake in a preheated 350°F oven until the chicken is cooked throughout, about 15 minutes on the grill or 25 minutes in the oven. Bring the remaining marinade to a boil in a small saucepan over medium heat. Reduce the heat to maintain a simmer and cook until the sauce begins to reduce and thicken. While grilling, baste the meat with the thickened sauce. If basting on raw meat, bring the sauce to a boil again, then pour any remaining sauce over the cooked meat before serving.

Phase 1 Meal: None (moderate amount of honey in the sauce).

Phase 2 Meal: Serve over ⅓ cup cooked brown rice or quinoa with Jicama, Clementine, and Avocado Salad (page 260). **For Dessert:** A few strawberries and 1 Chocolate Truffle (page 314).

Calories: 658; Carbohydrate: 35%; Protein: 25%; Fat: 40%

Phase 3 Meal: Reduce the salmon to 1¼ pounds (or chicken to 1½ pounds, if making the chicken variation). Serve with ½ cup cooked brown or white rice and Jicama, Clementine, and Avocado Salad (page 260). **For Dessert:** A few strawberries and 1 Chocolate Truffle (page 314).

Calories: 638; Carbohydrate: 40%; Protein: 22%; Fat: 38%

Pesto Baked Fish (All Phases)

With the pesto made ahead, you'll have this impressive dish done in minutes.

Preparation time: 5 minutes

Total time: 20 to 30 minutes

Makes 4 servings

- 1¼ to 1½ pounds white-fleshed fish fillets, such as cod, scrod, or hake
- ½ cup Basil Walnut Pesto (page 297)

Preheat the oven to 350°F.

Rinse the fish and pat dry. Spread a layer of the pesto, evenly distributed, on the top of each fillet. Place in a baking dish, pesto-side up.

Bake for 15 to 25 minutes, or until the fish is opaque and flakes easily. It will take less time for thin fillets and more time for fillets over 1 inch thick. Serve immediately. (See photo insert page 5.)

Calories: 228
Carbohydrate: 1 g
Protein: 29 g
Fat: 12 g

Variations

Substitute salmon for the white-fleshed fish. Spread pesto on the top and edges of the salmon and rub a bit of oil on the skin side. Preheat a cast-iron skillet in the oven, then put the fish in the pan, skin-side up to allow the skin to get a bit crispy, and bake as directed. Broil for the last 5 minutes for even crispier skin.

Substitute Lime Cilantro Pesto (page 298), Cilantro Chimichurri (page 300), or Parsley Chimichurri (page 301) for the Basil Walnut Pesto.

Add slices of ripe tomato on top of the pesto before baking.

Phase 1 Meal: Serve with a bowl (2 cups) of Minestrone Soup (page 248) drizzled with 1 teaspoon olive oil, and Zucchini with Garlic and Greens (page 212). **For Dessert:** 1 Chocolate Truffle (page 314) with 1 tablespoon Coconut Cardamom Macadamia Butter (page 57). **If using salmon:** Omit the olive oil on the soup and reduce the nut butter to 1½ teaspoons.

Calories: 665; Carbohydrate: 25%; Protein: 25%; Fat: 50%

Phase 2 Meal: Serve with 1 cup Sicilian Fava Bean Soup (page 244) and Millet Tabbouleh (page 234). **For Dessert:** Orange Chocolate Pudding (page 317). **If using salmon:** Substitute 1 cup raspberries for dessert.

Calories: 667; Carbohydrate: 35%; Protein: 24%; Fat: 41%

Phase 3 Meal: Use 4 ounces fish per serving. Serve with Artichoke Kalamata Olive Ragout (page 220) over 1 cup cooked pasta. **For Dessert:** 1 Coconut BonBon (page 316). **If using salmon:** Use 1 pound salmon and substitute 3 or 4 Chocolate-Dipped Strawberries (page 313) for dessert.

Calories: 691; Carbohydrate: 40%; Protein: 20%; Fat: 40%

Drunken Marinated Shrimp Kebabs (All Phases)

Rich and sweet, this classic Asian-style marinade pairs perfectly with shrimp and vegetables. Whether you are grilling for a summertime party or planning a simple dinner at home, these elegant kebabs are sure to please.

Preparation time: 10 minutes plus a few hours marinating

Total time: 35 minutes

Makes 4 servings

Miso-Sake Marinade

- 2 tablespoons dark miso paste, such as barley, red, or hearty brown rice
- 2 tablespoons sake, or 1 tablespoon mirin
- 1 to 2 tablespoons soy sauce (depending on the saltiness of the miso)
- 2 to 3 tablespoons water

Kebabs

- 1½ pounds medium shrimp, peeled and deveined
- 1 red bell pepper, zucchini, or other vegetables of your choice, cut into large chunks
- 1 small onion, cut into large chunks
- 8 ounces baby bella/cremini mushrooms, halved
- 1 teaspoon toasted sesame oil

Soak 8 to 12 bamboo skewers in water for 30 minutes to prevent burning, then drain.

Make the marinade: Combine all the marinade ingredients in a bowl and whisk until well mixed, or place in a wide-mouthed glass jar or cup that will fit an immersion blender without splashing and blend until smooth.

Make the kebabs: Place the shrimp and marinade in a shallow baking dish or in a zip-top bag, stirring or shaking the sealed bag to cover each shrimp with marinade. Set aside to marinate while making the vegetables, or, for best results, refrigerate for up to a few hours.

Preheat the oven to 400°F.

Toss the bell pepper, onion, and mushrooms with the sesame oil and spread them in a single layer in a baking dish or on a rimmed baking sheet. Bake for 5 to 10 minutes, or until vegetables begin to soften but are still bright in color. Remove from the oven; keep the oven on.

Thread the shrimp and lightly cooked vegetables onto the bamboo skewers, reserving any excess marinade. Place the skewers on the same baking sheet and bake for 5 to 8 minutes, or until the shrimp are opaque throughout and the vegetables are softened.

Place the remaining marinade in a small pot. Bring to a boil, then reduce the heat to low and simmer for about 5 minutes or until the sauce thickens a bit.

Arrange the skewers on a platter. Drizzle the sauce over the skewers and serve. (See photo insert page 6.)

Calories: 184
Carbohydrate: 10 g
Protein: 27 g
Fat: 4 g

Variations

Use ½ cup Basil Walnut Pesto (page 297) or other favorite sauce in place of the Miso-Sake Marinade. If the sauce is a paste instead of a liquid, skip the last step that thickens the sauce.

Grill on a lightly oiled grill instead of baking.

Phase 1 Meal: Serve with Miso Soup (page 258) and Cauliflower Couscous (page 211), drizzled with 1½ teaspoons toasted sesame oil and tossed with Seasoned Shiitake Mushrooms (page 217). **For Dessert:** ½ ounce square dark chocolate (at least 70% cacao) with 2½ tablespoons Coconut Cardamom Macadamia Butter (page 57).

Calories: 678; Carbohydrate: 26%; Protein: 24%; Fat: 50%

Phase 2 Meal: Serve with Miso Soup (page 258) and ½ cup cooked brown rice topped with Seasoned Shiitake Mushrooms (page 217). **For Dessert:** 2 or 3 Almond Coconut Macaroons (page 312).

Calories: 679; Carbohydrate: 38%; Protein: 25%; Fat: 37%

Phase 3 Meal: Serve with 1 ounce (dry) brown rice udon noodles cooked and tossed with a teaspoon of toasted sesame oil and Seasoned Shiitake Mushrooms (page 217).
For Dessert: ½ cup blueberries and 2 or 3 Almond Coconut Macaroons (page 312; Chocolate Chip Variation).

Calories: 668; Carbohydrate: 37%; Protein: 22%; Fat: 41%

Mussels in Garlic White Wine Broth (All Phases)

Mussels are easy and inexpensive to make—no reason to enjoy them at restaurants only. This impressive dish can serve as an appetizer while you prep any last-minute foods for a dinner party or as a quick main dish anytime.

Preparation time: 5 minutes

Total time: 25 minutes

Makes 4 servings

- 2 tablespoons extra-virgin olive oil
- 1 shallot, diced
- 3 cloves garlic, minced
- 1 teaspoon crushed red pepper flakes
- 1 cup dry white wine
- ¼ to ½ teaspoon salt
- 2 pounds mussels, cleaned (see Sidebar)
- ½ cup chopped fresh parsley

Heat the olive oil in a deep saucepan over medium heat. Add the shallot and garlic. Cook, stirring, until translucent, 3 to 5 minutes.

Add the crushed red pepper flakes, wine, and salt. Bring to a boil.

Add the mussels and parsley. Reduce the heat to medium-low, cover, and steam, gently stirring or shaking the pan with the lid on occasionally to keep the bottom shells from getting overcooked, for 10 minutes, or until all the mussels have opened. Discard any mussels that don't open.

Serve hot, with a portion of the broth in each bowl.

Calories: 277
Carbohydrate: 11 g

Protein: 27 g
Fat: 12 g

Phase 1 Meal: Serve with a Greek Salad (page 259). **For Dessert:** 1 Chocolate Truffle (page 314).

Calories: 631; Carbohydrate: 25%; Protein: 25%; Fat: 50%

Phase 2 Meal: Serve with a Greek Salad (page 259; Phase 2 Variation). **For Dessert:** ½ cup blueberries.

Calories: 645; Carbohydrate: 34%; Protein: 25%; Fat: 41%

Phase 3 Meal: Serve a side of salad greens and chopped raw vegetables tossed with 1 to 2 teaspoons Greek Dressing (page 285) and a thick slice of crusty sourdough bread (about 2 ounces). **For Dessert:** 1 Coconut BonBon (page 316).

Calories: 638; Carbohydrate: 36%; Protein: 22%; Fat: 42%

Chef Dawn's Tasty Tip

Perfect Mussels Every Time

Mussels and other shellfish like clams and oysters are typically live when you buy them and can have small bits of sand or debris in their shells. But the remedy is simple. Place them in a bowl with water, add 1 cup ice cubes, and let sit for 30 minutes to 1 hour to allow the shellfish to release any grit. Drain, rinse, and scrub any that still have dirt or grit on the outside. They can be stored in the refrigerator in a dry bowl, covered with a clean damp cloth and with a zip-top bag filled with ice placed on top of the cloth. To ensure that mussels are fresh, discard any that aren't closed when you buy them or haven't opened after you cook them. Some mussels will have a scrubby "beard" of threads peeking out of their shell. Remove the beard by holding the shell and pulling the threads toward the hinge and out.

BEEF AND PORK

Slow Cooker Shredded Beef or Pulled Pork (All Phases)

Rich and satisfying, Shredded Beef can be the base for so many recipes. It's delicious on its own, or spice it up with barbecue or other sauces. Use as a main protein with lower fat meals, or add it to salads to make a complete meal.

Preparation time: 15 to 20 minutes

Total time: 8+ hours (slow cooker)

Makes 6 servings (about 3 cups)

- 2¼ pounds beef chuck roast or pork shoulder roast
- 1½ tablespoons All-Purpose Seasoned Salt (page 283), or ½ teaspoon salt
- 1 teaspoon olive oil
- ½ cup water, unsalted beef stock, or Bone Broth (page 58)
- 2 teaspoons Sugar-Free Worcestershire Sauce (page 284)

Rub all sides of the roast evenly with the seasoned salt. Set aside.

Heat the olive oil in a slow cooker on the sauté setting or in a large Dutch oven or stovetop-safe slow cooker insert over medium heat. Add the roast and brown on all sides, about 15 minutes total. Remove the roast and set aside on a plate.

Add the water and scrape up any browned bits on the bottom of the pan. Bring to a boil.

Return the roast to the slow cooker, or transfer the roast and liquid from the pan to the slow cooker. Add the Worcestershire. Cover and cook on low or medium for 8 to 10 hours, or according to the manufacturer's instructions for roasts, until the meat is fully cooked and tender. (Alternatively, return the roast to the Dutch oven, cover, and transfer it to the oven. Bake at 275°F for 4 to 6 hours, or until the meat is fully cooked and tender.)

Shred the meat in the slow cooker or pot, using two forks and pulling along the grain to create thin strands. Heat the shredded meat, stirring frequently, until the liquid and spices have been absorbed. Serve immediately or cool and store in the refrigerator for 3 to 4 days or in the freezer for up to 6 months.

Calories: 371   Protein: 35 g
Carbohydrate: 1 g   Fat: 24 g

Phase 1 Meal: Serve with Artichoke Kalamata Olive Ragout (page 220), a side of salad greens and chopped raw vegetables tossed with 1 to 2 teaspoons Creamy Peppercorn Vinaigrette (page 286). **For Dessert:** 1 cup strawberries.

Calories: 655; Carbohydrate: 26%; Protein: 27%; Fat: 47%

Phase 2 Meal: Stir in 2 tablespoons Barbecue Sauce (page 290). Serve with a small baked sweet potato with 1 to 2 teaspoons butter, and Perfect Cucumber-Tomato Salad (page 261). **For Dessert:** 1 cup blueberries.

Calories: 649; Carbohydrate: 33%; Protein: 25%; Fat: 42%

Phase 3 Meal: Serve slightly smaller portions of Shredded Beef, and stir in 2 to 3 tablespoons Barbecue Sauce (page 290). Serve on a whole wheat bun with mustard, lettuce, sliced pickles, red onion, and tomato, 1 cup Creamy Millet Vegetable Soup (page 255), and sweet potato fries. **For Dessert:** 2 Chocolate-Dipped Strawberries (page 313).

Calories: 678; Carbohydrate: 39%; Protein: 21%; Fat: 40%

Beef, Bison, or Turkey Meatballs (All Phases)

A great appetizer or main dish, these little meatballs are sure to please. Make them simple with just meat, or add chickpea bread crumbs for a lighter, more balanced recipe. Serve on their own or with your favorite dipping sauces.

Preparation time: 15 minutes

Total time: 35 minutes

Makes 4 servings (about 30 mini meatballs)

- 1 small onion
- 1 small carrot
- 18 to 20 sprigs cilantro or parsley (about 1 ounce), coarsely chopped
- 1 clove garlic
- 1 to 2 teaspoons All-Purpose Seasoned Salt (page 283), or ½ teaspoon salt
- ¼ teaspoon ground black pepper
- ½ cup Chickpea Bread Crumbs (page 196; optional)
- 1¼ pounds ground beef (90% lean), ground buffalo, or ground turkey
- 1 tablespoon Sugar-Free Worcestershire Sauce (page 284)
- 3 tablespoons neutral-tasting oil, such as avocado oil

Place the onion, carrot, cilantro, garlic, seasoned salt, pepper, and Chickpea Bread Crumbs (if using) in a food processor. Process until the vegetables are finely minced.

Place meat in a large bowl. Stir in the minced vegetables and the Worcestershire until well combined. Form into mini (about 1-inch) meatballs or ovals for appetizers or to use in wraps, or into larger (2- to 3-inch) meatballs for a main dish.

Heat the oil in a large skillet over medium heat. Add the meatballs (work in batches, if necessary). Cover, reduce the heat to medium-low, and cook, turning occasionally, until browned on all sides and cooked through, 15 to 20 minutes. (See photo insert page 10.)

Serve with Lemon Aioli (page 298), Chimichurri (pages 300 and 301), Tzatziki (page 304), or any of your favorite sauces for dipping. Alternatively, wrap in large lettuce leaves or in Socca Wraps (page 198), top with Pickled Turnips (page 67) or other fermented vegetables, and drizzle with your favorite sauces.

Tip: Turkey and buffalo are generally leaner than beef and are best served with fattier dipping sauces.

Calories: 327 (Beef)   Protein: 31 g
Carbohydrate: 11 g   Fat: 17 g

Variations

Form into 4 to 6 large patties to create burgers.

Substitute ground lamb for the beef, and serve with lower-fat sauces and desserts.

Add cheese and different herbs or spices to create a variety of flavors. For example, for a spicy jalapeño burger, add lime, cilantro, jalapeño, and Monterey Jack cheese; for a Greek burger, add feta cheese, oregano, and basil.

Vegetarian version: Substitute 1 pound tempeh for the beef and ½ cup chickpea flour for the Chickpea Bread Crumbs; increase the All-Purpose Seasoned Salt to 1 tablespoon and add an extra teaspoon Sugar-Free Worcestershire Sauce. Steam the tempeh for 10 minutes, then add it to the food processor with the vegetables. Panfry the tempeh balls or patties as directed in the recipe, or deep-fry as directed in Tofu Vegetable Balls (page 171).

For Phase 2: Heat a cup or two of cooked brown rice or other cooked whole grain in the drippings left in the pan after cooking the meat.

Phase 1 Meal: Serve 7 or 8 mini or 2 or 3 large meatballs with 2 tablespoons Lemon Aioli (page 298), ½ cup Ful Mudammas (page 222), and Perfect Cucumber-Tomato Salad (page 261). **If using lamb (higher-fat meat):** Reduce the Aioli to 1 tablespoon, and use the lower amount of oil in the Ful Mudammas recipe. **For Dessert:** ½ cup blueberries.

Calories: 656; Carbohydrate: 26%; Protein: 24%; Fat: 50%

Phase 2 Meal: Place 7 or 8 mini meatballs in a Socca Wrap (page 198) with ¼ cup Cooked Quinoa (page 231), lettuce, cucumber, and sliced tomato, and ⅓ cup Tzatziki (page 304), and roll or fold to seal. **If using lamb (higher-fat meat):** Omit the Socca Wrap, serve with ½ cup quinoa, and ¼ cup Tzatziki (page 304). **For Dessert:** 1 cup blueberries.

Calories: 640; Carbohydrate: 36%; Protein: 27%; Fat: 37%

Phase 3 Meal: Place 7 or 8 mini meatballs in a 4-inch whole wheat pita with lettuce, cucumber, sliced tomato, Pickled Cabbage or Carrots (page 66), and 1 heaping tablespoon Lemon Aioli (page 298). **If using lamb (higher-fat meat):** Use about 6 meatballs, and substitute ½ cup Tzatziki (page 304) for the Lemon Aioli. **For Dessert:** 1 cup diced mango.

Calories: 628; Carbohydrate: 36%; Protein: 23%; Fat: 42%

Meat Loaf with Smoked Paprika Ketchup (Phases 2 and 3, with Phase 1 Variation)

Another retro recipe with a modern twist, this rich meat loaf with smoky ketchup will leave you deeply satisfied.

Preparation time: 5 minutes

Total time: 1½ hours

Makes 4 servings

- 1 medium onion, cut into large chunks
- 1 small carrot, cut into large chunks
- 1 stalk celery, cut into large chunks
- 2 cloves garlic, minced
- ½ cup Chickpea Bread Crumbs (page 196)
- 1 teaspoon extra-virgin olive oil (3 tablespoons for turkey or buffalo)
- 2 tablespoons tomato paste
- 2 teaspoons Sugar-Free Worcestershire Sauce (page 284)
- 1 egg, beaten, or 1 tablespoon ground chia seeds mixed with ¼ cup water
- ½ cup whole milk or unsweetened soy milk
- ¾ to 1 teaspoon salt
- ¼ teaspoon ground black pepper
- 1¼ pounds ground beef (85% lean), ground turkey, or ground buffalo
- 1 cup Smoked Paprika Ketchup (page 291)

Preheat the oven to 350°F.

Place the onion, carrot, celery, garlic, and Chickpea Bread Crumbs in a food processor. Process until the vegetables are finely minced.

Heat the olive oil in a medium skillet over medium heat. Add the minced vegetables and cook, stirring, until soft, about 5 minutes.

In a large bowl, combine the tomato paste, Worcestershire, egg, milk, salt, and pepper and mix until well combined. Add the meat and the vegetable mixture. Stir until well combined.

Spread the meat mixture into an even layer in a 9-inch square baking dish and top with a layer of Smoked Paprika Ketchup.

Bake for 1 hour. Set aside for about 15 minutes before slicing and serving.

Tip: Depending on the fat and water content of the meat, there may be some liquid left around the edges of the meat in the pan. Drizzle some of it on each slice before serving. If you have leftover meat loaf, this liquid will naturally reabsorb as the meat loaf is refrigerated.

Calories: 566   Protein: 35 g
Carbohydrate: 43 g   Fat: 29 g

Variations

For Phase 1: Substitute ⅔ cup Moroccan Sauce (page 292) for the Smoked Paprika Ketchup, which has honey.

For Phase 3: Substitute a few slices of stale sourdough bread (about 4 ounces), torn into pieces, lightly toasted, and crumbled, or ½ cup unseasoned bread crumbs for the Chickpea Bread Crumbs.

Phase 1 Meal: Use the Phase 1 Variation. Serve with cucumber and tomato slices seasoned with salt, pepper, and lemon juice. **For Dessert:** 1 cup blueberries.

Calories: 662; Carbohydrate: 26%; Protein: 21%; Fat: 54%

Phase 2 Meal: Serve with cucumber and tomato slices seasoned with salt, pepper, and lemon juice. **For Dessert:** ½ cup blueberries topped with 2 tablespoons plain whole-milk Greek yogurt.

Calories: 658; Carbohydrate: 35%; Protein: 23%; Fat: 42%

Phase 3 Meal: Use the Phase 3 Variation. Serve with cucumber and tomato slices seasoned with salt, pepper, and lemon juice. **For Dessert:** ½ cup diced mango.

Calories: 655; Carbohydrate: 39%; Protein: 22%; Fat: 39%

Grab-and-Go Meat Pies (All Phases)

Inspired by a combination of traditional Australian and French-Canadian meat pies, these little gems are perfect for a lunch or dinner on the run. Make them on Prep Day for a complete meal anytime. Our recipe testers in the United States liked extra vegetables, whereas those in the U.K. preferred mainly meat. See which you prefer, or try the vegan version.

Preparation time: 30 minutes

Total time: 1 hour

Makes 6 servings

- 1 medium carrot, cut into large chunks
- 1 small bulb fennel, cut into large chunks (optional)
- 1 medium onion, cut into large chunks
- 1 clove garlic
- 1 teaspoon extra-virgin olive oil
- ½ teaspoon salt
- ¼ teaspoon ground black pepper
- ⅛ teaspoon freshly grated nutmeg
- 1½ pounds ground beef (90% lean)
- ½ teaspoon All-Purpose Seasoned Salt (page 283), or a pinch of salt
- 1 to 2 tablespoons Sugar-Free Worcestershire Sauce (page 284)
- 2 tablespoons chickpea flour (see Tip, page 91)
- 3 tablespoons tomato paste
- 1 cup unsalted beef broth, Bone Broth (page 58), or water
- 2 recipes Grain-Free Piecrust dough (page 206)

Preheat the oven to 350°F.

Place the carrot, fennel (if using), onion, and garlic in a food processor. Process until the vegetables are finely minced.

Heat the olive oil in a large skillet over medium heat. Add the minced vegetables, salt, pepper, and nutmeg. Cook, stirring, until the vegetables are translucent, 3 to 5 minutes.

Add the beef, seasoned salt, and Worcestershire. Cook, stirring, until the beef begins to brown, about 5 minutes.

Stir in the chickpea flour and cook, stirring, for 5 minutes to lightly brown the flour and finish cooking the meat.

Stir in the tomato paste and broth. Simmer for 5 minutes. Taste and adjust the seasonings.

Roll out each round of pie dough into a thick log, then cut each into two parts, one larger than the other (the bottom crusts will need to be larger than the top crusts). Cut each log into 12 equal pieces (for muffin tins) or 6 pieces (for 6-inch individual pie tins). Roll out each piece between sheets of parchment paper to a size that will fit the bottom and top for each pie.

Press the rolled dough into each of 6 or 12 tins. (No need to oil the tins.) Add the filling to the raw dough, evenly distributing it among the tins. Place a piece of rolled out top crust dough on top of each of the pies, forming a dome shape over the filling, and tuck the top over the bottom crust. Seal the edges by pressing the overlapped top and bottom crusts together in the tins to form a contained mini pie.

Bake for 20 to 25 minutes, or until crusts are golden. Let cool for 5 to 10 minutes in the tins, then transfer to a plate.

Serve hot, or refrigerate for a quick grab-and-go meal or snack.

Calories: 600
Carbohydrate: 36 g

Protein: 35 g
Fat: 34 g

Variations

Vegan version: Substitute 1 recipe Crumbled Tempeh (page 192), or 1 recipe Basic Seitan (page 72), minced, plus 2 tablespoons olive oil for the beef. Add mushrooms with the vegetables for additional flavor. Omit the salt or season with salt to taste.

For a single pie, use a 9-inch pie plate.

Phase 1 Meal: Serve with a small square (about ½ ounce) dark chocolate (at least 70% cacao).

Calories: 682; Carbohydrate: 25%; Protein: 22%; Fat: 53%

Phase 2 or 3 Meal: Serve with a small pear.

Calories: 693; Carbohydrate: 34%; Protein: 21%; Fat: 45%

Slow-Cooked Beef Chuck Pot Roast with Parsnips (All Phases)

Modernize your pot roast with a few sweet, creamy parsnips in place of potatoes. This classic slow-cooked meat is easy to get ready in the morning for a satisfying dinner when you get home.

Preparation time: 25 minutes

Total time: 8 hours (slow cooker)

Makes 8 servings

- 2½ to 3 pounds nicely marbled chuck roast
- 1 teaspoon salt
- 2 to 3 teaspoons All-Purpose Seasoned Salt (page 283), or ½ to 1 teaspoon additional salt
- 1 teaspoon ground black pepper
- 1 tablespoon extra-virgin olive oil
- 1 large onion, diced
- 5 or 6 large cloves garlic, minced
- 1 cup water, unsalted beef stock, or Bone Broth (page 58)
- 1 cup dry white wine or additional water or stock
- 2 medium carrots, cut into large chunks
- 3 medium parsnips, cut into large chunks
- 3 tablespoons chickpea flour (see Tip, page 91)
- ¼ cup water

Rub the roast thoroughly on all sides with the salt, seasoned salt, and pepper.

Heat the olive oil in a slow cooker on the sauté setting or in a stovetop-safe slow cooker insert, or Dutch oven over medium heat. Add the roast and brown well on all sides, about 15 minutes. Remove the roast and set aside on a plate.

Add the onion and garlic to the pot and cook, stirring, until the onion is translucent, 3 to 5 minutes. Scoop the onion and garlic out and place on the plate, then put the roast back in the pot or into the slow cooker. Return the insert to the slow cooker, if necessary.

Mix the water and wine in a measuring cup and pour over the meat. Pour the sautéed onion and garlic back over the roast as well. Add the carrots and parsnips on top of and around the roast. Cover and cook on high for 5 to 6 hours or low for 8 to 9 hours, or according to the manufacturer's instructions. (Alternatively, return the meat, onion, and garlic to the Dutch oven and simmer on the stovetop, covered, for 2½ to 3 hours, adding the carrots and parsnips 40 minutes to 1 hour from the end of the cooking time.)

Carefully remove the roast from the pot when it is done. It should be fall-apart tender.

Mix chickpea flour and water in a measuring cup with an immersion blender to make a slurry.

Quickly whisk the slurry into the liquid in the pot and cook for about 5 minutes, or until the mixture thickens to a gravy consistency.

Slice the roast and spoon the sauce onto each portion as you serve it.

Calories: 454	Protein: 32 g
Carbohydrate: 13 g	Fat: 29 g

Phase 1 Meal: Serve with 1 cup Minestrone Soup (page 248), a side of salad greens and chopped raw vegetables tossed with 1 to 2 teaspoons Creamy Peppercorn Vinaigrette (page 286). **For Dessert:** 1 cup strawberries topped with 1 heaping tablespoon Cardamom Whipped Cream (page 324).

Calories: 674; Carbohydrate: 26%; Protein: 23%; Fat: 51%

Phase 2 Meal: Serve with 1 cup Minestrone Soup (page 248), Butternut Sage Puree (page 219), and sliced cucumbers and tomato seasoned with salt, pepper, and lemon juice. **For Dessert:** 1 cup strawberries.

Calories: 662; Carbohydrate: 33%; Protein: 24%; Fat: 43%

Phase 3 Meal: Serve with a small baked potato with 1 tablespoon sour cream, and sliced cucumbers and tomato seasoned with salt, pepper, and lemon juice. **For Dessert:** ½ small apple, cored, drizzled with ½ teaspoon honey.

Calories: 680; Carbohydrate: 36%; Protein: 22%; Fat: 42%

Beef Stroganoff (All Phases)

The smooth, creamy texture and rich flavor of this traditional Russian dish has made it a favorite around the world. Our version is simple to make vegetarian or dairy-free as well.

Preparation time: 15 minutes

Total time: 45 minutes

Makes 4 servings

- 1¼ pounds beef sirloin or other tender cut of beef, cut into ¼-inch-thick strips
- ¾ to 1 teaspoon salt
- ½ teaspoon ground black pepper
- 1 tablespoon extra-virgin olive oil
- 1 large onion, diced
- 2 cloves garlic, minced
- 16 ounces baby bella/cremini mushrooms, sliced
- 2 teaspoons Sugar-Free Worcestershire Sauce (page 284)
- ½ cup white wine
- ¾ cup sour cream or Dairy-Free Sour Cream (page 306)
- Fresh dill, chopped, for garnish

Season the beef with ½ teaspoon of the salt and the pepper.

Heat the olive oil in a large, deep skillet over medium heat. Add the beef and brown on each side, 3 to 5 minutes total. Remove the beef and set aside on a plate.

Add the onion, garlic, mushrooms, and ¼ to ½ teaspoon salt, to taste, to the pan, cover, and cook, stirring regularly, for 10 to 15 minutes, until the mushrooms have released their juices.

Return the beef and any juices from the plate to the pan, then add the Worcestershire and wine. Cover and cook, stirring regularly, until the beef is fully cooked, about 10 minutes.

Stir in the sour cream. Simmer, uncovered, until the sauce is bubbling and thickened, 5 to 10 minutes. Taste and adjust the seasonings.

Garnish with dill and serve.

Calories: 446
Carbohydrate: 12 g
Protein: 33 g
Fat: 29 g

Variations

Use ground beef (85% lean) in place of the sirloin strips and leave in the pot when sautéing the vegetables.

Vegetarian version: Substitute 1 recipe Panfried Tempeh (page 193) or Crumbled Tempeh (page 192) for the beef, and reduce the olive oil to 1 teaspoon; or substitute 1 recipe Basic Seitan (page 72) and increase the olive oil to 3 tablespoons. Add the tempeh or seitan after sautéing the onion mixture. Omit salt, or season with salt to taste.

Phase 1 Meal: Serve over a bed of spinach (1 to 2 ounces per serving), with a side of salad greens and chopped raw vegetables tossed with 1 to 2 teaspoons Creamy Peppercorn Vinaigrette (page 286). **For Dessert:** 1 cup blueberries topped with 1 tablespoon heavy cream.

Calories: 652; Carbohydrate: 26%; Protein: 22%; Fat: 52%

Phase 2 Meal: Serve over ½ cup cooked brown rice or whole buckwheat, with the same salad as for the Phase 1 Meal. **For Dessert:** ½ cup blueberries.

Calories: 673; Carbohydrate: 33%; Protein: 22%; Fat: 45%

Phase 3 Meal: Serve slightly smaller portions of the stroganoff over 1 cup cooked egg noodles, with the same salad as for the Phase 1 Meal. **For Dessert:** ½ cup blueberries.

Calories: 671; Carbohydrate: 39%; Protein: 22%; Fat: 39%

Slow Cooker Barbecue Ribs (Phases 2 and 3)

Melt-in-your-mouth tender with the smoky-sweet flavor of barbecue sauce. Marinate the ribs overnight, then leave them cooking all day in the slow cooker for a delicious, hassle-free dinner.

Preparation time: 15 minutes

Total time: 8+ hours (slow cooker)

Makes 4 servings

- 1 full rack of ribs (about 3½ pounds beef back ribs or about 2½ pounds St. Louis–style pork ribs)

BBQ Ma-rub-nade

- 2 tablespoons powdered red chile, such as New Mexican, ancho, or chile de árbol
- 1 tablespoon ground cumin
- 1 tablespoon onion powder
- 1 tablespoon garlic powder
- 1½ teaspoons ground ginger
- 1 tablespoon paprika
- 1 teaspoon smoked paprika
- ½ teaspoon cayenne pepper
- 1 teaspoon ground cinnamon (optional)
- 2 teaspoons salt
- 1½ teaspoons ground black pepper
- 2 tablespoons honey
- 2 tablespoons water

Glaze

- ½ cup Barbecue Sauce (page 290; optional)

Cut down the full rack of ribs into sections that will fit into your slow cooker or a roasting pan.

Make the ma-rub-nade: Combine all the ma-rub-nade ingredients in a medium bowl. (This can be made ahead and stored in the refrigerator until ready to use, up to 2 weeks.) Cover the ribs completely in the ma-rub-nade. For a more flavorful dish, place the ribs in a large baking dish or a gallon-size zip-top bag and cover or seal. Marinate in the refrigerator for 3 hours or up to overnight before cooking. The ribs will release some moisture as they marinate.

Transfer the ribs and any juices to a slow cooker, cover, and cook on low for 8 to 9 hours, or according to the manufacturer's instructions based on the size and weight of the ribs. Check for tenderness: The meat should be fully cooked and melt-off-the-bone tender. (Alternatively, wrap the ribs in heavy-duty aluminum foil and seal well. Put them in a roasting pan and bake at 275°F for 3½ hours. Carefully open the foil, watching for escaping steam.)

If desired, glaze the ribs: Preheat the oven to 400°F.

Brush the ribs evenly with the Barbecue Sauce. Place on a large baking sheet and bake for 10 to 15 minutes until the ribs reach the desired crispy glazed texture.

Calories: 437 (Beef)   Protein: 28 g
Carbohydrate: 22 g   Fat: 28 g

Calories: 451 (Pork) Protein: 37 g
Carbohydrate: 22 g Fat: 24 g

Phase 2 Meal: Serve with 1 cup Minestrone Soup (page 248) and a side of salad greens, chopped raw vegetables, and ⅓ cup Cooked Quinoa (page 231) tossed with 1 to 2 teaspoons Creamy Sun-Dried Tomato Dressing (page 287). **For Dessert:** ½ cup blueberries.

Calories: 688; Carbohydrate: 36%; Protein: 21%; Fat: 43%

Phase 3 Meal: Serve with a small baked potato with 1 heaping tablespoon sour cream. **For Dessert:** ½ small apple, cored, topped with 1 heaping tablespoon plain whole-milk Greek yogurt and drizzled with ½ teaspoon honey.

Calories: 675; Carbohydrate: 38%; Protein: 20%; Fat: 42%

LAMB

Slow-Cooked Moroccan Lamb Stew (All Phases)

Transport yourself to Morocco as the sweet spices fill the house and the recipe cooks itself. This rich stew will remind you of a slow cooked tagine with its sumptuous flavors and creamy textures.

Preparation time: 15 minutes

Total time: 8+ hours (slow cooker)

Makes 4 servings

- 1¼ pounds lamb meat (shoulder works well, but measure weight without bone), cut into chunks
- 1 recipe Moroccan Sauce (page 292)
- 2 tablespoons extra-virgin olive oil
- 1 large onion, cut into large chunks
- 2 large carrots, cut into large chunks
- 7 or 8 prunes or dried apricots (Phases 2 and 3) or 3 or 4 fresh apricots, quartered and pitted (Phase 1)
- 1 bay leaf
- 1 cinnamon stick (optional)
- 1 cup water or broth

Place the lamb in a baking dish or zip-top bag and add the Moroccan Sauce, making sure it covers all the pieces. Cover the dish or seal the bag and place in the refrigerator to marinate for at least 1 hour or up to overnight (or cook immediately if you have less time).

Heat the olive oil in a slow cooker on the sauté setting or in a stovetop-safe slow cooker insert, Dutch oven, or pressure cooker over medium heat.

Remove the lamb from the sauce (reserve the sauce) and add to the oil. Cook, turning regularly, until lightly browned on all sides, about 10 minutes total. Remove the lamb and set aside on a plate.

Add the onion to the pot and cook, stirring, until it begins to soften, 3 to 5 minutes. Return the lamb and any juices that have collected on the plate to the pot, then add the reserved sauce, carrots, prunes, bay leaf, cinnamon stick (if using), and water. Bring to a boil.

If using a slow cooker, return the insert to the slow cooker, if necessary, cover, and cook on low for about 8 hours or medium for 4 to 5 hours.

If using a Dutch oven, cover and simmer over low heat for about 2 hours.

If using a pressure cooker, cover and bring to high pressure according to the manufacturer's instructions. Pressure cook for 20 minutes. Allow the pressure to release naturally. Remove the lid, reduce the heat to low, and simmer for about 30 minutes, or until the liquid has reduced to a nice thick sauce.

Serve hot.

| Calories: 455 | Protein: 30 g |
| Carbohydrate: 20 g | Fat: 29 g |

Variations

Substitute pork, chicken thigh, or beef cubes for the lamb.

Vegetarian version: Substitute 1½ pounds extra-firm tofu, drained, pressed with an absorbent towel, and crumbled, and increase the salt to taste, or 1 recipe Basic Seitan (page 72) plus 2 additional tablespoons olive oil, for the lamb.

Sweet Potato Variation: Add 1 medium sweet potato, cut into large chunks, with the vegetables.

| Calories: 481 | Protein: 31 g |
| Carbohydrate: 26 g | Fat: 29 g |

Phase 1 Meal: Serve the Phase 1 version on top of Cauliflower Couscous (page 211). Serve with 1 cup Split Pea Soup (page 251) and ½ small cucumber, sliced and drizzled with 1 teaspoon Creamy Sun-Dried Tomato Dressing (page 287). **For Dessert:** ¼ cup strawberries topped with 1 heaping tablespoon Cardamom Whipped Cream (page 324).

Calories: 675; Carbohydrate: 27%; Protein: 24%; Fat: 49%

Phase 2 Meal: Serve the Sweet Potato Variation on top of Cauliflower Couscous (page 211). Serve with 1 cup Split Pea Soup (page 251) and ½ small cucumber, sliced and drizzled with 1 teaspoon Creamy Sun-Dried Tomato Dressing (page 287). **For Dessert:** ¼ cup strawberries.

Calories: 702; Carbohydrate: 34%; Protein: 24%; Fat: 42%

Phase 3 Meal: Serve with ⅓ cup cooked whole wheat couscous. Serve with 1 cup Split Pea Soup (page 251), ½ small cucumber, diced, ½ small tomato, diced, chopped parsley, and a squeeze of lemon juice. **For Dessert:** ¼ cup strawberries.

Calories: 694; Carbohydrate: 37%; Protein: 24%; Fat: 39%

Souvlaki (All Phases)

George Brown College culinary students Rebecca Moutoussidis and Jacqueline Zolis created this Greek classic as part of their *Always Hungry?* book class project. Serve the souvlaki with Tzatziki (page 304) or on its own as a side dish when you need a flavorful source of protein without a lot of fat.

Preparation time: 10 minutes plus optional overnight marinating

Total time: 45 minutes

Makes 4 servings

Marinade

- ⅔ cup fresh lemon juice
- ¼ cup extra-virgin olive oil
- 6 cloves garlic
- 2 tablespoons dried oregano
- 1 teaspoon salt
- 1 teaspoon ground black pepper

Souvlaki

- 1½ pounds lamb shoulder or stew meat or pork tenderloin, cut into 1-inch cubes
- 1 (1- to 1½-pound) eggplant, cut into ½-inch-thick rounds
- 4 medium red bell peppers, kept whole
- 1 tablespoon extra-virgin olive oil, for garnish (2 tablespoons with pork), plus more for the grill
- 1 recipe Tzatziki (page 304)

Make the marinade: Combine all the marinade ingredients in a wide-mouthed glass mason jar or cup that will fit an immersion blender without splashing. Blend, working the blender into the mixture until garlic is coarsely chopped. (The marinade can be made ahead and refrigerated for up to 1 month.)

Make the souvlaki: Place the meat in a large baking dish or a large zip-top bag, add the marinade, seal or cover, and refrigerate for at least 3 hours or up to overnight.

Thirty minutes before you plan to cook the meat, soak eight bamboo skewers in water to prevent burning, then drain.

Evenly distribute the cubes of meat among the skewers and set aside on a plate. Place the reserved marinade in a pot and bring to a boil over medium heat. Put the eggplant and bell peppers in a baking dish and pour half the hot marinade over the vegetables, tossing to completely coat, then set them aside to marinate. Set aside the remaining marinade for basting the meat.

Heat a grill pan over medium-high heat or heat a grill to medium-high. Brush the pan or grill grates with oil.

Lay the skewers in a single layer on the grill or grill pan. Cook, turning regularly and basting with the reserved marinade, until the meat is browned on the outside and the juices run clear, about 10 minutes. Transfer to a platter.

Grill the eggplant slices until softened and lightly charred, 3 to 4 minutes on each side. Transfer to the platter with the meat. Grill the bell peppers, turning and cooking until charred on all sides. Peel off the charred skin, remove the seeds, and slice the flesh into ½-inch-thick strips.

Alternatively, the souvlaki and vegetables can be cooked in the oven: Preheat the oven to 425°F.

Arrange the skewers on a baking sheet and bake, turning once, for 12 to 20 minutes, or until meat reaches desired doneness. Transfer to a platter and turn the oven to broil.

Cut the peppers in half and remove the seeds. Arrange in a single layer on a baking sheet, cut-sides down, and broil about 4 inches from the heat for 15 to 20 minutes, or until the skin is lightly charred and the peppers are soft. Turn once to ensure the peppers are cooked on both sides. Transfer to a bowl, cover with plastic wrap, and set aside to steam while you cook the eggplant. Set the oven to 425°F.

Line one or two baking sheets with parchment paper. Arrange the eggplant slices on the baking sheet(s), slightly overlapping. Bake for 20 to 25 minutes, or until soft.

Uncover the peppers, peel off the charred skin, and slice the flesh into ½-inch-thick strips.

To serve, arrange the grilled eggplant on each plate. Lay 2 souvlaki sticks on the eggplant. Top with red pepper strips and Tzatziki. Drizzle with the olive oil just before serving.

Calories: 530
Carbohydrate: 30 g
Protein: 48 g
Fat: 25 g

Variations

Vegetarian version: Substitute 1½ pounds Deep-Fried Tofu or 1 pound Deep-Fried Tempeh cubes (page 170) or Panfried Tempeh (page 193) for the lamb or pork. No need to cook these, as they are already cooked. Reduce the olive oil in the marinade to 1 tablespoon, and omit the olive oil garnish. Or substitute 1 recipe Basic Seitan (page 72) for the lamb (reduce salt to ⅛ teaspoon, and marinate and cook as directed even though the seitan is precooked) and serve with a higher-fat sauce like Lemon Aioli (page 298).

Substitute boneless, skinless chicken thighs cut into 1-inch cubes for the lamb or pork.

For Phase 3: Use 1 pound lamb or pork.

Phase 1 Meal: Serve with 6 or 7 Greek olives per person, tossed with fresh rosemary and orange zest, then warmed in a covered skillet over medium-low heat, stirring regularly, for about 5 minutes. **For Dessert:** 1 Chocolate Truffle (page 314).

Calories: 679; Carbohydrate: 23%; Protein: 27%; Fat: 50%

Phase 2 Meal: Serve with 3 or 4 Greek olives, warmed with herbs and zest as in the Phase 1 Meal, then tossed with ¼ cup Cooked Quinoa (page 231). **For Dessert:** ½ medium apple, cored, sliced, and drizzled with ½ teaspoon honey.

Calories: 675; Carbohydrate: 33%; Protein: 28%; Fat: 39%

Phase 3 Meal: Use the Phase 3 Variation. Serve with Millet Tabbouleh (page 234). **For Dessert:** 2 Chocolate-Dipped Strawberries (page 313).

Calories: 679; Carbohydrate: 37%; Protein: 23%; Fat: 40%

Mustard Peppercorn Roasted Rack of Lamb (All Phases)

Forget the mint jelly—this roasted rack of lamb has all the flavor it needs roasted with a simple sauce. The sauce will also turn roasted pork chops or pork tenderloin into an impressive restaurant-quality meal. A hearty meal for nights when you don't have much time to cook!

Preparation time: 10 minutes

Total time: 45 minutes

Makes 4 servings

- 2 or 3 large cloves garlic
- 2 to 3 teaspoons whole black peppercorns
- ¼ cup Dijon, German, or spicy brown mustard
- ¾ to 1 teaspoon salt
- ¼ cup water
- 1½ to 2 pounds rack of lamb (1 large or 1½ small racks), frenched (ask your butcher to do this)

Place the garlic, peppercorns, mustard, salt, and water into a wide-mouthed glass mason jar or cup that will fit an immersion blender without splashing. Blend until the peppercorns are coarsely ground.

Spread the sauce over the lamb on all sides. You can cook the lamb immediately, or place it in a zip-top bag and marinate in the refrigerator for 3 hours or up to overnight.

Arrange the lamb, covered in sauce, fatty-side up in an ovenproof skillet or baking pan. Bake for 25 to 30 minutes, or until a meat thermometer registers 130 to 140°F for medium-rare in the center of the rack (or to your desired doneness).

If desired, use a broiler-safe pan, turn on the broiler, and broil for a minute or two at the end of cooking for a crispier result.

Remove from the oven and let it rest for about 10 minutes, loosely covered with a lid or foil, before carving and serving.

Calories: 226	Protein: 27 g
Carbohydrate: 2 g	Fat: 13 g

Variations

Substitute about 1⅓ pounds bone-in pork chops for lamb.

Substitute 1 to 1¼ pounds pork tenderloin or beef rump roast for the lamb. Add 1 tablespoon oil to the marinade, and cook until done, depending on the thickness of the meat.

Phase 1 Meal: Serve with 1 cup Sicilian Fava Bean Soup (page 244), Sautéed Mushrooms (page 216) over Cauliflower Couscous (page 211), and 4 to 6 spears asparagus, steamed and drizzled with 1 teaspoon olive oil and a squeeze of lemon juice. **For Dessert:** 1 Chocolate Truffle (page 314).

Calories: 625; Carbohydrate: 25%; Protein: 25%; Fat: 50%

Phase 2 Meal: Serve with 1 cup Sicilian Fava Bean Soup (page 244), baked sweet potato (about 1 cup) with 1 heaping teaspoon butter, and 4 to 6 spears asparagus, steamed and drizzled with ½ teaspoon olive oil and a squeeze of lemon juice. **For Dessert:** 2 Chocolate-Dipped Strawberries (page 313).

Calories: 649; Carbohydrate: 37%; Protein: 24%; Fat: 39%

Phase 3 Meal: Serve with a small baked potato (about 1 cup) with 1 heaping teaspoon butter, and 4 to 6 spears asparagus, steamed and drizzled with ½ teaspoon olive oil and a squeeze of lemon juice. **For Dessert:** 1 cup blueberries with 3 tablespoons Pear Cinnamon Cashew Butter (page 58).

Calories: 617; Carbohydrate: 42%; Protein: 21%; Fat: 37%

VEGETARIAN

Chef Dawn's Tasty Tip

Out of the Pan, Into the Fire: The Art of Deep-Frying

Cast-iron cookware works well for deep-frying, as it holds and distributes heat more consistently than other metals. Woks, because of their shape, are also an effective choice. When oil is hot enough, whatever you are cooking should sink to the bottom of the pot or fryer and then rise to the top. If it never sinks, the oil is too hot. If it sinks and stays there for more than 5 to 7 seconds, the oil is not hot enough.

Sage Walnut Lentil Loaf (Phases 2 and 3, with Phase 1 Variation)

A flavorful and satisfying take on an old classic that is sure to please vegetarians and meat eaters alike. The lentils and mushrooms come together to create the perfect meaty texture, while our Smoked Paprika Ketchup will leave you wondering why you ever settled for sugary, store-bought ketchups.

Preparation time: 15 minutes

Total time: 1 hour 45 minutes

Makes 6 servings

- 1 cup dried green or brown lentils
- ¼ cup dried red lentils (or additional green or brown lentils)
- 2½ cups water
- 1 bay leaf
- 2 teaspoons salt
- 2 medium cloves garlic
- 1 medium onion, cut into large chunks
- 1 stalk celery, cut into large chunks
- ½ teaspoon ground black pepper
- 1 teaspoon ground dried sage
- 2 tablespoons extra-virgin olive oil, plus more for the pan
- Olive oil spray (optional)
- 8 ounces baby bella/cremini mushrooms, coarsely chopped
- 1 egg
- 2 egg whites
- ½ cup plain whole-milk Greek yogurt
- 2 teaspoons Sugar-Free Worcestershire Sauce (page 284)
- 1 tablespoon tahini
- 2 to 3 teaspoons chopped fresh sage (about 5 large leaves)
- ½ cup walnuts, coarsely chopped
- ½ cup Chickpea Bread Crumbs (page 196)
- 1 cup Smoked Paprika Ketchup (page 291)

Sort through the lentils and remove any stones or grit. Rinse well. Place in a pot with the water and bay leaf. Bring to a boil. Skim off any foam that rises to the top. Reduce the heat to low, cover, and simmer for 25 to 30 minutes, until the lentils are soft and the water has been absorbed. Stir 1 teaspoon of the salt into the cooked lentils. (This makes about 3 cups cooked lentils and can be done ahead of time for more efficiency. Set aside until ready to use or cool and store in the refrigerator for up to a week or in the freezer for up to 6 months.)

Place the garlic, onion, celery, remaining 1 teaspoon salt, the pepper, and the ground sage in a food processor and pulse until the vegetables are finely chopped.

Preheat the oven to 350°F. Grease a 9-inch square baking pan with oil or coat with olive oil spray.

Heat the olive oil in a large skillet over medium heat. Add the chopped vegetables (set the processor bowl aside—no need to wash it) and the mushrooms. Cook, stirring, until the mushrooms are soft and the liquid has been absorbed, about 15 minutes.

Transfer the vegetable-mushroom mixture back to the food processor bowl and add the egg, egg whites, yogurt, cooked lentils, Worcestershire, tahini, fresh sage, walnuts, and Chickpea Bread Crumbs. Pulse until fully combined but still chunky; do not process into a paste.

Spread the lentil mixture into an even layer in the prepared baking pan. Gently spread the ketchup evenly over the top. Bake for about 45 minutes, or until the loaf is bubbling. Remove from the oven and let the casserole rest for 5 minutes, then cut and serve or cool and store in the refrigerator for up to a week or wrap tightly in plastic wrap and store in the freezer for up to 3 months.

Tip: To reheat leftovers without drying out the loaf, place in a steamer basket and steam for about 5 minutes.

Calories: 430   Protein: 19 g
Carbohydrate: 53g   Fat: 18 g

Variations

Egg-free version: Substitute 8 ounces extra-firm tofu, drained, pressed with an absorbent towel, and finely crumbled, in place of the egg and yogurt.

For Phase 1: Replace the Smoked Paprika Ketchup topping with 1 recipe (about ⅔ cup) Moroccan Sauce (page 292).

Phase 1 Meal: Use Phase 1 variation. Serve with Miso Soup (page 258), a sliced hard-boiled egg drizzled with 1 teaspoon olive oil and sprinkled with salt and pepper, and ⅓ to ½ cup Tzatziki (page 304). **For Dessert:** A cup of your favorite herbal tea.

Calories: 695; Carbohydrate: 28%; Protein: 21%; Fat: 51%

Phase 2 or 3 Meal: Serve each portion with a side of salad greens, chopped raw vegetables, a slice of Smoke-Dried Tomato Seitan (page 73) or other vegetarian protein, and a sliced hard-boiled egg tossed with 1 to 2 teaspoons Greek Dressing (page 285). **For Dessert:** ½ cup strawberries and 2 tablespoons plain whole-milk Greek yogurt.

Calories: 689; Carbohydrate: 38%; Protein: 22%; Fat: 40%

Deep-Fried Tofu or Tempeh (All Phases)

Ever wonder how restaurants can turn tofu into perfectly golden, crispy cubes? Now that we're no longer afraid of fat, Deep-Fried Tofu is easy to make at home and tempeh is a crispy, meaty treat. Use it in stir-fries, soups, sauces, as a topping on salads, or a main ingredient in Buddha Bowls (page 263). These little cubes pair perfectly with a wide variety of sauces, soaking up and enhancing each nuanced flavor.

Preparation time: 5 minutes

Total time: 25 minutes

Makes 4 servings

- Neutral-tasting oil, such as high-oleic safflower or avocado oil, for deep-frying
- 1½ pounds extra-firm tofu, or 1 pound tempeh
- 1 to 2 teaspoons soy sauce

Pour 2 inches of oil into a deep fryer, heavy-bottomed pot, or wok. Heat the oil to 325 to 350°F. See Chef Dawn's Tasty Tip on deep-frying (page 167).

If using tofu, wrap the tofu in an absorbent towel and press gently between two cutting boards or heavy plates to remove any excess water. (Removing excess water will keep the tofu from causing the hot oil to spatter.) Cut the tofu into 1-inch cubes.

If using tempeh, cut into cubes to use for skewers. Or, for general use, cut the tempeh in half lengthwise to make a thinner block, then into 3-inch squares, and finally into triangles.

Working in batches as needed to avoid crowding the pan, gently place the tofu or tempeh in the hot oil and deep-fry, turning occasionally, until golden brown and crispy on all sides, 3 to 5 minutes total. Tofu cubes may stick together at the edges, but you can easily break them apart as you turn them. Remove from the oil with a mesh skimmer or tongs. Place on a plate lined with paper towels or covered with a bamboo sushi mat to drain. Transfer to a bowl and toss with the soy sauce while still hot.

Tip: Use these in place of any chicken, beef, lamb, or fatty fish ingredients in recipes.

Calories: 266 (Tofu) Protein: 25 g
Carbohydrate: 2 g Fat: 17 g

Calories: 281 (Tempeh) Protein: 23 g
Carbohydrate: 9 g Fat: 19 g

Tofu Vegetable Balls (All Phases)

For vegetarian families on the go, these protein packs are sure to please parents and kids alike. As part of their *Always Hungry?* book class project, George Brown College culinary students Olga Ni and Kang Lei made these irresistible bites, which are versatile enough to serve as a snack or a main dish.

Preparation time: 5 minutes

Total time: 30 minutes

Makes 4 servings (about 32 balls or patties)

- 3 small onions, cut into large chunks
- 2 medium carrots, cut into large chunks
- 1 cup packed fresh parsley, stems and leaves coarsely chopped (2 ounces)
- 6 cloves garlic
- 1 (½-inch) piece fresh ginger, peeled and thinly sliced
- 1 tablespoon extra-virgin olive oil
- 1⅓ pounds firm tofu, drained and pressed with an absorbent towel
- 6 tablespoons chickpea flour (see Tip, page 91)
- ¾ teaspoon salt
- 1 teaspoon soy sauce
- Neutral-tasting oil, such as high-oleic safflower or avocado oil, for deep-frying
- 1 lime, cut into wedges, for garnish

Place the onions, carrots, parsley, garlic, and ginger in a food processor and pulse until finely chopped.

Heat the olive oil in a skillet over medium heat. Add chopped vegetables and cook, stirring, until the vegetables are soft, about 5 minutes.

Crumble the tofu into a large bowl and mash with a fork into small pieces. Stir in the chickpea flour, salt, and soy sauce. Add the sautéed vegetables and combine well. Taste and adjust the seasonings.

Pour 2 inches of oil into a deep fryer, heavy-bottomed pot, or wok. Heat the oil to 325 to 350°F. See Chef Dawn's Tasty Tip on deep-frying (page 167).

Form the tofu mixture into 1½-inch-diameter balls, wetting your hands as needed to keep the mixture from sticking.

Gently place the tofu balls in the oil, working in batches as needed to avoid crowding the pan, and deep-fry, turning occasionally, until golden brown and crispy on all sides, 5 to 7 minutes total. Remove from the oil with a mesh skimmer or tongs. Place on a plate lined with paper towels or covered with a bamboo sushi mat to drain.

Serve with lime wedges.

Calories: 317
Carbohydrate: 14 g
Protein: 21 g
Fat: 20 g

Phase 1 Meal: Serve with 1 tablespoon Ginger Tahini Dressing (page 288), and a side of salad greens, chopped vegetables, and ½ cup edamame tossed with 1 to 2 teaspoons Creamy Sun-Dried Tomato Dressing (page 287). **For Dessert:** ½ small apple, cored and sliced, topped with 1 heaping tablespoon plain whole-milk Greek yogurt and 2 tablespoons peanuts.

Calories: 654; Carbohydrate: 23%; Protein: 23%; Fat: 54%

Phase 2 Meal: Serve with Fresh Quinoa Salad with Pomegranates (page 262) tossed with ⅓ cup edamame. **For Dessert:** 1 small apple, cored and sliced, topped with 2 to 3 tablespoons plain whole-milk Greek yogurt and 1 tablespoon peanuts.

Calories: 626; Carbohydrate: 34%; Protein: 22%; Fat: 44%

Phase 3 Meal: Serve with 1 to 2 ounces (dry) soba noodles, cooked according to the package directions, then sautéed with 1 teaspoon toasted sesame oil, 1 cup chopped vegetables, and 1 to 2 tablespoons of the Miso-Sake Marinade from Drunken Marinated Shrimp Kebabs (page 144). **For Dessert:** ½ small apple, cored and sliced, topped with 1 tablespoon Cashew Crème (page 323).

Calories: 634; Carbohydrate: 40%; Protein: 20%; Fat: 40%

Crispy Tofu Fries (All Phases)

We discovered these by accident one evening while frying chicken. Too much batter, not enough chicken, and a little quick thinking resulted in the birth of this remarkable recipe. Crispy Tofu Fries have become our favorite way to eat tofu, and they make a better vehicle for sauces than any store-bought chip! These little fries may remind you of those ubiquitous carb-laden snacks at street fairs. You'll be surprised at just how fabulous tofu can be.

Preparation time: 10 minutes

Total time: 20 to 30 minutes

Makes 8 servings

- 1½ pounds extra-firm tofu, drained and pressed with an absorbent towel
- 2 tablespoons soy sauce
- ½ cup neutral-tasting oil with a high smoke point, such as high-oleic safflower or avocado oil, or more as needed
- ½ cup chickpea flour (see Tip, page 91)
- ⅛ teaspoon garlic powder
- ½ teaspoon salt
- ⅛ teaspoon ground black pepper

Preheat the oven to 200°F.

Cut the tofu into ¾-inch-thick slices, then into 3 logs per slice. Place in a baking dish and cover evenly with the soy sauce. Set aside to marinate while you prepare the other ingredients or place in the refrigerator to marinate for a few hours or up to overnight.

Heat the oil in a large cast-iron skillet. The oil should be ¼ to ⅓ inch deep in the skillet and hot enough that it sizzles when the tofu is added, about 325°F.

Combine the chickpea flour, garlic powder, salt, and pepper in a shallow dish or pie plate. Dredge the tofu sticks in the chickpea mixture to completely cover, shaking off any excess.

Working in batches as needed to avoid overcrowding the pan, gently place the tofu sticks in the hot oil in a single layer. Cook until the bottom is browned and crispy, then flip and cook until browned and crispy on all sides, about 10 minutes total. Remove from the pan and place on a plate lined with paper towels or covered with a bamboo sushi mat to drain. Transfer to a baking sheet and keep warm in the oven until ready to serve. Skim any bits of flour from the oil with a mesh strainer or slotted spoon and discard. Add oil to the pan as needed and reheat. Repeat to fry the remaining tofu.

Serve with Lemon Aioli (page 298), Smoked Paprika Ketchup (page 291), or your other favorite sauces for dipping. (See photo insert page 9.)

Calories: 188
Carbohydrate: 5 g

Protein: 14 g
Fat: 12 g

Phase 1 Meal: Serve with 1 to 2 tablespoons Lemon Aioli (page 298), Baby Lima Beans in Creamy Shiitake Gravy (page 224), and The Perfect Cucumber-Tomato Salad (page 261) tossed with 2 to 3 tablespoons plain whole-milk Greek yogurt. **For Dessert:** 1 to 2 tablespoons roasted peanuts.

Calories: 643; Carbohydrate: 29%; Protein: 21%; Fat: 50%

Phase 2 Meal: Serve with 2 tablespoons Smoked Paprika Ketchup (page 291) and Savory Adzuki Beans (page 223), and toss together ¼ cup cooked brown rice, 1 cup blanched or steamed vegetables, and 1 heaping tablespoon Ginger Tahini Dressing (page 288). **For Dessert:** ¼ cup plain whole-milk Greek yogurt topped with 2 tablespoons roasted peanuts.

Calories: 639; Carbohydrate: 38%; Protein: 21%; Fat: 41%

Phase 3 Meal: Serve with 2 tablespoons Smoked Paprika Ketchup (page 291), 1½ ounces (dry) brown rice udon noodles, cooked and tossed with Seasoned Shiitake Mushrooms (page 217), 1 cup blanched or steamed vegetables, and 1 heaping tablespoon Ginger Tahini Dressing (page 288). **For Dessert:** ¼ cup plain whole-milk Greek yogurt topped with 2 tablespoons roasted peanuts.

Calories: 674; Carbohydrate: 40%; Protein: 19%; Fat: 41%

Chef Dawn's Tasty Tip

Poutine Will Never Be the Same

One of the George Brown College culinary school teams, Yingxin Ma and Yi-Ling Chen, used these tofu fries for an innovative Asian fusion take on poutine—the Canadian dish of French fries covered in gravy and cheese curds. I was impressed with the taste of this unique combination and craved it for weeks. Try it yourself: Sprinkle ½ to ¾ cup cottage cheese or cheese curds on the tofu fries, and top that all with kimchi, diced fresh tomatoes, and scallions. The spicy kimchi with the cool, creamy curds and fresh tomatoes made the perfect addition to these crispy tofu fries. Yum!

Marinated Baked Tofu (All Phases)

Tofu absorbs flavors well, making it a versatile vehicle for sauces, especially when it is marinated ahead of time. Baked tofu will keep for a week or more in the refrigerator and can be served warm or cold as a filling in wraps, a topping for salads, or a hearty main dish. No need to spend money on packages of expensive preseasoned tofu—now you can make your own.

Preparation time: 5 minutes

Total time: 35 to 55 minutes

Makes 4 to 6 servings

- 1½ pounds extra-firm tofu, drained and pressed with an absorbent towel
- 1 recipe Lemon Thyme Marinade (page 296), or any of your favorite marinades or sauces from pages 284 to 306
- Salt

Preheat the oven to 350°F.

Cut the tofu into ¼-inch-thick slices or 1-inch cubes. Place the tofu in a baking dish, pour over the marinade, and cover with plastic wrap, or put the tofu and marinade in a zip-top bag and seal the bag, making sure the marinade covers the tofu. (If the marinade is very thick, whisk it with ¼ cup water before using.) Tofu requires more salt than other proteins in order to remain flavorful, so if the sauce is on the less salty side, add salt to taste. Marinate in the refrigerator for at least 1 hour and up to overnight (or cook the tofu immediately if you have less time).

If you used a zip-top bag, transfer the tofu with the marinade to a baking dish or rimmed baking sheet in a single layer. Bake for 30 to 45 minutes, until the tofu is cooked through and the marinade has mostly been absorbed. Serve warm, or cool and store in the refrigerator for up to a week. Tofu does not freeze well, as freezing changes the texture to a spongy consistency. (See photo insert page 8.)

Tip: Make a bit extra to use throughout the week. When you increase the tofu to 2 pounds, use the same amount of marinade, just increase the salt a bit. There is plenty of flavor in these marinades to accommodate the increased amount of tofu.

Based on 4 servings
Calories: 267

Carbohydrate: 3 g
Protein: 24 g

Fat: 17 g

Variations

Substitute other sauces for the Lemon Thyme Marinade: ½ cup Fresh Turmeric Garlic Marinade (page 295), Cilantro Chimichurri (page 300), Parsley Chimichurri (page 301), Basil Walnut Pesto (page 297), Miso-Sake Marinade from Drunken Marinated Shrimp Kebabs (page 144), Lime Cilantro Pesto (page 298), Greek Dressing (page 285); or, for Phase 2, ¾ cup Barbecue Sauce (page 290) or Citrus Teriyaki (page 293), or 1 cup Spicy Asian Marinade (page 294; Tofu Variation).

Portobello or Baby Bella Pizzas (All Phases)

You won't even miss the crust with these satisfying little pizza bites. If you have meat eaters in the group, add a slice or two of pepperoni in place of the tempeh and you'll have a meal that meets everyone's tastes.

Preparation time: 5 minutes

Total time: 35 minutes

Makes 4 servings

- 12 large baby bella/cremini mushrooms or 6 large portobello mushrooms
- 2 tablespoons extra-virgin olive oil
- 1 small onion, diced
- 2 cloves garlic, minced
- ½ teaspoon Italian seasoning
- ½ teaspoon salt
- ⅛ teaspoon ground black pepper
- 1 cup Crumbled Tempeh (page 192) or Deep-Fried Tempeh (page 170)
- 1 to 2 cups packed chopped arugula or baby spinach (2 to 4 ounces)
- 3 ounces tomato paste (about ½ small can)
- 6 ounces mozzarella cheese, cut into 6 to 12 slices, depending on the number of mushrooms you use

Preheat the oven to 400°F.

Rinse or wipe the mushrooms. Pull off the stems and scoop the gills out of the mushroom caps; chop the stems and gills into small pieces and set aside.

Using 1 tablespoon of the olive oil, rub the outside of each mushroom cap. Place them on a rimmed baking sheet, gill-side up, and bake for 10 minutes. Remove from the oven and pour off any juice that has accumulated on the baking sheet. Set aside.

Heat the remaining 1 tablespoon olive oil in a skillet over medium heat. Add the diced mushroom stems and gills, the onion, garlic, Italian seasoning, ⅛ teaspoon of the salt, and the pepper. Cook, stirring, until the onion is translucent, 3 to 5 minutes.

Add the tempeh, arugula, and tomato paste. Cook, stirring, for 1 minute, or until the arugula is wilted.

Evenly distribute the tempeh mixture among the mushroom caps. Bake for about 20 minutes, adding a slice of mozzarella on top of each mushroom in the last 10 minutes of cooking.

Serve hot.

Calories: 356
Carbohydrate: 17 g
Protein: 23 g
Fat: 24 g

Variations

Meat version: Use any cooked meat in place of the tempeh, or omit the tempeh and top with pepperoni.

Phase 1 Meal: Serve with 1 cup Sicilian Fava Bean Soup (page 244). **For Dessert:** ½ cup fresh raspberries and ½ cup plain whole-milk Greek yogurt.

Calories: 617; Carbohydrate: 28%; Protein: 25%; Fat: 47%

Phase 2 Meal: Serve with Garlicky White Beans with Broccoli Rabe (page 221). **For Dessert:** 1 cup raspberries and ¼ cup plain whole-milk Greek yogurt.

Calories: 630; Carbohydrate: 34%; Protein: 23%; Fat: 43%

Phase 3 Meal: Use a 6-inch whole wheat pita or 4 mini pitas for the crust, and cut up and sauté mushrooms with the other ingredients as topping. **For Dessert:** Apple Pie Parfait (page 319).

Calories: 690; Carbohydrate: 40%; Protein: 21%; Fat: 39%

Falafel (All Phases)

Even if you've never tried falafel, you're going to want to give this one a go. There's no single flavor that overpowers the rest, and with both sides crisp from the fryer, these falafel are the perfect companion for our Tzatziki (page 304) or a bit of tahini with lemon juice.

Preparation time: 20 minutes (plus overnight soaking time)

Total time: 45 minutes

Makes 6 to 8 servings (about 36 patties)

- 1 cup dried chickpeas
- ½ cup packed fresh parsley, stems and leaves coarsely chopped (1 ounce)
- ½ cup packed fresh cilantro, stems and leaves coarsely chopped (1 ounce)
- 1 medium onion, cut into large chunks
- 2 large cloves garlic
- 1 teaspoon ground cumin
- ½ teaspoon ground coriander
- ¼ teaspoon powdered red chile, such as New Mexican, ancho, or chile de árbol
- ¼ teaspoon ground black pepper
- ½ teaspoon salt
- 2 to 3 tablespoons chickpea flour (see Tip, page 91), plus more if needed
- ½ teaspoon baking powder (optional, for lighter falafel)
- ½ cup neutral-tasting oil, such as high-oleic safflower or avocado oil, for frying

Sort through the chickpeas and remove any stones or grit. Rinse well. Put them in a large bowl, add water to cover by 3 to 4 inches, and set aside to soak for 8 hours or up to overnight. Drain the chickpeas and discard the soaking water.

Place the parsley, cilantro, onion, garlic, spices, and salt in a food processor. Pulse until well mixed. Add the chickpeas and pulse until the chickpeas are ground to a very fine meal but not quite to a paste. If you have time, set the mixture aside in the refrigerator for 1 to 2 hours to allow the flavors to fully develop.

Combine chickpea flour with baking powder (if using) and stir into the chickpea mixture right before using.

Heat the oil in a large cast-iron skillet over medium heat until a wooden spoon bubbles when touched to the bottom of the pot (325 to 350°F). The oil should not smoke before adding the falafel. (Alternatively, to deep-fry the falafel, use enough oil to fill a deep fryer, heavy-bottomed pot, or wok by about 2 inches. See Chef Dawn's Tasty Tip on deep-frying on page 167.)

Gently form the chickpea mixture into patties or balls using 1 heaping tablespoon of the mixture at a time. To ensure light, fluffy falafel, don't overhandle or tightly compact the mixture. The patties should hold together on their own. If not, stir in more chickpea flour, 1 tablespoon at a time.

Place the falafel close together in the pan, leaving room to turn them but cooking as many as possible. (If deep-frying, only add a few at a time and avoid crowding the pot.) Fry until they are well browned, about 5 minutes, turning only once to keep them from falling apart. Carefully remove from the pan and place on a plate lined with paper towels or covered with a bamboo sushi mat to drain. Transfer to a baking sheet and keep warm in a 200°F oven until ready to serve. Repeat with the remaining falafel.

Falafel are best served fresh, but can be refrigerated for up to a week or frozen for up to 6 months and reheated in the oven at 375°F for 10 minutes or until heated through.

Based on 6 servings (about 6 patties per serving)	Calories: 231 Carbohydrate: 25 g	Protein: 8 g Fat: 12 g

Phase 1 Meal: Serve with Tzatziki (page 304), sliced tomatoes seasoned with salt and lemon juice, and Deep-Fried Tofu (page 170) or Marinated Baked Tofu (page 175). **For Dessert:** 2 Chocolate-Dipped Strawberries (page 313). **For a meat-based meal:** Substitute ½ cup Shredded Chicken (page 110) or ⅓ cup Shredded Beef (page 148) for the tofu and drizzle 1 to 3 teaspoons olive oil on the Tzatziki and tomatoes.

Calories: 670; Carbohydrate: 25%; Protein: 26%; Fat: 49%

Phase 2 Meal: Serve with Tzatziki (page 304) and ½ serving Ful Mudammas (page 222), a few slices of Marinated Baked Tofu (page 175) or ⅓ cup Shredded Chicken (page 110). **For Dessert:** ½ Mango Lassi (page 311).

Calories: 676; Carbohydrate: 33%; Protein: 28%; Fat: 39%

Phase 3 Meal: Serve with Tzatziki (page 304) and Ful Mudammas (page 222). **For Dessert:** ½ Mango Lassi (page 311).

Calories: 687; Carbohydrate: 41%; Protein: 20%; Fat: 39%

Cabbage Kofta in a Tomato Tadka (All Phases)

Kofta are satisfying little patties of vegetables bound together with chickpea flour, usually simmered in a savory sauce. This recipe also makes use of *tadka*, a simple technique in Indian cooking for sautéing spices in hot oil until fragrant. Doing this allows the spices to release their full flavors into the dish as they infuse the oil with rich aromas. Together, these two Indian favorites create a wonderfully delicious dish.

Preparation time: 20 minutes

Total time: 50 minutes (less if sauce is prepped ahead)

Makes 4 servings

Kofta

- 1 pound cabbage or cauliflower, cut into large chunks (about 4 cups)
- 18 sprigs cilantro, coarsely chopped (about ¼ cup packed)
- 1 small chile (choose a mild to medium spicy chile to fit your taste preference), seeded, or a dash of cayenne pepper, or to taste
- 1 (½-inch) piece fresh ginger, peeled and cut into thin rounds, or ⅛ teaspoon ground ginger
- 1 cup chickpea flour (see Tip, page 91)
- 1 teaspoon ground turmeric
- 1 teaspoon garam masala or curry powder (see Tip)
- 1 teaspoon ground cumin
- 1 teaspoon baking powder
- ¾ teaspoon salt
- ¼ teaspoon ground black pepper

Sauce

- 1 tablespoon neutral-tasting oil, such as high-oleic safflower or avocado oil, or ghee, melted
- 1 large onion, diced
- 1 large clove garlic, minced
- 1 (½-inch) piece fresh ginger, peeled and minced (see Tip, page 289)
- 1 to 2 teaspoons garam masala (see Tip), or to taste
- ½ teaspoon ground cumin

- ½ teaspoon ground coriander
- ¾ teaspoon salt
- ¼ teaspoon ground black pepper
- 1 (14.5-ounce) can diced tomatoes, with their liquid
- ½ cup neutral-tasting oil, such as high-oleic safflower or avocado oil, for frying
- ¼ cup chopped fresh cilantro, for garnish

Make the kofta: Place the cabbage, cilantro, fresh chile, and fresh ginger in a food processor. (If using cayenne, add it to the chickpea flour with the other dried spices.) Pulse until finely minced. Set aside.

In a large bowl, combine the chickpea flour, turmeric, garam masala, cumin, baking powder, salt, pepper, and cayenne (if using). Set aside.

Make the sauce: Heat the oil in a pot or deep skillet over medium-high heat until very hot but not smoking. Add the onion, garlic, ginger, garam masala, cumin, coriander, salt, and pepper. Cook, stirring, until the onion is translucent and the spices are fragrant, about 5 minutes. The onion keeps the spices from burning as they infuse the oil with flavor.

Stir in the tomatoes with their liquid. Bring to a boil. Reduce the heat to low, cover, and simmer, stirring regularly, for 10 minutes to allow the flavors to fully incorporate.

Blend directly in the pot with an immersion blender until the sauce is still a bit chunky but well combined. (If the sauce is not deep enough to fully immerse the blender and prevent splattering, carefully transfer the sauce to a deep bowl or jar to blend. Return to the pan after blending.) Taste and adjust the seasonings. Leave on the stove on low to simmer for 5 to 10 minutes more, or until the kofta are ready. (The sauce can be made ahead and stored in a jar or other airtight container in the refrigerator for up to 1 week, then reheated for quicker prep. This also allows the flavors to fully develop.)

Cook the kofta: Combine the minced cabbage mixture with the chickpea-spice mixture, gently stirring with a spatula or your hands until all the flour has been absorbed.

Heat the oil in a large cast-iron skillet over medium heat until a wooden spoon bubbles when touched to the bottom of the pot (325 to 350°F). The oil should not smoke before adding the kofta. (Alternatively, to deep-fry the kofta, use enough oil to fill a deep fryer, heavy-bottomed pot, or wok by about 2 inches. See Chef Dawn's Tasty Tip on deep-frying on page 167.)

Gently form the kofta dough into balls, patties, or ovals, using about 3 tablespoons of dough for each patty. To ensure a light kofta, be sure to handle them gently without packing them too tightly, and cook them immediately. You should end up with about 16 kofta.

Place the kofta close together in the pan, leaving room to turn them but cooking as many as possible. (If deep-frying, only add a few at a time and avoid crowding the pot.) Fry until they are well browned on all sides, 5 to 10 minutes total. Remove from the pan and place on a plate lined with paper towels or covered with a bamboo sushi mat to drain. Transfer to a baking sheet and keep warm in a 200°F oven until ready to serve. Repeat with the remaining kofta.

Serve the kofta with the sauce poured over the top and garnished with fresh cilantro.

Kofta are best served fresh, but can be refrigerated for up to a week or frozen for up to 6 months and reheated in the oven at 375°F for 10 minutes or until heated throughout.

Tip: Garam masala and curry powder are Indian spice mixtures that vary in ingredients from region to region and even from cook to cook. There are several brands commercially available at the grocery store or your local Indian market. Try a few different combinations to find the ones you love best. Some may have more coriander or more cumin or other spices that are particularly tasty depending on your preferences. If you can find the whole spices mixed together in a bag, it is easy to grind a batch in a spice mill or coffee grinder. Freshly ground spices are more flavorful.

Calories: 286   Protein: 9 g
Carbohydrate: 27 g   Fat: 16 g

Phase 1 Meal: Serve with Indian Raita (page 303) and Deep-Fried Tofu (page 170). **For Dessert:** ½ cup strawberries. **For a meat-based meal:** Substitute ½ cup Shredded Chicken (page 110) for the tofu and add 2 tablespoons heavy cream to the berries, or substitute ⅓ cup Shredded Beef (page 148) for the tofu.

Calories: 648; Carbohydrate: 24%; Protein: 25%; Fat: 51%

Phase 2 Meal: Serve with ⅓ cup cooked brown rice, Indian Raita (page 303), and a smaller portion of Deep-Fried Tofu (page 170) or other proteins from the Phase 1 Meal. **For Dessert:** ½ cup strawberries.

Calories: 664; Carbohydrate: 34%; Protein: 22%; Fat: 44%

Phase 3 Meal: Serve with ⅓ cup cooked brown or white rice and Indian Raita (page 302). **For Dessert:** Mango Lassi (page 311).

Calories: 632; Carbohydrate: 41%; Protein: 19%; Fat: 40%

Quinoa Enchilada Casserole (Phases 2 and 3, with Phase 1 Variation)

George Brown College culinary students John Loui Ricardo and Julius De Guia wowed us with this tasty casserole from their *Always Hungry?* book class project. This casserole is quick and easy because components can be made ahead and assembled in a matter of minutes…but it tastes like it came from a fine restaurant.

Preparation time: 10 minutes

Total time: 1 hour

Makes 4 servings

Enchilada Sauce

- 1 tablespoon extra-virgin olive oil
- 1 tablespoon chili powder, or to taste
- ½ teaspoon dried Mexican oregano or regular oregano
- ½ teaspoon ground cumin
- ½ teaspoon garlic powder
- ½ teaspoon onion powder
- 1 (14.5-ounce) can diced tomatoes
- ¼ teaspoon salt, or to taste
- ¼ teaspoon ground black pepper, or to taste

Casserole

- 2 cups Cooked Quinoa (page 231)
- 3 tablespoons chopped Anaheim or other mild chile (about ½ chile)
- 2 cups cooked beans (see Do-It-Yourself Beans, page 74) or drained and rinsed canned beans, such as black beans, chickpeas, pinto beans, or a combination
- 8 or 9 sprigs cilantro, chopped
- ½ teaspoon ground cumin
- ½ teaspoon chili powder
- ¼ teaspoon salt, or more as needed
- ¼ teaspoon ground black pepper, or to taste
- 1 cup shredded cheese, such as cheddar or mozzarella
- 1 avocado, diced, for garnish
- 2 Roma (plum) tomatoes, diced, for garnish

Preheat the oven to 375°F.

Make the enchilada sauce: Heat the olive oil in a medium pot over medium heat. Stir together the chili powder, oregano, cumin, garlic powder, and onion powder in a bowl. Add the spices to the hot oil all at once. Cook, stirring, for a few seconds to allow the spices to become fragrant and infuse the oil with flavor without burning.

Add the tomatoes, salt, and pepper. Bring to a boil. Reduce the heat to low, cover, and simmer for 10 minutes. Puree directly in the pot with an immersion blender. (If the sauce is not deep enough to fully immerse the blender and prevent splattering, carefully transfer the sauce to a deep bowl or jar to blend. Return to the pan after blending.) Simmer for 5 minutes more to slightly reduce the sauce. Taste and adjust the seasonings. Set aside. (This sauce can be made ahead and stored in an airtight container in the refrigerator for up to 2 weeks and reheated for quicker prep.)

Make the casserole: In a 9-inch square casserole dish, combine the quinoa, enchilada sauce, chile, beans, cilantro, cumin, chili powder, salt, pepper, and ¾ cup of the cheese. Adjust the seasonings. Sprinkle the remaining ¼ cup cheese evenly over the top.

Bake until bubbling and the cheese has melted, about 15 minutes. (See photo insert page 11.)

Serve immediately, garnished with the avocado and fresh tomato.

Calories: 478
Carbohydrate: 54 g
Protein: 20 g
Fat: 21 g

Variations

For Phase 1: Substitute 1 pound extra-firm tofu, drained, pressed with an absorbent towel, crumbled, and seasoned with ¾ teaspoon salt, or 2 cups cottage cheese for the quinoa.

Calories: 487
Carbohydrate: 38 g
Protein: 30 g
Fat: 25 g

Phase 1 Meal: Use the Phase 1 Variation, garnished with 2 tablespoons plain whole-milk Greek yogurt. **For Dessert:** 1 Chocolate Truffle (page 314).

Calories: 636; Carbohydrate: 28%; Protein: 23%; Fat: 49%

Phase 2 or 3 Meal: Serve with ½ serving Baked Tofu (page 175; Chimichurri Variation). **For Dessert:** 1 cup strawberries.

Calories: 668; Carbohydrate: 39%; Protein: 20%; Fat: 41%

Summer Squash Casserole (All Phases)

This is a cheese lover's delight! Hearty and delicious, this simple casserole can be eaten as is, or personalized with your favorite herbs, spices, or chiles.

Preparation time: 15 minutes

Total time: 55 minutes

Makes 4 servings

- 1 tablespoon butter or olive oil
- 3 cloves garlic, minced or pressed
- 1 large onion, halved and sliced into half-moons
- 4 large summer squash like zucchini or yellow squash, sliced into ¼-inch-thick rounds
- ½ teaspoon salt
- ¼ to ½ teaspoon ground black pepper

Creamy Cheese Sauce

- ½ cup half-and-half
- ½ cup heavy cream
- 2 eggs
- ⅓ cup grated Parmesan cheese
- 2 heaping tablespoons chickpea flour (see Tip, page 91)
- 1 teaspoon garlic powder
- ¼ teaspoon salt
- ¼ teaspoon ground black pepper, or to taste
- 1 cup shredded cheddar cheese

Preheat the oven to 350°F.

Melt the butter in a large skillet over medium heat. Add the garlic, onion, squash, salt, and pepper. Stir well, then cover and let the vegetables sweat for a few minutes. Uncover and cook, stirring, until the vegetables are soft and the liquid has mostly evaporated, about 15 minutes.

Meanwhile, make the creamy cheese sauce: Stir together the half-and-half, cream, eggs, Parmesan, chickpea flour, garlic powder, salt, and pepper in a medium bowl.

When squash is ready, add the cream sauce, stirring thoroughly and fairly quickly, as the mixture will start to thicken. Stir in ¾ cup of the cheddar cheese. Adjust the seasonings.

Transfer the mixture to a 9-inch square casserole dish or ovenproof skillet. Sprinkle the remaining ¼ cup cheddar evenly over the top.

Bake for 30 to 35 minutes, or until set and the cheese has browned lightly.

Calories: 429
Carbohydrate: 22 g
Protein: 18 g
Fat: 31 g

Variations

Substitute 1 large head cauliflower, cut into florets, boiled, and drained, for the squash.

Tofu Variation: Add 8 ounces tofu, crumbled and seasoned with ½ teaspoon salt, or 1 cup cottage cheese with the squash. Serve with berries and plain whole-milk Greek yogurt for a complete Phase 1 Meal.

Calories: 496
Carbohydrate: 23 g
Protein: 26 g
Fat: 34 g

For Phases 2 and 3: Use ¾ cup half-and-half and ¼ cup heavy cream.

Calories: 396
Carbohydrate: 22 g
Protein: 18 g
Fat: 27 g

Phase 1 Meal: Serve with 2 slices Smoke-Dried Tomato Seitan (page 73) or similar higher-protein, lower-fat side (see Equivalents Table, page 49), and a side of salad greens and chopped raw vegetables tossed with 1 to 2 teaspoons Greek Dressing (page 285). **For Dessert:** ½ cup blueberries.

Calories: 656; Carbohydrate: 26%; Protein: 22%; Fat: 52%

Phase 2 Meal: Use the Phases 2 and 3 Variation. Serve with 2 slices Smoke-Dried Tomato Seitan (73) or similar higher-protein, lower-fat side (see Equivalents Table, page 49), and 1 cup cooked broccoli with a squeeze of lemon juice. **For Dessert:** ½ apple, cored, sliced, and drizzled with ½ teaspoon honey.

Calories: 635; Carbohydrate: 34%; Protein: 24%; Fat: 42%

Phase 3 Meal: Use the Phases 2 and 3 Variation. Serve with 1 slice Smoke-Dried Tomato Seitan (page 73) or similar higher-protein, lower-fat side (see Equivalents Table, page 49), and 1½ cups cooked broccoli with a squeeze of lemon juice. **For Dessert:** 1 cup diced mango or other tropical fruit.

Calories: 670; Carbohydrate: 38%; Protein: 19%; Fat: 43%

Creamy Green Chile Casserole (All Phases)

Rich, creamy, and easy to make dairy-free! You can adjust this casserole to any level of spiciness by choosing milder or hotter peppers. The smoky flavor of the green chiles combined with the luscious texture of the casserole make this dish a year-round favorite.

Preparation time: 10 minutes

Total time: 1 hour

Makes 6 to 8 servings

- 1 or 2 large cloves garlic
- 1 large onion, cut into large chunks
- 1 medium leek, halved lengthwise, cut into large pieces, and rinsed well
- 2 medium carrots, cut into large chunks
- 1 tablespoon neutral-tasting oil, such as high-oleic safflower or avocado oil
- 2 pounds extra-firm tofu, drained, pressed with an absorbent towel, and crumbled
- 1 teaspoon salt
- 2 tablespoons water
- 1 recipe Green Chile Cream Sauce (page 305)
- 1 large zucchini, thinly sliced
- ½ cup shredded cheese, such as Monterey Jack or cheddar
- 8 ounces fresh spinach (about 4 cups packed)

Preheat the oven to 375°F.

Place the garlic, onion, leek, and carrots in a food processor. Pulse until finely minced. Set aside.

Heat the oil in a large skillet over medium heat. Add the tofu and salt. Cook, stirring regularly, for about 5 minutes. Stir in the water to help incorporate the salt into the tofu.

Add the minced vegetables to the pan and cook, stirring, for 5 minutes more, then cover and cook until the vegetables are tender but still bright in color, 2 to 3 minutes.

In a 9 x 13-inch casserole dish, layer 1 cup of the chile cream sauce, a thin layer of the zucchini, and then one-third of the tofu mixture. Repeat until all tofu and zucchini have been used, using about 2 cups sauce between the layers.

Top with the remaining sauce, then the cheese. Bake until the casserole is bubbling and the top is golden brown, 30 to 40 minutes.

Serve on top of a bed of spinach. The spinach will begin to wilt under the heat of the casserole. Serve immediately.

Based on 6 servings   Carbohydrate: 31 g   Fat: 25 g
Calories: 474   Protein: 32 g

Variations

Soy-free version: Substitute 4 cups cottage cheese for the tofu and layer in without cooking the cottage cheese.

Dairy-free version: Omit the cheese and use an unsweetened, nondairy milk for the Green Chile Cream Sauce (page 305).

For Phase 3: Reduce the cheese to ¼ cup. Add two or three layers of corn tortillas (about 12 tortillas) and increase the servings to 8 per casserole.

Based on 8 servings   Carbohydrate: 41 g   Fat: 19 g
Calories: 432   Protein: 25 g

Phase 1 Meal: Serve with a side of salad greens and chopped raw vegetables topped with a sliced hard-boiled egg, and 2 to 3 teaspoons of Greek Dressing (page 285). **For Dessert:** ½ cup berries and 1 tablespoon plain whole-milk Greek yogurt.

Calories: 674; Carbohydrate: 26%; Protein: 24%; Fat: 50%

Phase 2 Meal: Decrease the portion size to serve 8 instead of 6. Serve with ⅓ cup Mexican Rice (page 227), and a side of salad greens and chopped raw vegetables topped with a sliced hard-boiled egg, and 2 to 3 teaspoons Greek Dressing (page 285). **For Dessert:** ¾ cup berries and 1 tablespoon plain whole-milk Greek yogurt.

Calories: 687; Carbohydrate: 35%; Protein: 21%; Fat: 44%

Phase 3 Meal: Use the Phase 3 Variation. Serve with a side of salad greens and chopped raw vegetables topped with a sliced hard-boiled egg, and 2 to 3 teaspoons Greek Dressing (page 285). **For Dessert:** ½ cup berries and ½ cup diced mango or pineapple.

Calories: 667; Carbohydrate: 39%; Protein: 20%; Fat: 41%

Fennel Rutabaga Gratin (All Phases)

Rutabaga might not be the first vegetable you think of when planning dinner for your family, but their tender, creamy texture makes the perfect base for this gratin. You'll never even miss the potatoes. This casserole is even better the next day, once the flavors have had time to fully mingle—a real crowd-pleaser.

Preparation time: 15 minutes

Total time: 1¼ hours

Makes 6 to 8 servings

- 1 tablespoon extra-virgin olive oil
- 1 medium onion, diced
- 1 large clove garlic
- ¼ cup chickpea flour (see Tip, page 91)
- 1 to 1½ teaspoons salt, or more to taste
- ½ to 1 teaspoon ground black pepper, or to taste
- 2½ cups whole milk or unsweetened soy milk
- ½ cup heavy cream
- 1 medium rutabaga, thinly sliced
- 1 medium fennel bulb, thinly sliced, fennel fronds chopped and reserved for garnish
- 1 cup grated cheddar or other mild cheese

Preheat the oven to 350°F.

Heat the olive oil in a medium skillet over medium heat. Add the onion and garlic and cook, stirring, until translucent, 3 to 5 minutes.

Add the chickpea flour, salt, and pepper and stir until the flour has been absorbed by the oil. Cook, stirring until the mixture turns a light golden color, 5 to 7 minutes.

Combine the milk and cream. Add it to the skillet, whisking continuously until very smooth. Bring to a boil. Reduce the heat to low and simmer, stirring regularly, for 10 minutes to thicken the sauce. Remove from the heat.

Pour a small amount of the sauce into a 9-inch square baking dish to just cover the bottom. Add a layer of rutabaga, then a layer of fennel slices, and finally a layer of cheese. Repeat until all the ingredients have been used, ending with a layer of cheese. Do not overfill the casserole dish. Leave ½ inch of room to allow for bubbling and to prevent spilling over while baking.

Bake for 30 to 45 minutes or until the filling is bubbling and the cheese is melted. Remove from the heat.

Garnish with the fennel fronds and serve.

| Based on 6 servings | Carbohydrate: 19 g | Fat: 20 g |
| Calories: 285 | Protein: 10 g | |

Variations

Use thinly sliced cauliflower in place of the fennel and rutabaga.

Dairy-free version: Increase the olive oil to ⅓ cup, and use 3 cups unsweetened soy milk pureed with 8 ounces tofu and seasoned with ½ teaspoon salt in place of the milk, cream, and cheese.

| Based on 6 servings | Carbohydrate: 15 g | Fat: 17 g |
| Calories: 256 | Protein: 12 g | |

Phase 1 Meal: Serve with 1 cup Minestrone Soup (page 248), 2 or 3 slices Smoke-Dried Tomato Seitan (page 73) or Crispy Tofu Fries (page 173), or 2 to 3 ounces Deep-Fried Tempeh (page 170), 1 tablespoon Lemon Aioli (page 298) for dipping the protein, and Spicy Pickled Vegetables (page 68). **For Dessert:** ½ cup strawberries and 2 tablespoons plain whole-milk Greek yogurt.

Calories (Seitan): 680; Carbohydrate: 28%; Protein: 26%; Fat: 46%

Calories (Tempeh or tofu): 679; Carbohydrate: 26%; Protein: 19%; Fat: 55%

Phase 2 Meal: Serve with a bowl (2 cups) of Miso Soup (page 258), a side of salad greens and chopped raw vegetables tossed with 2 slices Smoke-Dried Tomato Seitan (page 73) or similar higher-protein, lower-fat meat substitute (see Equivalents Table, page 49), ¼ cup Cooked Quinoa (page 231), and 1 to 2 teaspoons Ginger Tahini Dressing (page 288). **For Dessert:** ½ cup blueberries topped with 1 heaping tablespoon plain whole-milk Greek yogurt.

Calories: 654; Carbohydrate: 36%; Protein: 25%; Fat: 39%

Phase 3 Meal: Serve with a bowl (2 cups) of Minestrone Soup (page 248; Phase 3 Variation), a side of salad greens and chopped raw vegetables tossed with 1 to 2 teaspoons Cashew Balsamic Dressing (page 286), and a few triangles (about 1 ounce) Deep-Fried Tempeh (page 170). **For Dessert:** ¼ cup blueberries topped with 1 tablespoon Cashew Crème (page 323).

Calories: 662; Carbohydrate: 43%; Protein: 17%; Fat: 40%

Mediterranean Quinoa (Phases 2 and 3)

Unlike other vegetarian proteins, seitan is a higher-protein, lower-fat choice for a meal. If you are not gluten-sensitive, it provides a versatile option to increase protein, allowing for a wider variety of higher-fat side dishes and desserts. Gluten-free variations are included on page 192.

Preparation time: 10 minutes

Total time: 35 minutes

Makes 4 servings

- 3 tablespoons olive oil
- 1 medium onion, diced
- 2 cloves garlic, minced
- ¼ teaspoon salt
- ¼ teaspoon ground black pepper
- 1 recipe Smoke-Dried Tomato Seitan (page 73), cut into small pieces
- 30 Kalamata olives, pitted and chopped
- 1 (14-ounce) can artichoke hearts, drained and cut into thin pieces
- 1 cup cooked chickpeas (see Do-It-Yourself Beans, page 74) or drained and rinsed canned chickpeas
- 1 large bunch kale, spinach, or other leafy greens (10 to 12 ounces), chopped (about 5 cups)
- 2 to 3 tablespoons water
- 2 cups Cooked Quinoa (page 231)
- 1 scallion, thinly sliced, for garnish

Heat the olive oil in a large skillet over medium heat. Add the onion, garlic, salt, and pepper and cook, stirring, until translucent, 3 to 5 minutes.

Add the seitan, olives, artichoke hearts, and chickpeas. Cook, stirring, for 5 to 10 minutes to allow the flavors to meld.

Add the kale and water. Cover and steam until the kale begins to wilt, 2 to 4 minutes. Stir in the quinoa. Cover and simmer for 2 to 3 minutes more.

Serve hot, garnished with the scallion.

Calories: 621
Carbohydrate: 59 g
Protein: 40 g
Fat: 26 g

Variations

Gluten-free version: In place of the Smoke-Dried Tomato Seitan, soak 4 or 5 sun-dried tomatoes (unsalted) in ½ cup warm water with ½ teaspoon smoked paprika and ½ to 1 teaspoon salt in a glass mason jar until reconstituted, about 30 minutes. Blend until smooth with an immersion blender. Transfer to a saucepan and add 1½ pounds diced tofu or chicken tenders. Cook over medium heat until the water has been absorbed and the protein is cooked through. Season with salt to taste.

For Phase 3: Use ¾ recipe Smoke-Dried Tomato Seitan (page 73). Substitute 8 ounces cooked whole wheat pasta for the quinoa.

Phase 2 Meal: Serve with ½ cup strawberries and 1 tablespoon Cardamom Whipped Cream (page 324) or Cashew Crème (page 323).

Calories: 669; Carbohydrate: 38%; Protein: 24%; Fat: 38%

Phase 3 Meal: Use the Phase 3 Variation. Serve with ½ cup diced pineapple and 1 tablespoon Cardamom Whipped Cream (page 324) or Cashew Crème (page 323).

Calories: 669; Carbohydrate: 40%; Protein: 23%; Fat: 37%

Crumbled Tempeh (All Phases)

This tempeh has a rich, meaty texture that substitutes well for ground meat in any of your favorite recipes. Make enough to use all week, and store it in the refrigerator to create a quick meal anytime.

Preparation time: 5 minutes

Total time: 25 minutes

Makes 4 servings

- 3 tablespoons extra-virgin olive oil
- 1 teaspoon salt
- 1 pound tempeh, minced or crumbled

Oven method: Preheat the oven to 350°F.

In a large bowl, stir together the oil, salt, and tempeh until well distributed. Transfer the tempeh to a 9 x 12-inch baking pan. Bake for 20 to 30 minutes, stirring regularly, until the tempeh is browned and crispy on all sides.

Stovetop method: Heat the oil in a large cast-iron or other heavy-bottomed skillet over medium heat. Add the salt and tempeh. Cook, stirring frequently and breaking up larger pieces into smaller crumbles with a spatula, until the tempeh is browned and fully cooked, about 20 minutes. Add water as needed to keep from burning or sticking. (See photo insert page 8.)

Calories: 279
Carbohydrate: 13 g

Protein: 22 g
Fat: 16 g

Panfried Tofu or Tempeh (All Phases)

This basic recipe provides an easy way to prepare tempeh or tofu for use in your favorite recipes. Serve it in place of any of the meats used in the meal plans. Make enough on Prep Day to last the whole week. It keeps well in the refrigerator in an airtight container.

Preparation time: 5 minutes

Total time: 20 minutes

Makes 4 servings

- 2 tablespoons extra-virgin olive oil
- 1 pound tempeh, cut lengthwise into ¼-inch-thick strips, or 14 to 16 ounces extra-firm tofu, drained, gently pressed with an absorbent towel, and cut into ¼-inch-thick strips
- 1 tablespoon soy sauce
- 3 tablespoons water
- ¼ teaspoon garlic powder

Heat the olive oil in a large cast-iron skillet or griddle over medium-high heat. Arrange the tempeh or tofu in a single layer in the skillet and cook until browned and crispy on the bottom, 5 to 7 minutes. Turn the strips over and cook on the second side until browned and crispy. Reduce the heat to low.

In a small bowl, combine the soy sauce, water, and garlic powder. Pour the sauce over the browned tempeh or tofu. For tempeh, cover and simmer for 3 minutes more on each side. For tofu, simmer, uncovered, for 1 minute or less on each side.

Serve immediately, or refrigerate for up to 10 days to use in other recipes. Reheat in a cast-iron skillet or in the toaster oven to restore the crispy texture. (See photo insert page 8.)

Calories: 169 (Tofu)
Carbohydrate: 2 g

Protein: 16 g
Fat: 13 g

Calories: 251 (Tempeh)   Protein: 22 g
Carbohydrate: 14 g   Fat: 13 g

Variations

Add fresh ginger or other herbs or spices to the sauce.

My *Always Delicious* Story

In January 2016, I had a very discouraging visit to my nurse practitioner. My weight was 230 pounds, my blood pressure was 148/88 and my HgA1c was 6.4 percent. Cholesterol numbers were all bad. The nurse practitioner told me that there was very little she could do to help me get healthy unless I took responsibility myself. So I dusted off my workout clothes and started the old-standard calorie-restriction diet. The gym workouts sucked and I only made progress by starving myself.

By May, I'd lost eighteen pounds and some of the labs showed a small improvement. But a trip to Las Vegas and the births of two grandchildren interrupted my workout routine and dieting. Every trip through a checkout line was an excuse for a candy bar or two. At my September checkup, my HgA1c was 6.5 percent, higher than ever.

Then a friend on Facebook told me about *Always Hungry?* The "science" of it made sense, and my wife was willing to join me, so we jumped into Phase 1 at the end of October. I started walking, too—as it turns out, there are miles of trails in the hills near our house. Now I'm up to five or six miles most mornings. My energy level has gone through the roof, a significant non-scale victory (NSV).

Today's visit to the nurse practitioner was amazing. Weight 192 pounds, blood pressure 115/70, and HgA1c 5.2 percent, a *huge* NSV! Cholesterol numbers are perfect. By the way, my wife's HgA1c dropped from 6.5 percent in November to 5.9 percent this January!!!

We're about 99 percent Phase 1, except for my wine. We weathered Thanksgiving, Christmas, and a family vacation in January without much difficulty. And luckily, the few times we fell off the wagon didn't trigger cravings for more of the same. *Always Hungry?* has been life-changing!

Gary M., age 65, Orcutt, California

CHAPTER 7

Chickpea Flour & Revisionist Foods

Although we recommend finding delicious dishes that don't require revision in order to meet your health needs, there are times you might want to use higher quality ingredients, such as grain-free flours, to re-create an old favorite. Our recipes have more balanced macronutrients than typical recipes using white flour or sugar, but will still satisfy your desire for familiar flavors. Take a moment to learn about the properties of a few of the grain-free flours we use.

Chickpea flour (also known as garbanzo bean flour, gram flour, or besan, and sometimes labeled that way at your grocery store) is versatile, producing a texture that can resemble wheat flour. Because it is gluten-free, the dough needs to be fairly thick to create a structure that will rise. Adding eggs, ground chia or flaxseeds (see Egg Substitutes, page 92), Greek yogurt, pureed vegetables like sweet potatoes, or other ingredients to thicken the batter will help produce the right structure. Depending on the recipe, baking powder, baking soda, carbonated water, or beaten egg whites might also be needed to form a lighter dough. Chickpea flour requires less oil and can be used as a binder or filler in recipes that call for flour.

Almond flour may also be substituted for wheat flour and works well in sweet recipes or as a filler or binder. Naturally higher in fat, almond flour also requires less oil than other flours. Its texture is less creamy than chickpea flour; combine them for a more neutral flavor in dessert crusts.

Coconut flour's distinct flavor works best in recipes that call for...coconut. The texture is less smooth and more gritty than other flours, and it absorbs much more liquid, complicating its use as a substitute. However, with some care, coconut flour can provide a delightful, light, fluffy texture in baking, especially when using eggs as a leavening agent.

Easy Chickpea Bread Crumbs (All Phases)

Readers regularly ask for bread crumb substitutes, and this one is the best. It can make so many recipes healthier and more satisfying. These bread crumbs store well in an airtight jar in the cupboard and can be used in a variety of recipes, from Meat Loaf (page 152) to Meatballs (page 149) and even as a panko breading substitute to fry fish or chicken.

Preparation time: 10 minutes plus overnight soaking

Total time: 40 minutes

Makes about 2¼ cups

- 1 cup dried chickpeas
- 1 teaspoon extra-virgin olive oil
- ¼ teaspoon salt

Sort through the chickpeas and remove any stones or grit. Rinse well. Place the chickpeas in a bowl and add enough water to cover by a few inches. Cover with a bamboo mat or a towel. Set aside at room temperature to soak overnight or for at least 8 hours.

Preheat the oven to 350°F. Line a baking sheet with parchment paper.

Drain the chickpeas well. Spread them on an absorbent towel and pat dry with another towel.

Place them in a food processor and pulse until you have a fine bread crumb or fine couscous consistency. You want finely ground crumbs, but you don't want a paste.

Toss the chickpea crumbs with the olive oil and salt, then spread on the prepared baking sheet.

Bake for 30 to 40 minutes, being sure to remove from the oven to check and stir every 5 to 10 minutes.

Remove from the heat or cook longer to reach a golden brown, dry bread crumb consistency. Sift out any large chunks or return the mixture to the food processor, and process until it reaches a small crumble consistency.

Make sure bread crumbs are dry and cooled. Store in an airtight container in the cupboard for up to 3 months.

Calories: 22 (Per 1 tablespoon)   Protein: 1 g
Carbohydrate: 4 g   Fat: 1 g

Variations

Use 2 to 2½ cups canned chickpeas in place of dry chickpeas. Drain, rinse, and pat dry with a towel. Toss chickpeas with salt and oil. Spread the whole chickpeas on a parchment paper–lined baking sheet and bake for 20 minutes, stirring once, then let cool and process in the food processor as described above. Return the crumbs to the baking sheet and bake for 5 to 8 minutes more, or until they reach a golden brown, dry bread crumb consistency.

Add herbs or spices with the oil and salt to create seasoned bread crumbs for your favorite recipes.

Socca Crepes (All Phases)

Sparkling water creates a light, lacy crepe that doesn't even need baking powder. Fill with savory or sweet fillings and serve as a main dish, snack, or dessert.

Preparation time: 5 minutes

Total time: 35 to 40 minutes

Makes 4 to 6 servings (6 crepes)

- 1 cup chickpea flour (see Tip, page 91)
- 1 cup sparkling water
- 1 tablespoon extra-virgin olive oil, plus more for the pan
- 1 egg
- ¼ teaspoon salt

Place all the ingredients in a wide-mouthed glass mason jar or cup that will fit an immersion blender without splashing. Blend until smooth. Use right away so that the sparkling water brings a lighter texture to the crepe.

Heat a 10- to 12-inch cast-iron skillet over medium-high heat. Brush ¼ to ½ teaspoon of the oil onto the hot skillet and adjust the heat as necessary—the pan should be hot, but the oil should not smoke.

Pour about ⅓ cup of the batter onto the hot oiled skillet, tilting the pan in a circular motion as you pour so the batter coats the surface evenly.

Cook until the edges brown and lift easily from the skillet, about 3 minutes. Turn and brown on the other side, 2 to 3 minutes. Remove from the heat and use immediately or refrigerate and reheat to soften before using.

Fill with your favorite sweet or savory ingredients as desired.

Tip: This batter is best used right away. The sparkling water will become flat if stored for too long.

Based on 4 servings   Carbohydrate: 14 g   Fat: 6 g
Calories: 137   Protein: 7 g

Variations

Get creative with adding herbs and spices to the batter to make a more flavorful savory or sweet crepe.

Vegan version: Omit the egg and increase the oil to 2 tablespoons.

Based on 4 servings   Carbohydrate: 13 g   Fat: 9 g
Calories: 149   Protein: 5 g

Basic Socca Wrap (All Phases)

These wraps are a go-to favorite in the Ludwig home. Keeping a jar of batter in the refrigerator means you can make a wrap anytime for a quick snack or picnic lunch. Use in place of tortillas or wheat-based sandwich wraps.

Preparation time: 5 minutes

Total time: 30 minutes

Makes 4 to 6 servings (6 wraps)

- 1 cup chickpea flour (see Tip, page 91)
- ¼ teaspoon baking powder (optional)
- 1 cup water
- 2 tablespoons extra-virgin olive oil, plus more for the pan
- ¼ teaspoon salt

Place all the ingredients in a wide-mouthed glass jar or cup that will fit an immersion blender without splashing. Blend until smooth. Cover the jar and refrigerate until ready to use, up to 1 week.

Heat a 10- to 12-inch cast-iron skillet over medium to medium-high heat. Brush ¼ to ½ teaspoon of the oil onto the skillet.

Pour ¼ to ⅓ cup of the batter onto the hot skillet, tilting the pan in a circular motion as you pour so the batter coats the surface evenly.

Cook until the edges brown and lift easily from the skillet, about 3 minutes. Turn and brown on the other side, 2 to 3 minutes. Remove from the heat and use immediately, or refrigerate and reheat to soften before using.

Fill as desired to make a lunch or breakfast wrap.

Based on 6 servings	Carbohydrate: 9 g	Fat: 6 g
Calories: 100	Protein: 3 g	

Variations

Add an egg for a heartier batter.

For Phase 3: Substitute buckwheat flour for half of the chickpea flour.

Shredded Chicken Quesadilla (All Phases)

Eating quesadillas is now a reality in Phases 1 and 2! This quick-and-easy Latin-style sandwich makes a great grab-and-go lunch, snack, or even breakfast. Get creative with different fillings to please all the tastes and food preferences in your family.

Preparation time: 5 minutes

Total time: 15 minutes

Makes 2 servings

- 2 Basic Socca Wraps (page 198)
- 3 tablespoons shredded cheddar cheese
- ¾ cup Shredded Chicken (page 110)
- 2 tablespoons Fresh Salsa (page 302)
- ⅓ cup Refried Beans (page 225)
- 1 tablespoon sour cream or Dairy-Free Sour Cream (page 306)
- ¼ avocado, sliced

Heat a cast-iron skillet or griddle over medium-high heat. Warm one Socca Wrap on one side for about 15 seconds, then flip. Reduce the heat to medium. Sprinkle half the cheese evenly over the warm wrap. Layer on the chicken, salsa, and remaining cheese, evenly distributing them over the wrap.

Spread the beans evenly over one side of the second Socca Wrap. Place it bean-side down on top of the fillings in the first wrap. Flip the entire quesadilla using a large spatula and cook on the other side until lightly browned, 1 to 2 minutes.

Carefully remove from skillet and place on a large cutting board to cool, 2 to 3 minutes.

Cut into 6 wedges, and garnish with sour cream and avocado before serving.

Calories: 397	Protein: 31 g
Carbohydrate: 24 g	Fat: 20 g

Variations

Vegetarian version: Substitute ⅔ cup Crumbled Tempeh (page 192) or other vegetarian protein for the chicken, substitute 3 tablespoons plain whole-milk Greek yogurt for the sour cream, and omit the avocado to accommodate the higher fat and lower protein content of the tempeh.

Phase 1 Meal: For Dessert: 2 Chocolate Truffles (page 314).

Calories: 499; Carbohydrate: 25%; Protein: 26%; Fat: 49%

Phase 2 Meal: Serve with Mexican Rice (page 227). **For Dessert:** ½ cup strawberries.

Calories: 535; Carbohydrate: 38%; Protein: 25%; Fat: 37%

Phase 3 Meal: Substitute two 10-inch whole wheat tortillas for the socca wraps. Reduce the chicken to ½ cup. **For Dessert:** 1 Chocolate Truffle (page 314).

Calories: 567; Carbohydrate: 40%; Protein: 20%; Fat: 40%

Chickpea Cheddar Crisps (All Phases)

Rich and crisp: Your quest for a delicious, grain-free cracker has ended! Serve as an appetizer or snack with your favorite dips or spreads.

Preparation time: 15 minutes

Total time: 35 minutes

Makes 6 servings (24 crisps)

- 1 cup shredded sharp cheddar cheese, at room temperature
- 4 tablespoons (½ stick) salted butter, very well softened
- ½ cup chickpea flour (see Tip, page 91)

- ½ teaspoon baking powder
- ½ teaspoon salt
- ½ teaspoon garlic powder
- ¼ teaspoon cayenne pepper or other herbs or spices, or to taste

In a large bowl using an immersion blender, cream together the cheese and butter, pulsing with the blender until almost smooth and stopping to scrape down the sides of the bowl frequently.

In a separate bowl, combine the chickpea flour, baking powder, salt, garlic powder, and cayenne and mix well.

Add the flour mixture to the butter mixture, blending with a spatula until a crumbly dough forms, then quickly knead by hand until the dough is smooth.

Form the dough into a log about 2 inches wide. Wrap in plastic wrap and refrigerate for at least 1 hour or up to 3 hours or freeze until ready to use for up to 1 month.

Preheat the oven to 350°F.

Unwrap the dough and slice it crosswise into discs about ¼ inch thick (no need to thaw frozen dough before cutting). Arrange them on a baking sheet in a single layer. Bake for 20 to 25 minutes, or until lightly golden and crisp.

Store in an airtight container in the cupboard for up to 2 weeks.

Calories: 172	Protein: 7 g
Carbohydrate: 5 g	Fat: 14 g

Socca Cracker (All Phases)

The Italians call it *socca* or *farinata* and have been making it for decades. Crunchy and satisfying, this traditional, crispy European flatbread can be used with your favorite dips, spreads, or pâtés. Best made fresh, or used the same day, the batter can be stored in the refrigerator for a week and used any time you need a quick and easy cracker.

Preparation time: 5 minutes

Total time: 15 minutes

Makes 4 servings (about 4 large crackers)

- 1 cup chickpea flour (see Tip, page 91)
- 1 cup warm water
- ½ teaspoon salt
- ⅛ teaspoon ground black pepper, or to taste
- 1 to 2 teaspoons extra-virgin olive oil, plus more for the pan
- Fresh or dried herbs or spices, such as garlic powder, thyme, rosemary, basil, or oregano

Preheat the oven to broil.

Place all the ingredients in a wide-mouthed glass jar or cup that will fit an immersion blender without splashing. Blend until smooth. Cover the jar and refrigerate until ready to use, up to 1 week.

Heat a 12-inch cast-iron skillet over medium to medium-high heat. Brush a small amount of oil onto the skillet. Pour ⅓ to ½ cup of the batter (about ¼ of the total batter) onto the hot oiled skillet, tilting the pan in a circular motion so the batter coats the surface evenly.

Place under the broiler and cook until the cracker browns on top and lifts easily from the skillet, 3 to 5 minutes. Flip the cracker and broil on the other side until browned and crispy.

Remove from the heat and serve immediately, or place in an airtight container and reheat to a crispy texture under the broiler before serving. Repeat to make 4 crackers.

Calories: 104
Carbohydrate: 13 g
Protein: 5 g
Fat: 3 g

Rosemary Biscuits (All Phases)

These fluffy, lightly seasoned biscuits make the perfect base for our Breakfast Stacks (page 88) and are also delicious eaten as a side with soups, salads, or entrées. The combination of oil and Greek yogurt creates a light biscuit that's still dense enough to hold toppings.

Preparation time: 5 minutes

Total time: 15 minutes

Makes 4 servings

- 1 cup chickpea flour (see Tip, page 91)
- 1½ teaspoons baking powder
- ⅛ teaspoon garlic powder
- ⅛ teaspoon dried thyme
- ¼ teaspoon dried rosemary, or 1 teaspoon chopped fresh rosemary
- ⅛ teaspoon salt
- 2 tablespoons neutral-tasting oil, such as high-oleic safflower or avocado oil
- ⅓ cup plain whole-milk Greek yogurt
- Olive oil or olive oil spray, for the pan

Preheat the oven to 450°F.

Combine the chickpea flour, baking powder, garlic powder, thyme, rosemary, and salt in a large bowl. Mix the oil into the flour mixture until the oil is completely incorporated. Stir in the yogurt to form a thick, sticky dough. Set aside.

Heat a small cast-iron or other ovenproof skillet over medium heat, and brush or spray with olive oil. Remove from the heat once it is hot.

Divide the dough into four equal parts, scooping each part into the hot skillet to form a biscuit shape without overworking the dough. Space the biscuits evenly in the skillet. It is okay if the biscuits touch one another and/or touch the edges of the pan. This will help them keep their structure as they rise.

Place in the oven and bake for 8 to 10 minutes, or until golden brown. The biscuits will easily slide out of the pan with a spatula. Use immediately, or store in the refrigerator in an airtight container for up to 1 week. Reheat in the oven or toaster oven before serving.

Calories: 174
Carbohydrate: 15 g
Protein: 7 g
Fat: 10 g

Chile Cheese Fritters (All Phases)

This recipe was developed after we ran out of time in the middle of making stuffed chiles. We just mixed everything together. Fortunately, the fritters ended up being far easier and even more delicious than the original version. These also freeze well to reheat for a quick snack or side dish on a busy day.

Preparation time: 5 minutes

Total time: 30 minutes

Makes 6 servings

- 1 egg
- 1½ cups sparkling water or beer
- 1 teaspoon salt
- 2¼ cups chickpea flour (see Tip, page 91)
- 6 ounces sharp cheddar cheese, shredded
- 6 ounces New Mexican green chiles or other chiles of your choice, roasted, peeled, and chopped (or canned green chiles), or more to taste
- ¼ cup neutral-tasting oil, such as high-oleic safflower or avocado oil
- ½ cup Fresh Salsa (page 302)

Beat the egg with the sparkling water and salt in a large bowl. Add the chickpea flour and blend with a whisk or immersion blender until smooth. Stir in the cheese and chiles.

Heat the oil in a large cast-iron skillet over medium heat. Drop 2 tablespoons of the batter at a time to form mini fritters, or 3 tablespoons at a time for larger fritters, into the hot oil. Cook until browned on the bottom, then flip and cook until browned on the other side, 3 to 5 minutes per side. Remove with a spatula and transfer to a baking sheet. Keep warm in a 200°F oven until ready to serve. Repeat with the remaining batter.

Garnish the fritters with salsa and serve.

Calories: 359   Protein: 16 g
Carbohydrate: 25 g   Fat: 22 g

Variations

Add 1½ pounds cooked protein to the batter when you add the cheese and chiles. For example, add cooked ground beef, Shredded Chicken (page 110), or Crumbled Tempeh (page 192).

Phase 1 Meal: Serve with a heaping ⅓ cup Shredded Chicken (page 110) or 3 to 4 ounces of your favorite vegetarian protein and a side of salad greens and chopped raw vegetables tossed with 1 to 2 teaspoons Lime Cilantro Pesto (page 298). **For Dessert:** 1 cup strawberries topped with 1 heaping tablespoon Cardamom Whipped Cream (page 324).

Calories: 606; Carbohydrate: 26%; Protein: 26%; Fat: 48%

Phase 2 Meal: Serve with ⅓ cup Shredded Chicken (page 110) or 3 to 4 ounces of your favorite vegetarian protein and ⅓ cup Mexican Rice (page 227). **For Dessert:** 1 cup strawberries.

Calories: 622; Carbohydrate: 35%; Protein: 24%; Fat: 41%

Phase 3 Meal: Serve with a bowl (1¼ cups) of Cuban Black Bean Soup (page 253). **For Dessert:** ½ to 1 cup strawberries.

Calories: 620; Carbohydrate: 44%; Protein: 18%; Fat: 38%

Cornbread (Phase 3)

The cast-iron skillet creates a crisp bottom crust and an unbeatable "fresh from the griddle" flavor. Crisp edges give way to a tender, fluffy center in this remarkable, gluten-free version of traditional cornbread.

Preparation time: 10 minutes

Total time: 30 minutes

Makes 6 to 8 servings

- 1 cup chickpea flour (see Tip, page 91)
- ¾ cup stone-ground cornmeal
- 1 tablespoon baking powder
- ½ teaspoon salt
- 1 cup whole milk or unsweetened soy milk
- 2 eggs, beaten
- 1 teaspoon pure maple syrup
- 2 tablespoons plus 1 teaspoon extra-virgin olive oil

Preheat the oven to 400°F.

Combine the chickpea flour, cornmeal, baking powder, and salt in a large bowl.

In a separate medium bowl, combine the milk, eggs, maple syrup, and 2 tablespoons of the olive oil.

Stir the wet ingredients into the dry ingredients until well combined.

Heat a cast-iron skillet over medium heat. Brush the skillet with the remaining 1 teaspoon oil. Pour the batter into the pan, transfer to the oven, and bake for 15 to 20 minutes, or until the top is golden brown. Remove from the oven and set aside to cool for 2 to 3 minutes. Slide the cornbread out of the skillet using a spatula to loosen the bottom crust from the pan. Cut into slices and serve warm, or cool and store in an airtight container in the refrigerator for up to a week. Reheat in a toaster oven to serve.

Based on 6 servings   Carbohydrate: 26 g   Fat: 9 g
Calories: 216   Protein: 8 g

Variation

Egg-free version: In place of the eggs, use 8 ounces extra-firm tofu, drained and pressed with an absorbent towel. Using an immersion blender, blend the tofu with the other wet ingredients until smooth. Increase the salt to ¾ teaspoon.

Grain-Free Piecrust (All Phases)

This simple, gluten-free crust adds a surprisingly delightful flavor to any sweet or savory pie. A little flakiness, a little crumbliness, and just the right level of saltiness make for a perfect, mild crust.

Preparation time: 10 minutes

Total time: 15 to 30 minutes

Makes 6 to 12 servings (12 muffin-sized crusts or one 9-inch single piecrust)

- 1½ cups chickpea flour (see Tip, page 91)
- ¼ cup neutral-tasting oil, such as high-oleic safflower or avocado oil
- ⅛ teaspoon salt
- 2 to 4 tablespoons whole milk or unsweetened soy milk, or more as needed

Preheat the oven to 375°F.

Mix the chickpea flour, oil, and salt in a medium bowl until crumbly and fully incorporated. Add the milk 1 tablespoon at a time until the dough holds together in a ball and becomes smooth and pliable without being wet and sticky.

To use for a pie or quiche, form the dough into a ball. Roll the ball between two pieces of parchment paper and press the dough into a 9-inch pie plate or a 10-inch quiche pan. Press any cracks closed.

To use for muffin tin crusts, roll the dough into a log and cut it crosswise into 12 equal discs. Roll out each disc individually between two sheets of parchment paper and press the discs into the wells of a muffin tin. Press any cracks closed.

If the filling will be watery, prick the bottom of the crust(s) with a fork and prebake for 5 minutes.

Fill and bake according to the recipe instructions.

Tip: There is no harm in overmixing or overkneading this dough because it is gluten-free. The dough does not need to be refrigerated or set aside before using. Refrigerating will dry the dough and make it harder to use. If it is too crumbly, add a bit of milk a little at a time while kneading until it is smooth but not sticky.

| Based on 6 servings | Carbohydrate: 14 g | Fat: 11 g |
| Calories: 175 | Protein: 5 g | |

Variations

Substitute almond flour for half the chickpea flour and reduce the oil to 3 tablespoons.

Add 1 to 2 teaspoons pure maple syrup for a Phase 2 or 3 sweet pie.

For Phase 3: Use whole wheat or spelt flour and increase the oil to ⅓ cup.

| Based on 6 servings | Carbohydrate: 32 g | Fat: 13 g |
| Calories: 277 | Protein: 7 g | |

Grain-Free Pizza (All Phases)

Pizza night can now be a guilt-free part of your healthy lifestyle! We've given you examples of our favorite topping combinations, but this recipe lets everyone at the dinner table choose their favorites.

Preparation time: 20 minutes

Total time: 40 minutes

Makes 6 servings

Socca Pizza Crust

- ¾ cup whole milk or unsweetened soy milk
- ½ teaspoon salt
- ⅛ teaspoon ground black pepper, or to taste
- 1 clove garlic
- ¼ teaspoon dried oregano
- ¼ teaspoon dried basil, or 1 teaspoon chopped fresh basil
- 3 tablespoons extra-virgin olive oil
- 1 cup chickpea flour (see Tip, page 91)
- ½ cup packed coarsely grated zucchini (about ½ medium)

Easy Pizza Sauce

- 1 (6-ounce) can tomato paste
- ½ teaspoon Italian seasoning
- ½ teaspoon salt
- ¼ teaspoon ground black pepper

Toppings

- 2 cups packed chopped kale leaves or other leafy greens
- ½ recipe Sautéed Mushrooms (page 216)
- ¾ to 1 pound cooked protein, such as rotisserie chicken, Shredded Chicken (page 110), Shredded Beef (page 148), Crumbled Tempeh (page 192), or several slices of pepperoni
- 8 ounces mozzarella cheese, shredded

Preheat the oven to 400°F. Bring a small pot of water to a boil.

Make the crust: Combine the milk, salt, pepper, garlic, oregano, basil, and 2 tablespoons of the oil in a deep cup or mixing bowl and blend using an immersion blender until the garlic is minced. Add the chickpea flour and blend until no lumps remain. (The batter can be made ahead and stored in the refrigerator for up to 1 week and used as needed to make fresh crusts throughout the week.) Stir in the zucchini.

Heat a 12-inch cast-iron skillet over medium heat. Brush the skillet with ½ tablespoon of the oil (or use the remaining 1 tablespoon oil if using a large griddle for mini crusts). Spread 1 to 1¼ cups (about half) of the batter into the hot oiled skillet. (Alternatively, use about ¼ to ⅓ cup of the batter to make 5-inch round mini pizza crusts. These small crusts are easier to flip and store after cooking. Make several of these on a large griddle.)

Cook until well browned and crispy on the bottom, 8 to 10 minutes. Flip the crust(s) and cook until well browned and crispy on the other side. Remove from the heat and set aside. Repeat with the remaining batter to make a second crust (or additional smaller crusts).

For a crispier texture, place the cooked crust in the hot oven directly on the oven rack for 5 to 10 minutes while cooking the second crust. Repeat with the second crust.

Make the sauce: Combine the tomato paste, Italian seasoning, salt, and pepper in a small bowl until well mixed. Set aside.

Assemble the pizzas: Place kale leaves in the boiling water ½ to 1 cup at a time and blanch for about 45 seconds, or a shorter time for less hearty greens like spinach or arugula. Remove the leaves with a mesh strainer or slotted spoon and spread onto a plate covered with a bamboo sushi mat to cool and drain. Repeat with the remaining greens.

Spread the sauce evenly over the crusts. Layer the mushrooms, kale, and protein evenly over the crusts. Top evenly with the cheese.

Place the pizzas on a baking sheet and bake for 5 minutes, or until the cheese is melted. For crispy, browned cheese, switch the oven to broil and broil for up to 1 minute at the end to reach the desired texture.

Calories: 429
Carbohydrate: 20 g
Protein: 34 g
Fat: 24 g

Phase 1 Meal: For Dessert: ½ cup blueberries and 1 Chocolate Truffle (page 314).

Calories: 574; Carbohydrate: 26%; Protein: 25%; Fat: 49%

Phase 2 Meal: Serve with Fresh Quinoa Salad with Pomegranates (page 262).
For Dessert: ¾ cup blueberries.

Calories: 572; Carbohydrate: 35%; Protein: 25%; Fat: 40%

Phase 3 Meal: Substitute whole wheat, thin-crust pizza crust for the Socca Crust. Use ¾ pound protein. **For Dessert:** ½ cup blueberries and 1 Chocolate Truffle (page 314).

Calories: 588; Carbohydrate: 41%; Protein: 22%; Fat: 37%

My *Always Delicious* Story

I've had type 1 diabetes since early adulthood and learned how to achieve tight control on an insulin pump. But my last blood test was astounding—my hemoglobin A1c was 4.6 percent!!! I didn't even know "normal" (nondiabetic) values went that low! At first my doctor was *sure* that I'd had a ton of low blood sugars to get that number. But I have the kind of pump my doctor can plug in to look back at months of results. And he had to admit that there were few highs or lows, just mostly a continuous state between 80 and 120. Beyond cutting back on processed carbs, I think the most important thing about the *Always Hungry?* program is that it helped me listen to my body and respond flexibly to my needs.

—*Peggy A., age 51, Salt Lake City, Utah*

CHAPTER 8

Side Dishes

VEGETABLES

Cauliflower Couscous (All Phases)

Riced cauliflower has become a popular grain substitute—however, true rice lovers might find the texture lacking. Recently, while tasting George Brown College culinary team recipes, we sampled a variation that really hit the mark. Samantha Jimenez and Tisha Riman used a more finely blended cauliflower, and the result was magic. Their Cauliflower Couscous has just the right texture to mimic the light fluffiness of couscous without all the processed carbs.

Preparation time: 5 minutes

Total time: 10 minutes

Makes 4 servings (4 to 5 cups)

- 1 medium (1- to 1½-pound) cauliflower, cut into large chunks
- 1 teaspoon olive oil
- 1 clove garlic, or more to taste, minced
- ¼ teaspoon salt
- ¼ teaspoon ground black pepper
- 2 tablespoons water

Place the cauliflower in a food processor and pulse until broken down to the texture of couscous.

Heat the olive oil in a large skillet over medium heat. Add the cauliflower, garlic, salt, pepper, and water. Cook, stirring, for 3 to 4 minutes, or until cauliflower is just tender without being mushy.

Serve warm. (See photo insert page 7.)

Calories: 47   Protein: 3 g
Carbohydrate: 7 g   Fat: 2 g

Zucchini with Garlic and Greens (All Phases)

Sautéed zucchini soaks up and holds any flavors you add, making each bite a delicious, juicy burst. We've paired it with garlic for richness and greens for structure, creating a dish to keep in the regular rotation. A Ludwig family favorite.

Preparation time: 5 minutes

Total time: 10 minutes

Makes 4 servings

- 1 tablespoon extra-virgin olive oil
- 1 large clove garlic
- 1 large zucchini, cut into ½-inch-thick half-moons
- ¼ teaspoon salt
- 1 small bunch greens, such as chard, kale, collards, mustard greens, spinach, or broccoli rabe (about 6 ounces), coarsely chopped (3 to 4 packed cups) (see Tip, page 137)

Heat the olive oil in a skillet over medium heat.

Add the garlic, zucchini, and salt. Cook, stirring, until the zucchini begins to soften, about 3 minutes.

Stir in the chopped greens. Cover and cook until the greens begin to wilt, about 1 minute. Alternate stirring and covering until the greens are wilted but still bright in color.

Remove from the skillet and serve hot.

Calories: 56   Protein: 2 g
Carbohydrate: 5 g   Fat: 4 g

Sautéed Bok Choy and Shiitake (All Phases)

Savory bok choy with shiitake is a common side dish in Asian cuisine, and it's easy to make at home. Mirin, Japanese cooking wine, adds an unmistakable depth of flavor. Serve with any of your favorite Asian meals.

Preparation time: 5 minutes

Total time: 15 minutes

Makes 4 servings

- 1 teaspoon toasted sesame oil
- 1 large clove garlic, minced
- 6 ounces fresh shiitake mushrooms, sliced (2 to 3 cups)
- 2 medium baby bok choy (about ½ pound), coarsely chopped
- 1 tablespoon mirin, or 2 tablespoons sake
- 1 to 2 teaspoons soy sauce

Heat the sesame oil in a deep skillet over medium heat.

Stir in the garlic and mushrooms. Cook, stirring, until the mushrooms are soft, about 5 minutes.

Stir in the bok choy, mirin, and soy sauce. Cover and simmer for a few minutes or until the bok choy is tender-crisp and still bright in color.

Transfer to a serving platter and serve warm. (See photo insert page 4.)

Calories: 60
Carbohydrate: 10 g
Protein: 4 g
Fat: 2 g

Herb Roasted Root Vegetables (All Phases)

Hearty and warming, these Phase 1 root vegetables make a great winter side dish. Get creative with different combinations and find your favorites. For Phase 2, include starchy vegetables like beets, sweet potato, or winter squash in the mix. Add your favorite marinated protein and cook on a large, rimmed baking sheet to create the perfect all-in-one sheet pan dinner.

Preparation time: 10 minutes

Total time: 55 minutes

Makes 4 servings

- 4 cups large chunks root vegetables, such as onion, carrot, rutabaga, parsnip, celeriac, kohlrabi, etc.
- 1 to 2 tablespoons extra-virgin olive oil
- ¼ teaspoon salt
- Leaves from 1 (3-inch) fresh rosemary sprig or other herbs of your choice, chopped
- 1 large clove garlic, minced or pressed

Preheat the oven to 425°F.

Toss the vegetables with the oil, salt, herbs, and garlic in a large bowl or 9 x 13-inch baking dish. Spread the vegetables evenly in the baking dish.

Roast for 30 to 45 minutes, stirring regularly, until the vegetables are tender in the center and slightly crisp or caramelized on the outside.

Calories: 113   Protein: 2 g
Carbohydrate: 16 g   Fat: 5 g

Summer Grilled or Roasted Vegetables (All Phases)

Fresh summer vegetables, juicy from the grill, make the perfect side dish for any protein. Season with any of your favorite dressings to make prep time a breeze. Whether you grill them outside, use a stovetop grill pan, or roast them in the oven, these veggies will enhance any summer meal or party. Cut vegetables in sizes that will cook at the same time; for example, eggplant can be cut smaller or thinner because it takes longer to cook, whereas broccoli and cauliflower can be left in larger florets.

Preparation time: 10 minutes

Total time: 35 minutes

Makes 4 to 6 servings

- 6 cups sliced or cubed summer vegetables, such as zucchini, cauliflower, bell peppers (any color), broccoli, eggplant, onions, asparagus, mushrooms, etc.
- ¼ to ⅓ cup Creamy Peppercorn Vinaigrette (page 286), Greek Dressing (page 285), or other dressing of your choice

Preheat the oven to 400°F.

Toss the vegetables with the vinaigrette in a large bowl.

Spread the vegetables evenly in a 9 by 13-inch baking dish or over a large baking sheet. Roast, stirring or turning every 10 to 15 minutes, until vegetables are tender, 20 to 30 minutes total, depending on the vegetables.

Alternatively, heat an outdoor grill to medium or a stovetop grill pan over medium heat.

Transfer the vegetables to a stainless-steel grilling tray or mesh grill basket, or onto the hot grill pan. Grill, stirring or tossing regularly, until the vegetables are tender.

Based on 4 servings	Carbohydrate: 12 g	Fat: 10 g
Calories: 144	Protein: 3 g	

Variations

Use Basil Walnut Pesto (page 297), Lime Cilantro Pesto (page 298), or Chimichurri (page 300) in place of the vinaigrette.

Add your favorite marinated quick cooking protein like shrimp or small cubes of marinated chicken or tofu and cook on a large, rimmed baking sheet to create the perfect all-in-one sheet pan dinner.

Sautéed Mushrooms (All Phases)

One of our most versatile recipes, this simple dish can be served as a topping on steak, pork chops, or any grilled meats. Enhance whole grains like Millet Mashed Fauxtatoes (page 236), brown rice, or Cooked Quinoa (page 231). Use them to top pizzas or as filling in crepes or wraps.

Preparation time: 5 minutes

Total time: 20 minutes

Makes 4 servings

- 2 tablespoons extra-virgin olive oil
- 1 large clove garlic
- 16 ounces baby bella/cremini mushrooms, sliced
- ¼ teaspoon salt

Heat the olive oil in a large skillet over medium heat. Add the garlic and cook, stirring, to infuse the oil, about 1 minute.

Add the mushrooms and salt. Cook, stirring regularly, until the mushrooms are soft and all the liquid has been absorbed, 10 to 15 minutes.

These are delicious made ahead and will keep in an airtight container in the refrigerator for up to 1 week.

Calories: 86   Protein: 3 g
Carbohydrate: 5 g   Fat: 7 g

Variation

Use less oil or 2 tablespoons water to sauté if serving with a higher-fat meat or meal.

Seasoned Shiitake Mushrooms (All Phases)

We're talking umami—that rich, savory flavor now considered the fifth basic taste. Use these as filling for wraps, as additions to stir-fries, or as toppings for meats, whole grains, or Buddha Bowls (see pages 263 to 269).

Preparation time: 5 minutes

Total time: 20 minutes

Makes 4 servings

- 1 tablespoon neutral-tasting oil, such as high-oleic safflower or avocado oil
- 16 ounces fresh shiitake mushrooms, cut into ¼-inch pieces (5 to 6 cups)
- 2 tablespoons sake, or 1 tablespoon mirin
- 2 tablespoons soy sauce

Heat the oil in a large skillet over medium heat. Add the mushrooms and cook, stirring, for 2 to 3 minutes, until the mushrooms begin to soften.

Add the sake and soy sauce. Cook, stirring regularly, until all the liquid has been absorbed and reduced to a thick coating, 10 to 15 minutes.

Calories: 77
Carbohydrate: 8 g
Protein: 3 g
Fat: 4 g

Braised Cabbage with Apples (Phases 2 and 3)

Sweet, tart, and melt-in-your-mouth delicious. The soft texture of cabbage, tanginess of the balsamic, and sweetness of the apples with cinnamon make this a dish you won't want to miss. Serve with a higher-protein/moderate-fat main dish (see Equivalents Table, page 49).

Preparation time: 10 minutes

Total time: 35 minutes

Makes 4 servings

- 2 tablespoons extra-virgin olive oil
- 2 tablespoons butter or extra-virgin olive oil
- 1 medium red onion, halved and thinly sliced into half-moons
- ½ teaspoon salt
- 1 medium head cabbage, shredded (about 6 cups)
- ⅔ cup white balsamic vinegar
- ½ teaspoon ground black pepper
- 1 teaspoon ground cinnamon
- 1 large apple, unpeeled, halved, cored, and thinly sliced

Heat the olive oil in a large pot or Dutch oven over medium heat, then add the butter (to keep butter from burning) and let melt.

Add the onion and a pinch of the salt. Cook, stirring, until the onion starts to soften, about 3 minutes. Add the cabbage in handfuls, and stir to coat with the oil and butter. Cover and allow cabbage to wilt for 1 to 2 minutes.

Stir in the vinegar, remaining salt, and the pepper. Reduce the heat to low, cover, and cook, stirring regularly, until cabbage is wilted and soft, 15 to 18 minutes.

Stir in the cinnamon and apple. Cook, covered, until the apple is soft, 3 to 5 minutes.

Calories: 245   Protein: 3 g
Carbohydrate: 33 g   Fat: 13 g

Butternut Sage Puree (Phases 2 and 3)

Sage isn't just for the holidays anymore. This delicate puree is simple to make and sure to please. Serve it as a flavorful complement to higher-fat meals.

Preparation time: 5 minutes

Total time: 15 minutes

Makes 4 servings

- 2 cups peeled butternut squash wedges
- ⅛ teaspoon salt
- 4 or 5 large (3-inch) fresh sage leaves, or more to taste
- 1 teaspoon extra-virgin olive oil

Place 1 inch of water in the bottom of a pot. Insert a steamer basket and place the squash inside. Bring the water to a boil, cover, and reduce the heat to medium-low, then steam until the squash is tender throughout when poked with a fork, about 10 minutes.

Transfer the squash to a bowl that will fit an immersion blender without splashing. Add the remaining ingredients and puree until creamy.

Calories: 59
Carbohydrate: 12 g

Protein: 2 g
Fat: 1 g

Variations

Add 1 tablespoon butter or heavy cream if serving with a lower-fat meal.

Use other herbs or spices. Sweet spices like cinnamon, nutmeg, cardamom, or cloves go well with squash.

Add 1 to 2 tablespoons whole milk or unsweetened soy or almond milk for a creamier texture.

Calories: 83 (Variation with 2
  tablespoons whole milk)

Carbohydrate: 13 g
Protein: 2 g

Fat: 4 g

Artichoke Kalamata Olive Ragout (All Phases)

Similar to pasta primavera, this Mediterranean-inspired ragout touts a tangy bite from artichoke hearts and salty olives. Use as a side dish, or add a protein to create a full meal.

Preparation time: 5 minutes

Total time: 25 minutes

Makes 4 to 6 servings

- 1 tablespoon extra-virgin olive oil
- 1 large onion, diced
- 2 cloves garlic, minced or pressed
- 10 ounces baby bella/cremini mushrooms, sliced
- ¼ to ½ teaspoon dried oregano
- ¼ teaspoon salt
- ⅛ teaspoon ground black pepper
- 1 (14-ounce) can artichoke hearts, drained and quartered
- 10 to 12 Kalamata olives, pitted and chopped
- 1 (14.5-ounce) can diced tomatoes
- ¼ cup tomato paste (about 3 ounces)
- ¼ cup grated Parmesan cheese, for garnish (optional)

Heat the olive oil in a large skillet or Dutch oven over medium heat. Add onion, garlic, mushrooms, oregano, salt, and pepper. Cook, stirring, until the onion is translucent and the mushrooms are beginning to soften, about 5 minutes.

Add the artichoke hearts, olives, and tomatoes. Bring to a boil. Reduce the heat to medium and simmer, uncovered, for 5 minutes.

Stir in the tomato paste to thicken the sauce. Taste and adjust the seasonings.

Simmer for 5 minutes more, or as needed to cook off any excess liquid.

Serve warm on top of whole grains or Millet-Corn Polenta (page 236), or with fish, chicken, tofu, or other protein.

Based on 4 servings   Carbohydrate: 28 g   Fat: 6 g
Calories: 188   Protein: 7 g

BEANS

Garlicky White Beans with Broccoli Rabe (All Phases)

White beans and garlic team up to tame the bitter greens. This combination just shines.

Preparation time: 5 minutes

Total time: 45 minutes

Makes 4 servings

- 1 tablespoon extra-virgin olive oil
- 2 large cloves garlic
- 1¾ cups cooked white beans measured with cooking liquid (see Do-It-Yourself Beans page 74) or drained and rinsed canned beans measured with water
- ¼ teaspoon salt, or to taste
- 1 bunch broccoli rabe, mustard greens, or other bitter greens sliced into ½-inch pieces

Heat the olive oil in a large skillet over medium heat. Add the garlic and cook, stirring, for 30 seconds to infuse the oil with garlic flavor.

Stir in the beans with their cooking liquid and the salt (use more or less to taste depending on how salted the beans are). Cook until the beans are warm throughout, about 5 minutes.

Stir in the broccoli rabe. Cover and cook until the broccoli rabe is tender but still bright in color, 3 to 5 minutes.

Calories: 149
Carbohydrate: 21 g
Protein: 8 g
Fat: 4 g

Tip: If using canned beans measured with water, you may need to cook the beans longer before adding the greens for a creamy texture.

Ful Mudammas (Egyptian Fava Bean Stew) (All Phases)

A staple food in Egypt, this hearty stew highlights the unique flavor of fava beans in a warm, flavorful sauce. Serve as a robust side dish, or top with boiled eggs and olive oil for a vegetarian entrée. If you are using the small, dried favas, the skins do not need to be removed.

Preparation time: 5 minutes

Total time: 45 minutes

Makes 6 servings

- 3 to 4 tablespoons olive oil
- 4 cloves garlic, minced or pressed
- 1 large onion, diced
- 1 to 2 teaspoons ground cumin
- ¼ to ½ teaspoon ground black pepper
- 3 cups cooked fava beans measured with cooking liquid (see Do-It-Yourself Beans, page 74) or drained and rinsed canned beans measured with water (small fava beans work best)
- 1 cup cooked chickpeas measured with cooking liquid (see Do-It-Yourself Beans, page 74) or drained and rinsed canned chickpeas measured with water
- ½ to 1 teaspoon salt, or to taste
- 1 cup chopped fresh parsley
- 1 medium tomato, diced
- 3 tablespoons fresh lemon juice

Heat 2 tablespoons of the olive oil in a large skillet over medium heat. Add the garlic, onion, cumin, and pepper. Cook, stirring, until the onion is translucent, 3 to 5 minutes.

Add the beans with their cooking liquid and salt (use more or less to taste, based on the saltiness of the beans). Bring to a boil. Reduce the heat to medium-low and simmer, uncovered, for 15 to 30 minutes, or until the liquid has mostly cooked down and thickened a bit.

Stir in the parsley, tomato, and lemon juice. Simmer for 2 to 3 minutes more.

Serve warm, garnished with the remaining 1 to 2 tablespoons olive oil. (See photo insert page 12.)

Calories: 251
Carbohydrate: 32 g
Protein: 11 g
Fat: 10 g

Variations

Add a bit of cayenne or other ground chile for a spicy dish.

Garnish with tahini instead of or in addition to the olive oil.

Top each portion with 1 or 2 sliced hard-boiled eggs.

Savory Adzuki Beans (All Phases)

In Japanese cooking, adzuki beans are traditionally paired with sweet flavors. In this recipe, the classic combination of mirin and miso enhances the umami flavor—a splendid vegetarian alternative to beans cooked with a ham bone or other meat.

Preparation time: 5 minutes

Total time: 20 minutes

Makes 4 to 6 servings (about 2 cups)

- 2 cups cooked adzuki beans measured with cooking liquid (see Do-It-Yourself Beans, page 74) or drained and rinsed canned beans measured with water
- 2 tablespoons mirin
- 1 tablespoon dark miso paste, diluted in 2 tablespoons water
- 1 small leek, halved lengthwise, thinly sliced, and rinsed well
- Salt
- Scallions, chopped, for garnish

Place beans and mirin in a pot. Bring to a boil over medium-high heat. Reduce the heat to medium-low and simmer for 5 minutes.

Stir in the miso and leek until the miso is completely incorporated. Simmer, uncovered, for 10 minutes, or until the liquid has mostly been absorbed and thickened. Taste and adjust the seasonings, adding salt as needed.

Serve hot, garnished with scallions.

Based on 6 servings   Carbohydrate: 15 g   Fat: 0 g
Calories: 73   Protein: 4g

Baby Lima Beans in Creamy Shiitake Gravy (All Phases)

Healthy comfort food! The shiitake gravy makes a velvety, luscious sauce for the lima beans, and it's topped off with a generous touch of garlic.

Preparation time: 5 minutes

Total time: 50 minutes

Makes 8 servings

- 2 tablespoons extra-virgin olive oil
- 1 medium onion, diced
- 2 cloves garlic, minced or pressed
- 8 ounces fresh shiitake mushrooms, sliced (about 3 cups)
- 1 teaspoon salt
- ¼ teaspoon ground black pepper
- ¼ cup chickpea flour (see Tip, page 91)
- 2 cups cooked baby lima beans measured with cooking liquid (see Do-It-Yourself Beans, page 74) or drained and rinsed canned beans measured with water
- 1 to 2 tablespoons soy sauce
- Fresh parsley or scallions, chopped, for garnish

Preheat oven to 350°F. Heat the olive oil in a large ovenproof skillet or pot over medium heat. Add the onion, garlic, mushrooms, salt, and pepper. Cook, stirring, until the mushrooms soften, about 10 minutes.

Add the chickpea flour and cook, stirring, for 3 to 5 minutes to absorb liquid and lightly brown the flour. The flour will be clumpy on the vegetables but will evenly distribute into a thick gravy after the beans are added.

Add the beans and their cooking liquid and stir or whisk gently to allow the flour mixture to absorb the liquid. Cook, stirring, until the liquid begins to thicken. Stir in the soy sauce, using more or less to taste.

Cover, transfer to the oven, and bake for about 30 minutes, or until the casserole is creamy and bubbling throughout. Uncover for the last 10 minutes of baking.

Serve hot, garnished with parsley or scallions.

Calories: 208
Carbohydrate: 33 g
Protein: 11 g
Fat: 4 g

Refried Beans (All Phases)

This simple refried bean recipe adds a spicy flair to any savory dish. Spread on tacos, quesadillas, or salads for a Mexican meal at home.

Preparation time: 5 minutes

Total time: 20 minutes

Makes 6 servings (about 2 cups)

- 1½ tablespoons extra-virgin olive oil
- ½ to 1 jalapeño or other mild to medium chile pepper, seeded and chopped
- ½ teaspoon garlic powder
- 1 teaspoon ground cumin
- ½ teaspoon dried Mexican oregano or regular oregano
- 3 cups cooked pinto or black beans measured with cooking liquid (see Do-It-Yourself Beans, page 74) or drained and rinsed canned beans measured with water
- Salt
- ½ cup chopped fresh cilantro, for garnish

Heat the olive oil in a pot or deep skillet over medium heat. Add the chile, garlic powder, cumin, and oregano. Cook for 10 to 15 seconds to infuse the oil and bring out the flavor of the spices.

Stir in the beans. Bring to a boil. Reduce the heat to low and simmer, stirring regularly, for 5 to 10 minutes to allow the liquid to reduce and thicken a bit and the flavors to incorporate. (This may take longer for canned beans.) Taste and season with salt as needed.

Puree directly in the pot with an immersion blender and simmer for 2 to 3 minutes. (If the beans are not deep enough to fully immerse the blender and prevent splattering, carefully transfer them to a deep bowl or jar to blend. Return to the pan after blending.) The mixture will thicken even more as it cools.

Garnish with the cilantro and serve hot.

Calories: 156
Carbohydrate: 23 g
Protein: 8 g
Fat: 4 g

WHOLE GRAINS

Pressure-Cooked Brown Rice (Phases 2 and 3)

The flavor and texture of pressure-cooked short-grain brown rice is truly something special—smooth and creamy while retaining that toothy feel. This cooking method brings out the natural sweetness of rice. It pairs nicely with other hearty grains, beans, or nuts. For boiled rice, see the Guide to Cooking Whole Grains on page 333.

Preparation time: 5 minutes plus overnight soaking

Total time: 50 minutes

Makes 8 servings (about 4 cups)

- 2 cups uncooked short-grain brown rice
- 3 cups water
- ¼ teaspoon salt

Place the rice and water in a pot or bowl. Soak overnight or for about 8 hours. It is natural for the rice to absorb some of the water.

Transfer the rice and water to a pressure cooker and add the salt. Bring to pressure over medium heat.

Reduce the heat to low and cook at full pressure for 30 to 45 minutes, or according to the manufacturer's instructions. Allow the pressure to release naturally.

Serve hot.

Calories: 150	Protein: 3 g
Carbohydrate: 35 g	Fat: 2 g

Variations

Rice with Beans: Use 1 cup short-grain brown rice; ½ cup dried beans, such as chickpeas, adzuki beans, or black soybeans; and 2½ to 3 cups water.

Based on 6 servings	Carbohydrate: 34 g	Fat: 2 g
Calories: 163	Protein: 5 g	

Rice with Other Grains: Use 1 cup short-grain brown rice; ½ cup sweet rice, hulled barley, wheat berries, or other hearty whole grains; and 2¼ cups water.

Based on 6 servings	Carbohydrate: 37 g	Fat: 1 g
Calories: 160	Protein: 3 g	

Rice with Chestnuts: Use 1 cup short-grain brown rice; ½ cup peeled cooked chestnuts or ¼ cup dried chestnuts, reconstituted in ⅓ cup warm water; and an additional 1½ cups water. Use the chestnut soaking water when cooking the rice.

Based on 4 servings
Calories: 168

Carbohydrate: 39 g
Protein: 3 g

Fat: 2 g

Mexican Rice (Phases 2 and 3)

When plain rice starts to get boring, spice it up with this traditional Tex-Mex favorite. Used widely in the Southwestern United States and inspired by traditional Spanish and Mexican recipes, this seasoned rice spans cultures to delight diners across the world.

Preparation time: 5 minutes

Total time: 45 minutes

Makes 4 servings (about 3 cups)

- 1 tablespoon extra-virgin olive oil
- 1 cup uncooked brown basmati rice
- 1 small onion, finely diced
- 1 small red bell pepper, finely diced
- 1½ teaspoons chili powder
- ½ teaspoon garlic powder
- ¼ teaspoon salt
- ¼ teaspoon ground black pepper
- Dash of cayenne, or to taste (optional)
- 1 (14.5-ounce) can diced tomatoes
- 1½ cups water
- ¼ cup chopped cilantro

Heat the olive oil in a large skillet over medium heat. Add the rice and cook, stirring occasionally, for 5 minutes. Add the onion, bell pepper, chili powder, garlic powder, salt, black pepper, and cayenne. Cook, stirring, for 5 minutes, or until the vegetables soften.

Add the tomatoes and water. Bring to a boil. Reduce the heat to low and simmer, covered, for 30 to 45 minutes, or until all the liquid has been absorbed.

Fluff with a fork, garnish with cilantro, and serve hot.

Calories: 260
Carbohydrate: 43 g

Protein: 5 g
Fat: 9 g

Brown Rice "Tater" Tots (Phases 2 and 3)

When we served this dish to two seven-year-olds, one declared, "Oh, these are tater tots," and the name just stuck. These are a staple in the Ludwig home. We all have different preferred ways to eat them: dipped in Lemon Aioli (page 298), Smoked Paprika Ketchup (page 291), or regular ketchup; topped with nut butter; or simply as is.

Preparation time: 10 minutes

Total time: 30 minutes

Makes 4 servings

- Neutral-tasting oil, such as high-oleic safflower or avocado oil, for deep-frying
- 2 cups cooked short-grain brown rice
- Soy sauce or salt

Pour 2 to 3 inches of oil into a small heavy-bottomed pot (see Chef Dawn's Tasty Tip on deep-frying page 167). Heat the oil over medium heat to 325 to 350°F.

Set a bowl of water nearby for wetting your hands. Scoop 1 to 2 tablespoons of the rice into your hand. Work the ball in your hands, pressing tightly to form it into a cylinder or oval that holds together without being too sticky. Wet your hands as necessary to keep the rice from sticking to them.

Working in batches as necessary to avoid crowding the pot, gently place the rice balls into the hot oil. Cook, turning occasionally, for 3 to 5 minutes, or until lightly golden brown and crispy on the outside. The rice balls may stick together at the edges, but you can easily break them apart as you turn them.

Remove the rice balls from the oil with a mesh strainer and set on a plate lined with a paper towel or covered with a bamboo sushi mat to drain. Add a few drops of soy sauce or a sprinkle of salt to each one while they are hot to create a salty-on-the-outside taste. Transfer to a baking dish and keep warm in a 200°F oven if you won't be serving them immediately.

Serve hot. These can also be refrigerated for up to 1 week and reheated in the oven or toaster oven before serving. (See photo insert page 14.)

Tip: This recipe works best with cold leftover rice that is a bit on the sticky side, like Pressure-Cooked Brown Rice (page 226). If your rice is too dry to stick together, add a bit of cooked oats or other sticky grain to help bind it together without making it too wet.

Calories: 171   Protein: 2 g
Carbohydrate: 23 g   Fat: 8 g

For Meals: These pair well with higher-protein, lower-fat entrées, such as Parchment-Baked Fish (page 138).

Brown Rice Mushroom Risotto (Phases 2 and 3)

Short-grain brown rice and sweet brown rice, a stickier version of short-grain rice, both have a creamier texture than other brown rice varieties, making them the best options for risotto. The sticky quality of sweet rice adds an additional layer of richness and texture. Try this satisfying, whole-grain recipe as a side dish or add protein for a vegetarian entrée.

Preparation time: 5 minutes

Total time: 1 hour

Makes 4 servings

- 4½ cups water or broth
- 1 ounce dried porcini mushrooms
- 2 tablespoons extra-virgin olive oil
- ¾ cup uncooked brown rice
- ¼ cup uncooked sweet brown rice
- 1 large clove garlic
- 1 medium onion, diced
- ¼ to ½ teaspoon dried thyme
- ½ to ¾ teaspoon salt
- ¼ teaspoon ground black pepper
- ½ cup white wine
- 1 pound asparagus, green beans, blanched Brussels sprout halves, or other green vegetable
- 4 ounces Parmesan cheese, grated (optional)

Heat the water in a saucepan over medium-low heat.

Place the dried porcini in a bowl and pour over 1 cup of the hot water. Set aside to soften until you are ready to use them.

Heat the olive oil in a Dutch oven or deep skillet over medium heat. Add the brown rice and sweet rice and cook, stirring, for 5 minutes. Add the garlic, onion, thyme, salt, and pepper. Cook until the onion is translucent, 3 to 5 minutes.

Stir the wine into the rice, reduce the heat to medium-low, and cook until the wine has been absorbed, about 3 minutes.

Remove the soaked porcinis with a mesh strainer or slotted spoon, reserving the soaking liquid. Set the liquid aside to allow any sediment to sink to the bottom.

Coarsely chop the porcini. Stir the chopped porcini, the soaking liquid (leaving sediment at the bottom), and ½ cup of the hot water into the rice. Cook, stirring, until the liquid has been absorbed, 2 to 3 minutes.

Stir in 1½ cups of the hot water. Cover, reduce the heat to low, and cook until the water has been absorbed, about 20 minutes. Stir in the remaining 1½ cups hot water, cover, and cook for 20 minutes, or until the water has been absorbed.

Stir in asparagus and Parmesan (if using). Cover and simmer for about 5 minutes. Taste and adjust the seasonings.

Serve hot.

Tip: If you are using a tougher vegetable like Brussels sprouts, bring a pot of water to a boil, halve the vegetables, add them to the boiling water, and cook until tender but still bright in color, usually just a few minutes, then drain. No need to dip the vegetables in an ice bath to stop the cooking—just add them directly to the risotto after blanching (see Guide to Cooking Vegetables, page 329).

Calories: 191 (Without Parmesan)	Carbohydrate: 25 g Protein: 6 g	Fat: 8 g

| Calories: 310 (With Parmesan)
Carbohydrate: 29 g | Protein: 15 g
Fat: 16 g | |

Variations

Quick pressure cooker version: Put the rice in a bowl with 2 cups water and set aside to soak overnight. Sauté the vegetables, then add the wine and cook for 1 to 2 minutes. Add the rice and its soaking water (some of the water will have been absorbed by the rice). Bring to pressure and cook at high pressure for 40 minutes. Allow the pressure to release naturally. Chop the dried mushrooms. Stir the chopped mushrooms and asparagus into the hot rice. Cover and let sit for 5 minutes to allow the mushrooms to soften. Stir once again to incorporate the flavors. Taste and adjust the seasonings. Serve.

For Meals: This pairs well with higher-protein, lower-fat entrées, such as Parchment-Baked Fish (page 138).

Cooked Quinoa (Phases 2 and 3)

The distinct, nutty flavor of quinoa substitutes well for brown rice when you want more variety or a quicker-cooking grain. Mix this fluffy grain with a variety of dried fruits, vegetables, or spices to create cold or hot side dishes worth raving about.

Preparation time: 5 minutes

Total time: 25 minutes

Makes 6 to 8 servings (about 3 cups)

- 2 cups water
- ¼ teaspoon salt
- 1 cup uncooked quinoa, rinsed well

In a small saucepan, bring the water and salt to a boil. Add the quinoa and return the water to a boil. Reduce the heat to low, cover, and simmer for 20 to 30 minutes, or until all the water has been absorbed.

Transfer the quinoa to a large bowl and fluff with a fork.

Based on 6 servings
Calories: 111

Carbohydrate: 20 g
Protein: 4 g

Fat: 2 g

Quinoa Croquettes (Phases 2 and 3)

These easy vegetarian burgers make a satisfying appetizer, side dish, or vegetarian entrée. Use leftover vegetables without anyone knowing. This simple recipe is delicious as is, but is also great as a base for your own masterpiece dishes. Play around with various grains, beans, vegetables, and spices. The patties also freeze well for a quick savory snack.

Preparation time: 10 minutes

Total time: 30 minutes

Makes 8 to 10 servings (about 48 mini patties)

- 1 large carrot, cut into large chunks
- 2 stalks celery, cut into large chunks
- 1 small onion, cut into large chunks
- 4 or 5 collard green leaves, kale leaves, or other hearty greens, cut into large chunks
- 18 sprigs cilantro, coarsely chopped
- 8 to 10 sprigs parsley, coarsely chopped
- ½ teaspoon salt
- ⅛ teaspoon ground black pepper
- 3 cups Cooked Quinoa (page 231) or other cooked whole grain
- 3 cups cooked chickpeas or other beans, drained and rinsed (see Do-It-Yourself Beans, page 74) or drained and rinsed canned beans
- 1 to 1¼ cups chickpea flour (see Tip, page 91)
- ½ cup extra-virgin olive oil, for frying

Place the carrot, celery, onion, collards, cilantro, and parsley in a food processor. Pulse until finely chopped. Transfer the vegetables to a large bowl and add the salt, pepper, quinoa, and beans. Mix well with a fork, lightly smashing the beans until well combined.

Add 1 cup of the chickpea flour and stir well. The mixture should be stiff enough to hold together in patties. If it is not, add the remaining chickpea flour 1 tablespoon at a time until the desired consistency is reached. Set mixture aside.

Heat the olive oil in a shallow 12-inch cast-iron skillet (the oil should just cover the bottom of the skillet) over medium heat.

Form the vegetable mixture into 2- to 3-inch balls, then flatten them into patties. Gently place the patties close together in the pan, leaving room to turn them but cooking as many as possible. Fry until browned on both sides, turning only once they are fully browned on each side, 5 to 10 minutes total. Remove from the heat and set aside on a plate lined with a paper towel or bamboo sushi mat to drain. Repeat with the remaining vegetable mixture.

Serve with your favorite sauce, or wrap in a lettuce leaf with sauce drizzled over the top. (See photo insert page 13.)

Based on 8 servings (6 or 7 mini patties per serving)	Calories: 409 Carbohydrate: 56 g	Protein: 16 g Fat: 15 g

Variations

Add prepared mustard, chopped fresh chiles, or dried herbs or spices to create interesting ethnic flavors.

Phase 2 or 3 Meal: Serve with 2 tablespoons Lemon Aioli (page 298), sliced cucumbers seasoned with salt and lemon juice, and 2 slices Smoke-Dried Tomato Seitan (page 73) or a similar vegetarian protein (see Equivalents Table, page 49) or ⅓ cup Shredded Chicken (page 110). **For Dessert:** 1 cup raspberries topped with 2 tablespoons plain whole-milk Greek yogurt.

Calories: 663; Carbohydrate: 36%; Protein: 21%; Fat: 43%

Millet Tabbouleh (Phases 2 and 3, with Phase 1 Variation)

Quick, fresh, whole-grain tabbouleh satisfies on a summer day. Make ahead to allow the flavors to fully develop. Great for potlucks or parties.

Preparation time: 10 minutes

Total time: 25 minutes

Makes 4 to 6 servings

- 2 cups boiling water
- 1 cup uncooked millet, rinsed and drained
- ¼ teaspoon salt
- 3 to 4 ounces fresh parsley (1½ to 2 cups packed)
- 10 to 12 fresh mint leaves, or more to taste
- 1 small red onion or Pickled Red Onions (page 69), quartered
- 1 large tomato, finely diced

Dressing

- 3 tablespoons fresh lemon juice
- ¼ teaspoon salt
- ¼ teaspoon ground black pepper
- 1 to 2 tablespoons extra-virgin olive oil

Bring the water to a boil in a medium saucepan. Add the millet and salt. Bring back to a boil. Reduce the heat to low. Stir, cover, and cook for 25 minutes, or until all the water has been absorbed. Remove from the heat, transfer to a glass bowl, and fluff the millet with a fork a few times as it cools. (Alternatively, use 3 cups leftover cooked millet.)

While the millet cooks, combine the parsley, mint, and onion in a food processor and pulse until finely minced.

Make the dressing: Stir all the dressing ingredients together in a small bowl or jar. Set aside.

Once millet is completely cooled, stir in the parsley, mint, onion, and tomato. Toss with the dressing and refrigerate for at least 30 minutes for flavors to develop.

Tip: The most time-consuming part of this recipe is waiting for the millet to cook and cool. To save time, make the millet on Prep Day or while you are cooking another meal so it is ready to go when you want to make tabbouleh.

Based on 6 servings
Calories: 174

Carbohydrate: 28 g
Protein: 5 g

Fat: 5 g

Variations

Add dried currants or chopped raisins for a sweet addition.

Substitute quinoa for the millet.

For Phase 1: Substitute 3 cups Cauliflower Couscous (page 211) for the cooked millet and divide the tabbouleh into 4 servings instead of 6.

For Phase 3: Substitute 1½ cups bulgur wheat for the millet. Place the bulgur into 1½ cups boiling water. Cover and set aside for at least 5 minutes, or until the water has been absorbed.

Phase 1 Meal: Use the Phase 1 Variation. Serve with 4 ounces boneless, skinless diced cooked chicken and ¼ avocado. **For Dessert:** ½ cup blueberries and 1 Chocolate Truffle (page 314).

Calories: 532; Carbohydrate: 24%; Protein: 24%; Fat: 52%

Phase 2 or 3 Meal: Divide the tabbouleh into 4 servings instead of 6. Toss with 3 ounces skinless diced cooked chicken or equivalent protein (see Equivalents Table page 49). and ¼ avocado per serving. **For Dessert:** ½ Mango Lassi (page 311).

Calories: 586; Carbohydrate: 37%; Protein: 23%; Fat: 40%

Millet Mashed Fauxtatoes (Phases 2 and 3)

These "fauxtatoes" add whole grains to your diet in an impressive impersonation of the conventional potato-based dish. Top with Sautéed Mushrooms (page 216) or a drizzle of olive oil and serve alongside your favorite proteins.

Preparation time: 5 minutes

Total time: 40 minutes

Makes 6 servings

- 2 cups water
- ½ cup uncooked millet, rinsed and drained
- 1 medium head cauliflower, coarsely chopped
- 1 large clove garlic, minced
- 2 tablespoons extra-virgin olive oil
- ½ teaspoon salt
- ¼ teaspoon ground black pepper

Bring the water to a boil in a medium pot over medium-high heat. Stir in the millet, cauliflower, garlic, 1 tablespoon of the olive oil, the salt, and the pepper. Return to a boil. Reduce the heat to low, cover, and cook for 30 minutes, or until the water has been absorbed.

Puree directly in the pot with an immersion blender until smooth and creamy.

Serve warm, drizzled with the remaining 1 tablespoon olive oil as a garnish.

Calories: 128   Protein: 4 g
Carbohydrate: 17 g   Fat: 6 g

Soft Millet-Corn Polenta (Phases 2 and 3)

This whole-grain variation on classic polenta is easy to make and great for leftovers.

Preparation time: 5 minutes

Total time: 25 minutes

Makes 4 servings

- 2½ cups water
- ⅔ cup uncooked millet, rinsed and drained

- 3 tablespoons frozen or canned corn kernels, drained
- ¼ to ½ teaspoon salt
- Soy sauce or additional salt, for serving (optional)

Bring the water to a boil in a medium pot. Stir in the millet, corn, and salt and return the water to a boil. Stir briefly, reduce the heat to low, cover, and simmer until the water has been fully absorbed, 20 to 30 minutes.

Scoop a portion onto each plate and serve immediately, with a splash of soy sauce or light sprinkle of salt.

Alternatively, spread the hot millet into an 8- or 9-inch baking dish. Let cool, slice into squares, and serve like traditional polenta.

Tip: The texture is soft when warm, but thickens to a polenta consistency when cooled. Using an ice cream scoop to make rounded, evenly portioned scoops when it is warm will result in perfectly set mounds when cooled, or pressing into a baking dish will make it easy to cut into portions once cooled and then panfry in oil to crispy perfection.

Calories: 132   Protein: 4 g
Carbohydrate: 26 g   Fat: 1 g

Variations

Panfry the cooled millet squares in a cast-iron skillet with 1 to 2 tablespoons extra-virgin olive oil until brown and crispy on one side, then flip and brown on the second side.

Top with grated Parmesan or other cheese.

Add your favorite herbs or spices when you add the salt.

My *Always Delicious* Story

I've had fibromyalgia/chronic fatigue for twenty-five years. My problem has been sticking with an exercise plan, because the first fifteen minutes of any workout (even a slow hike) can be painful, especially in cold weather. After being on *AH* for eight months, I'd say that my symptoms are vastly improved. Preparing to go out for a walk now feels like fun. A workout feels like a privilege. I'm stuck at four pounds above my ideal weight (I know that sounds silly), but if that's my set point, then so be it. I love my food. I am delighted by the lack of hunger. But most of all, I am ever so grateful for being able to feel happily married to my physical self. My body isn't perfect, but it's no longer a burden—it's my greatest friend and ally.

Karyn K., age 52, Manhattan, New York

CHAPTER 9

Soups, Salads & Buddha Bowls

SOUPS

Thai Coconut Fish Soup (All Phases)

Coconut milk adds a soothing balance to the spicy red curry paste in this traditional Thai soup. A generous portion of napa cabbage makes all the big flavor burst in a juicy bite.

Preparation time: 10 minutes

Total time: 35 to 40 minutes

Makes 6 servings (about 12 cups)

- 1 stalk lemongrass or 6 to 7 drops of lemongrass essential oil (optional)
- 1 (2-inch) piece fresh ginger, peeled and thinly sliced (see Chef Dawn's Tasty Tip, page 289)
- 2 cloves garlic
- 4 to 5 tablespoons Thai red curry paste (choose a brand with no sugar added), or more to taste
- 2 (13.5-ounce) cans unsweetened coconut milk
- 2 to 2½ teaspoons salt, or to taste
- 1 tablespoon extra-virgin olive oil
- 1 large onion, diced
- 2 or 3 large stalks celery, thinly sliced on an angle
- 1 large carrot, cut into large chunks
- 4 to 5 cups water or unsalted broth
- 2 to 2½ pounds white-fleshed fish, such as cod, haddock, hake, etc., cut into large chunks

- 2 to 3 cups chopped napa cabbage or hearty green vegetable like kale or collards
- ½ cup chopped fresh cilantro, for garnish
- Fresh lime juice, for serving

Remove tough outer leaves of the lemongrass (if using) and cut it into thin rounds. Place the ginger, garlic, lemongrass, red curry paste, coconut milk, and salt in a blender. Blend until well combined. Set aside.

Heat the oil in a large stockpot or Dutch oven over medium heat. Add onion, celery, and carrot. Cook, stirring, until the vegetables soften, 3 to 5 minutes.

Pour the coconut milk mixture and water over the vegetables. Bring to a boil. Reduce the heat to low and simmer, covered, for 10 to 15 minutes.

Add the fish. Simmer, uncovered, until the fish is cooked through, about 10 minutes. Taste and adjust the seasonings, adding more salt or curry paste as desired.

Add the cabbage. Simmer, uncovered, for 2 to 3 minutes, or until the greens are tender but still bright in color. Serve garnished with fresh cilantro and lime juice.

Calories: 448   Protein: 34 g
Carbohydrate: 11 g   Fat: 31 g

Variations

Add 1 (2- to 3-inch) piece fresh turmeric, peeled, to the blender with the coconut milk mixture and blend until smooth.

Vegetarian version: Substitute 2 pounds extra-firm tofu, drained, pressed with an absorbent towel, and cut into small pieces for the fish.

Phase 1 Meal: Serve over Cauliflower Couscous (page 211). **For Dessert:** 1 cup blueberries topped with ¼ cup plain whole-milk Greek yogurt.

Calories: 641; Carbohydrate: 25%; Protein: 26%; Fat: 49%

Phase 2 Meal: Serve over ½ cup cooked brown rice. **For Dessert:** 1 cup diced mango.

Calories: 671; Carbohydrate: 36%; Protein: 22%; Fat: 42%

Phase 3 Meal: Serve over ⅔ cup cooked brown or white rice. **For Dessert:** 1 cup diced mango.

Calories: 684; Carbohydrate: 37%; Protein: 22%; Fat: 41%

Hot-and-Sour Soup (All Phases)

You can now make this exquisitely simple soup, a favorite in Chinese restaurants, at home.

Preparation time: 10 minutes

Total time: 30 to 40 minutes

Makes 6 servings (about 10 cups)

- 6 cups water or unsalted broth
- 4 dried shiitake mushrooms, left whole, or 8 to 10 fresh shiitakes, cut into small dice
- 1 (2-inch) piece fresh ginger, peeled and thinly sliced
- ¼ cup soy sauce
- 1 teaspoon red pepper flakes, or ¼ to ½ teaspoon cayenne pepper
- 2 tablespoons toasted sesame oil
- 8 ounces extra-firm tofu, drained, pressed with an absorbent towel, and cut into small pieces
- 2 stalks celery, finely diced
- 1 egg (optional)
- 1 egg white (optional)
- 2 cups napa cabbage, cut into 1-inch pieces
- ¼ cup red wine vinegar, or more to taste
- Dash of cayenne pepper, or to taste (optional)
- Scallions, chopped, for garnish

Bring the water to a boil in a large soup pot or Dutch oven and add the shiitake mushrooms. Reduce the heat to maintain a simmer for about 10 minutes. If using dried shiitakes, cook until they are soft enough to slice. Remove dried shiitakes with a slotted spoon and cut them into small chunks, then return them to the pot with the simmering cooking liquid and simmer 5 minutes more.

Place the ginger, soy sauce, red pepper flakes, and sesame oil in a wide-mouthed mason jar or cup that will fit an immersion blender without splashing. Blend well, working the blender into the thicker pieces of ginger until they are finely chopped.

Add the ginger mixture, tofu, and celery to the simmering shiitake cooking liquid. Bring back to a soft boil. If using eggs, beat the egg with the egg white and, while whisking vigorously, slowly pour into the boiling soup.

Reduce the heat to low and simmer, covered, for 5 to 10 minutes.

Add the cabbage and vinegar. Simmer for 5 to 10 minutes. Taste and adjust the seasonings, adding more soy sauce, vinegar, or a dash of cayenne to reach the desired flavor profile.

Serve hot, garnished with scallions.

Calories: 125
Carbohydrate: 5 g

Protein: 8 g
Fat: 8 g

Portuguese Seafood Stew (All Phases)

This hearty soup is a complete meal in one pot. The delicate aroma of wine enhances savory sausage and seafood to create magnificent depth of flavor. A simple dessert of fresh berries nicely rounds out the meal.

Preparation time: 5 minutes

Total time: 45 minutes

Makes 4 to 6 servings (12 cups)

- 6 cups water, unsalted broth, or Bone Broth (page 58)
- 2 tablespoons extra-virgin olive oil
- 1 medium onion, halved and thinly sliced into half-moons
- 3 cloves garlic, minced or pressed
- ¼ pound kielbasa or chorizo sausage, diced
- ½ to 1 teaspoon salt, or to taste
- ½ teaspoon ground black pepper, or to taste
- 1 (14.5-ounce) can diced tomatoes
- 30 Kalamata olives, pitted and coarsely chopped
- 1 bay leaf
- ½ cup dry white wine
- 1¼ pounds cod or other white-fleshed fish, cut into large chunks
- 8 to 16 mussels (see Chef Dawn's Tasty Tip, page 147), clams, peeled shrimp, or an additional ½ pound fish
- 4 to 5 cups packed, coarsely chopped kale, arugula, spinach, or other leafy greens like chard, collards, or mustard greens (see Tip, page 137)
- ¼ cup chopped fresh cilantro or parsley, for garnish

Bring the water to a boil in a kettle or pot.

In a separate soup pot, heat the oil over medium heat. Add the onion, garlic, sausage, salt, and pepper. Cook, stirring, until the onion is translucent, 3 to 5 minutes.

Add the tomatoes, olives, bay leaf, and wine. Cook, stirring, for 5 minutes more.

Add the boiling water from the kettle or pot. Bring back to a boil. Reduce the heat to medium-low and simmer, covered, for 10 minutes.

Gently place fish and shellfish into the simmering liquid. Add additional water, if needed, to reach the desired soup consistency. Bring back to a boil. Reduce the heat to medium-low and simmer, uncovered, until the fish or shrimp are opaque and the shellfish have opened, about 15 minutes or more, depending on the thickness and type of seafood used. Discard any unopened shellfish.

Stir in the kale, taste, and adjust the seasonings. Simmer for 5 minutes more to allow the kale to soften. Serve warm, distributing the seafood evenly among the portions. Garnish with the cilantro or parsley.

Based on 4 servings
Calories: 543

Carbohydrate: 17 g
Protein: 39 g

Fat: 33 g

Variations

Vegetarian or vegan version: Substitute ½ pound vegetarian chorizo or vegetarian Italian sausage for the kielbasa and 1½ pounds extra-firm tofu, drained, pressed with an absorbent towel, and cut into small pieces, for the seafood and increase salt to taste.

Phase 1 Meal: Serve with a side of salad greens and chopped raw vegetables tossed with 1 to 2 teaspoons Greek Dressing (page 285). **For Dessert:** 1 cup raspberries.

Calories: 672; Carbohydrate: 25%; Protein: 25%; Fat: 50%

Phase 2 Meal: Serve each portion over ½ cup cooked brown rice. **For Dessert:** Handful of raspberries.

Calories: 683; Carbohydrate: 31%; Protein: 25%; Fat: 44%

Phase 3 Meal: Reduce the fish in the recipe to ¾ pound. Serve each portion with a thick slice of crusty sourdough bread. **For Dessert:** 1 cup raspberries.

Calories: 661; Carbohydrate: 38%; Protein: 21%; Fat: 41%

Chicken or Turkey Soup on a Budget (All Phases)

Mom's answer to what ails you. This savory soup works just as well with leftover turkey or chicken but works best with pieces that have large bones that are easy to remove before serving. Prep is quick, and the soup cooks itself.

Preparation time: 10 minutes

Total time: 8 hours (slow cooker)

Makes 4 servings (about 12 cups)

- 8 cups water, or more to cover
- ½ chicken, or 2 turkey legs (about 2 pounds meat and bones)
- 1 large onion, diced
- 2 cloves garlic
- 3 stalks celery, diced
- 2 large carrots, cut into thick rounds
- 2 large parsnips or other root vegetables, such as rutabaga, celeriac, or turnip, diced
- 2 bay leaves
- 1 teaspoon dried thyme
- ½ teaspoon ground sage
- ½ teaspoon ground black pepper
- 1 teaspoon salt, or more to taste
- 3 to 4 cups packed chopped greens, such as kale, arugula, or spinach, (see Tip, page 137)

Slow Cooker: Place all the ingredients except the greens, with water just to cover, in a slow cooker with a sauté setting or in a stovetop-safe slow cooker insert or a Dutch oven on the stovetop. Bring to a boil. Transfer to the slow cooker, if necessary. Cover and cook on low for about 8 hours or on high for 4 to 5 hours, or according to the manufacturer's instructions, until the meat is cooked and falling off the bone.

Stovetop: Combine all the ingredients except the greens in a large pot, bring to a boil, reduce the heat to low, cover, and simmer for 3 to 4 hours, or until the meat is fully cooked.

Pressure Cooker: combine all the ingredients except the greens in the pressure cooker, cover, and bring to high pressure. Pressure cook for about 30 minutes, or according to the manufacturer's instructions for poultry. Allow the pressure to release naturally.

Remove any large bones, taste, and adjust the seasonings. Just before serving, stir in the chopped greens and heat until wilted. Serve.

Calories: 427   Protein: 31 g
Carbohydrate: 24 g   Fat: 23 g

Phase 1 Meal: Serve with Rosemary Biscuits (page 203). **For Dessert:** 2 Chocolate-Dipped Strawberries (page 313).

Calories: 654; Carbohydrate: 27%; Protein: 24%; Fat: 49%

Phase 2 Meal: Serve with ½ cup cooked brown rice or ½ cup Cooked Quinoa (page 231). **For Dessert:** ½ Mango Lassi (page 311).

Calories: 653; Carbohydrate: 36%; Protein: 25%; Fat: 39%

Phase 3 Meal: Serve the soup in smaller portions with 2 slices of Cornbread (page 205) and 1 teaspoon butter with each serving. **For Dessert:** ½ Poached Pear with Dried Plums (page 325).

Calories: 646; Carbohydrate: 38%; Protein: 20%; Fat: 42%

Sicilian Fava Bean Soup (All Phases)

Accented by a warm blend of tomato, fennel, and oregano, the fava bean's unique flavor has the starring role in this soup. Although the skin on large fava beans can be a bit too tough for some tastes, small favas have skins that add an interesting texture and do not need to be peeled.

Preparation time: 5 minutes

Total time: 1 hour (30 minutes, if beans are made ahead)

Makes 6 servings (about 10 cups)

- 3 cloves garlic, minced or pressed
- 1 medium onion, cut into large chunks
- 1 stalk celery, cut into large chunks
- 1 medium leek, halved lengthwise, cut into large chunks, and rinsed well
- 1 medium fennel bulb, cut into large chunks (about 2 cups)
- 2 tablespoons extra-virgin olive oil
- 1 teaspoon dried oregano, or 1 tablespoon fresh
- 1 teaspoon salt, or to taste
- ½ teaspoon ground black pepper

- 3 cups cooked fava beans measured with their cooking liquid (see Do-It-Yourself Beans, page 74; start with 1 cup small dried fava beans) or drained and rinsed canned fava beans measured with water
- 3 to 4 cups unsalted broth or water
- ½ (14.5-ounce) can diced tomatoes
- 1 scallion, chopped, for garnish
- 1 lemon, sliced, for garnish

Place the garlic, onion, celery, leek, and fennel in a food processor and pulse until finely chopped.

Heat the olive oil in a large soup pot or Dutch oven over medium heat. Add the chopped vegetables, oregano, salt, and pepper. Cook, stirring, until well softened, 5 to 10 minutes.

Add the beans, water, and tomatoes. Bring back to a boil. Reduce the heat to low, cover, and simmer for 20 to 30 minutes, or until the flavors meld.

Puree directly in the pot with an immersion blender until smooth and creamy. Simmer for about 5 minutes more to allow the flavors to further develop.

Serve warm, garnished with scallions and lemon slices.

Calories: 176
Carbohydrate: 26 g
Protein: 8 g
Fat: 5 g

Variations

Substitute pinto, lentils, or other beans if you can't find fava beans.

Polish White Borscht (Phases 2 and 3, with Phase 1 variation)

George Brown College culinary students Natasha Roy and Bernadeta Hopek brought their Polish roots to the *Always Hungry?* book class project with this savory borscht. Traditionally served as an Easter breakfast or lunch, this borscht will quickly become a favorite any time of year.

Preparation time: 20 minutes

Total time: 45 minutes

Makes 4 servings (about 8 cups)

- 4 cups water, unsalted broth, or Bone Broth (page 58)
- 3 or 4 cloves garlic, minced
- 1 medium onion, chopped
- 2 teaspoons chopped fresh thyme leaves, or ¾ teaspoon dried thyme
- 1 bay leaf
- ⅛ teaspoon dried marjoram
- ½ cup grated fresh horseradish root, or ½ to ¾ cup prepared horseradish
- ¼ pound ground turkey
- 1 teaspoon salt, or to taste
- 1 teaspoon ground black pepper, or to taste
- 4 medium golden beets, cut into 1-inch cubes
- 1 cup cooked white beans, such as cannellini or great northern (see Do-It-Yourself Beans, page 74) or drained and rinsed canned beans
- ½ cup sour cream or Dairy-Free Sour Cream (page 306)
- ½ cup half-and-half
- 4 eggs, hard-boiled, peeled, and sliced
- Fresh parsley or dill, for garnish

Combine the water, garlic, onion, thyme, bay leaf, marjoram, and horseradish in a large stockpot and bring to a boil over high heat. Reduce the heat to low. Cover and simmer while preparing the other ingredients.

Mix the ground turkey, ½ teaspoon of the salt, and ½ teaspoon of the pepper in a medium bowl and form into small meatballs. Add them to the simmering soup and cover the pot.

Fit a steamer basket in a separate pot. Add 1 to 2 inches of water to the bottom of the pot, just under the level of the basket. Place the beets in the steamer basket and bring the water to a boil. Cover and cook until the beets are tender throughout when poked with a skewer or fork, 10 to 15 minutes. Remove from the heat and set aside.

In a bowl deep enough to use the immersion blender without splashing, combine the beans and steamed beets and blend, adding water as needed, to create a smooth, thick puree. Stir in the sour cream and half-and-half. Pour this mixture into the simmering soup and bring back to a boil. Season with the remaining ½ teaspoon each salt and pepper, adding more as desired. Add water as needed to reach the desired consistency.

Stir in the egg slices. Simmer for 5 to 10 minutes more to allow the flavors to fully incorporate.

Serve hot, garnished with parsley or dill.

Calories: 320   Protein: 19 g
Carbohydrate: 25 g   Fat: 16 g

Variations

For Phase 1: Omit the beets, increase the ground turkey to ⅓ pound, and increase the half-and-half to ⅔ cup.

Calories: 325   Protein: 20 g
Carbohydrate: 20 g   Fat: 18 g

Phase 1 Meal: Use the Phase 1 Variation. Crumble 1 ounce cooked turkey bacon over each portion. **For Dessert:** Apple Pie Parfait (page 319; Phase 1 Variation).

Calories: 532; Carbohydrate: 23%; Protein: 27%; Fat: 50%

Phase 2 Meal: Crumble 1 ounce cooked turkey bacon over each portion. **For Dessert:** Apple Pie Parfait (page 319).

Calories: 537; Carbohydrate: 34%; Protein: 25%; Fat: 41%

Phase 3 Meal: Serve with Pear Cranberry Pie (page 320).

Calories: 557; Carbohydrate: 38%; Protein: 18%; Fat: 44%

Minestrone Soup (All Phases)

This delightful stew is a staple throughout Italy and beloved worldwide. Chock-full of fresh seasonal vegetables, minestrone can be made with whichever vegetables are left in the fridge. We use it often to round out our meal plans with slow-acting carbohydrate and a bit of protein.

Preparation time: 10 minutes

Total time: 1 hour

Makes 6 servings (about 12 cups)

- 1 tablespoon extra-virgin olive oil
- 1 medium onion, diced
- 2 cloves garlic, minced or pressed
- 1 stalk celery, thinly sliced
- 2 medium carrots, cut into large chunks
- 1 teaspoon dried basil
- ½ teaspoon dried thyme
- ½ teaspoon dried oregano
- 1 teaspoon salt, or to taste
- ¼ teaspoon ground black pepper, or to taste
- 1 (14.5-ounce) can diced tomatoes
- 1 bay leaf
- 3 cups water or unsalted broth
- 2½ to 3 cups Cooked Cannellini or Kidney Beans (see Do-It-Yourself Beans, page 74), measured with cooking liquid
- 1 medium zucchini, cut into small pieces
- 3 to 4 cups packed seasonal green vegetables like green beans, arugula, escarole, kale or other leafy greens, chopped
- A few sprigs parsley, chopped, for garnish

Heat the oil in a soup pot over medium heat. Add the onion and garlic. Cook, stirring, until translucent, 3 to 5 minutes.

Add the celery, carrots, basil, thyme, oregano, salt, and pepper. Cook, stirring, for 10 minutes more.

Add the tomatoes, bay leaf, water, and beans. Bring to a boil. Reduce the heat to low, cover, and simmer for 30 minutes to 1 hour. Taste and adjust the seasonings.

Add the zucchini and green vegetables. Simmer for 10 to 15 minutes more, or until the vegetables are tender.

Garnish with the parsley. Serve hot.

Calories: 168   Protein: 9 g
Carbohydrate: 27 g   Fat: 3 g

Variations

For Phase 3: Add 2 cups cooked whole wheat pasta, small shells, or elbows (about 4 ounces uncooked) when you add the zucchini and green vegetables.

Calories: 226   Protein: 11 g
Carbohydrate: 39 g   Fat: 3 g

Slow Cooker Chili (All Phases)

There's nothing like a steaming bowl of chili on a cold day. So satisfying, this hearty stew is even better the next day. This recipe makes a big batch to eat now and freeze for another meal.

Preparation time: 10 minutes

Total time: 8+ hours (slow cooker)

Makes 8 servings (about 12 cups)

- 2 cups dried beans (1½ cups pinto, ½ cup black or adzuki or any other combination)
- 1 tablespoon extra-virgin olive oil
- 1 large onion, diced
- 2 cloves garlic, minced
- 2 tablespoons chili powder
- 1½ teaspoons ground cumin
- 2½ pounds ground beef (85% lean)
- 8 cups water
- 4 ounces tomato paste
- 1½ teaspoons salt, or to taste
- 2 cups Fresh Salsa (page 302), or 1 jalapeño, seeded and pureed with 1 (14.5-ounce) can diced tomatoes
- 1 small red onion, minced
- 1 cup shredded cheddar or other mild cheese

Sort through the beans and remove any stones or grit. Rinse well. Place in a large pot or bowl with enough water to cover by a few inches. Soak for 8 hours or up to overnight. Drain the soaked beans and set aside.

Heat the olive oil in a slow cooker on the sauté setting or in a stovetop-safe slow cooker insert or pressure cooker over medium heat. Add the onion, garlic, chili powder, and cumin and cook, stirring, until the onion is translucent.

Add the meat and cook, stirring, for 5 minutes, or until the meat begins to brown. Add the soaked beans and the 8 cups fresh water. Bring to a boil.

If using a slow cooker, replace the insert, if necessary, cover, and cook on medium for 8 hours or according to the manufacturer's instructions, until the beans are tender.

If using a pressure cooker, cover, bring to high pressure, and cook for 25 minutes or according to the manufacturer's instructions, until the beans are tender.

Once beans are cooked, stir in the tomato paste, salt, and salsa. Simmer for 20 to 30 minutes more to allow the flavors to fully come together. Taste and adjust the seasonings, adding more chili powder, salt, or salsa as desired.

Serve hot, garnished with the red onion and cheese.

Calories: 576   Protein: 41 g
Carbohydrate: 39 g   Fat: 28 g

Variations

Stovetop version: Substitute 6 cups cooked beans measured with cooking liquid (see Do-It-Yourself Beans, page 74) and additional bean cooking liquid or water to reach 8 cups or canned beans, rinsed and drained, then measured with water to reach 8 cups total for the dried beans and water. Cook on the stovetop for 30 minutes or more.

Vegetarian version: In place of the beef, substitute 1½ pounds Crumbled Tempeh (page 192) sprinkled on the top at the end, or 2 pounds extra-firm tofu, drained, pressed with an absorbent towel, and crumbled, then cooked with the beans. Increase the salt and spices to taste to flavor the tofu or tempeh.

Substitute ground turkey or buffalo for the beef and increase the oil to ⅓ cup to account for the lower-fat meats.

For Phase 3: Use 2 pounds ground beef.

Phase 1 Meal: Serve with a side of salad greens with chopped raw vegetables and 1 to 2 teaspoons Creamy Peppercorn Vinaigrette (page 286). **For Dessert:** A few strawberries and 1 heaping tablespoon Cardamom Whipped Cream (page 324).

Calories: 688; Carbohydrate: 27%; Protein: 25%; Fat: 48%

Phase 2 Meal: Serve with a side of salad greens with chopped raw vegetables and 1 to 2 teaspoons Creamy Peppercorn Vinaigrette (page 286). **For Dessert:** ½ cup blueberries.

Calories: 680; Carbohydrate: 32%; Protein: 25%; Fat: 43%

Phase 3 Meal: Use the Phase 3 Variation. Serve with 1 slice of Cornbread (page 205) and 1 teaspoon butter or olive oil. **For Dessert:** ½ cup blueberries.

Calories: 699; Carbohydrate: 36%; Protein: 23%; Fat: 41%

Split Pea Soup (All Phases)

Delicious aromas wafting from your kitchen will entice family and friends. The rich, familiar texture this soup creates ensures everyone will enjoy every nourishing bite. It reheats beautifully and is even better the next day. Burdock creates an earthy depth of flavor that is worth a trip to the Asian grocery or natural foods store.

Preparation time: 10 minutes

Total time: 1 to 8 hours (depending on your cooking method)

Makes 8 servings (about 12 cups)

- 6 cups water or unsalted broth, plus more as needed
- 1 teaspoon extra-virgin olive oil
- 1 small onion, diced
- 1 clove garlic, minced
- 2 stalks celery, diced
- 2 medium carrots, parsnips, turnips, or other root vegetables, cut into ½-inch chunks
- 1 medium (12-inch) burdock root (2 to 3 ounces), sliced into thin rounds (optional)
- ½ teaspoon dried thyme or other favorite herbs
- 2 cups dried split peas (about 1 pound)
- 1 or 2 bay leaves
- 1 teaspoon salt, or to taste
- ½ teaspoon ground black pepper, or to taste
- Scallions or fresh parsley, chopped, for garnish

Bring the water to a boil in a kettle or pot.

Heat the olive oil in a soup pot, stovetop-safe slow cooker insert, or pressure cooker over medium heat. Add the onion, garlic, celery, carrots, burdock (if using), and thyme. Cook, stirring occasionally, until the vegetables soften, 5 to 10 minutes.

While the vegetables are cooking, rinse the dried peas until the water runs clear.

Add the peas, hot water, and bay leaves to the vegetables. Bring to a boil.

If using a soup pot, reduce the heat and simmer for 1 to 2 hours, or until the peas are creamy and soft.

If using a slow cooker, return the insert to the slow cooker, cover, and cook on low for 8 hours or on high for 3 to 4 hours, or according to the manufacturer's instructions.

If using a pressure cooker, cover and bring to pressure over medium-high heat, reduce the heat to low, and simmer at full pressure or according to the manufacturer's instructions for about 30 minutes. Allow the pressure to release naturally.

Once the peas are completely soft and creamy, add additional water, if needed, to reach a thick soup consistency. If desired, puree with an immersion blender for a creamier soup. Season with the salt and pepper. Simmer for 5 to 10 minutes more.

Serve warm, garnished with scallions or parsley.

Let any leftover soup cool, then store in an airtight container (or individual portion containers) in the refrigerator for up to a week or in the freezer for up to 3 months. The soup will thicken to a paste when cooled. Add water when reheating, and season to taste.

Tip: Burdock is the secret ingredient here. It adds a rich, earthy flavor that is unparalleled. If you can't find burdock, substitute another root vegetable like rutabaga or parsnips.

Calories: 202   Protein: 12 g
Carbohydrate: 36 g   Fat: 1 g

Variations

Add a ham bone or cubes of ham with the beans.

Cuban Black Bean Soup (All Phases)

The Cuban secret ingredient—a touch of vinegar—adds a delightful depth of flavor to this soup that tastes almost smoky and is hard to recognize as vinegar. You'll want to make extra to freeze. It's a crowd-pleasing favorite.

Preparation time: 10 minutes

Total time: 40 minutes

Makes 8 servings (10 cups)

- 3 to 4 cups water or unsalted broth
- 2 tablespoons extra-virgin olive oil
- 1 large onion, cut into large chunks
- 2 large stalks celery, cut into large chunks
- 2 or 3 cloves garlic
- 2 small carrots, cut into large chunks
- 1 red bell pepper, cut into large chunks
- 1 small jalapeño, poblano, or other mild or medium chile of your choice, seeded
- 1 teaspoon ground cumin
- 1 teaspoon paprika
- 1 teaspoon dried Mexican oregano or regular oregano
- ¼ teaspoon ground chipotle chile
- 1 bay leaf
- 6 cups cooked black beans measured with their cooking liquid (see Do-It-Yourself Beans, page 74; start with about 2½ cups/1 pound dried beans)
- 1½ to 2 teaspoons salt
- 2 tablespoons apple cider vinegar or fresh lime juice
- ½ cup packed, chopped fresh cilantro
- 1 lime, sliced into thin wedges, for garnish

Bring the water to a boil in a kettle or pot.

Heat the olive oil in a large soup pot or Dutch oven over medium heat.

Place the onion, celery, garlic, carrot, bell pepper, jalapeño, cumin, paprika, oregano, and chipotle in a food processor. Pulse until the vegetables are finely minced. Add the vegetable mixture and bay leaf to the hot oil and cook, stirring, until the vegetables soften, 5 to 10 minutes.

Add the beans, hot water, salt, and vinegar. Bring to a boil. Reduce the heat to low and simmer for 15 minutes or more to allow the salt to cook in and the flavors to marry. Taste and adjust the seasonings.

Remove the bay leaf and partially puree the soup directly in the pot with an immersion blender (pulse a few times to get a thick, chunky consistency—do not blend until smooth). Add more water, if needed, to reach the desired consistency. Simmer for 5 minutes more.

Serve hot, garnished with the cilantro and with lime wedges alongside for squeezing. (See photo insert page 11.)

Calories: 227   Protein: 12 g
Carbohydrate: 36 g   Fat: 4 g

Variations

Add a ham bone or cubes of ham when adding the beans.

Creamy Millet Vegetable Soup (Phases 2 and 3)

The sweet vegetables in this soup turn a simple whole grain into a nourishing comfort food.

Preparation time: 15 minutes

Total time: 45 minutes

Makes 4 servings (8 cups)

- 5 to 6 cups water
- 1 tablespoon extra-virgin olive oil
- 1 medium onion, diced
- ½ cup minced cabbage
- 1 cup chopped cauliflower
- 1 cup small chunks peeled winter squash, such as kabocha, butternut, buttercup, etc.
- ½ cup uncooked millet
- 1 bay leaf
- 1 teaspoon salt, or more to taste
- Ground black pepper

Bring the water to a boil in a kettle or pot.

In a separate soup pot, heat the olive oil over medium heat. Add the onion, cabbage, and cauliflower and cook, stirring, until the onion is translucent, about 5 minutes.

Add the squash, millet, bay leaf, salt, and hot water. Bring back to a boil. Cover, reduce the heat to low, and simmer for 30 to 40 minutes, until the vegetables are soft and the millet is creamy.

Season with pepper and more salt to taste. Add enough salt to bring out the naturally sweet taste of the vegetables without making the soup too salty.

Serve hot.

Tip: Millet will continue to absorb water as you cook it, so if you want it thicker and creamier, then cook it longer. The soup will also thicken when refrigerated and may need water added when you reheat it.

Calories: 155   Protein: 4 g
Carbohydrate: 25 g   Fat: 5 g

Broccoli Cheddar Soup (All Phases)

This time-tested pairing always satisfies. Now you can thicken it without the wheat flour and enjoy in any phase.

Preparation time: 15 minutes

Total time: 45 minutes

Makes 8 servings (about 8 cups)

Roux

- 3 tablespoons butter
- 1 tablespoon extra-virgin olive oil
- 5 tablespoons chickpea flour (see Tip, page 91)

Soup

- 2 cups half-and-half
- 3 cups unsalted chicken broth, Bone Broth (page 58), or water
- Pinch of freshly grated nutmeg, or to taste
- ½ teaspoon salt, or to taste
- Ground black pepper, to taste
- 2 broccoli crowns, chopped into small florets, stalks peeled and thinly sliced (about 6 cups)
- 2 to 3 cups freshly grated sharp cheddar cheese (about 10 ounces)

Make the roux: Melt the butter with the olive oil in a large stockpot or Dutch oven over medium heat. Stir in the chickpea flour and cook, stirring continuously, until the mixture bubbles and turns a darker golden brown, 2 to 3 minutes.

Make the soup: Combine the half-and-half, broth, nutmeg, salt, and pepper to taste in a jar or bowl. Add this mixture to the roux, whisking continuously as you pour it in. Stir with the whisk until the mixture comes to a simmer.

Add the broccoli. Bring back to a simmer, stirring frequently. Cover and cook, stirring regularly, for 15 to 20 minutes, or until the broccoli is tender. Once the soup starts to thicken, begin adding the cheese. Any clumps will smooth out and blend into the soup as it cooks. Taste and adjust the seasonings.

Serve hot.

Tip: Some pregrated cheeses can contain starches or powders (to prevent clumping) that will cause your soup to overthicken. Grate your own or choose grated cheese without additives.

Calories: 309   Protein: 13 g
Carbohydrate: 10 g   Fat: 25 g

Variations

For Phases 2 and 3: Substitute whole milk for the half-and-half.

Calories: 272   Protein: 13 g
Carbohydrate: 10 g   Fat: 20 g

Phase 1 Meal: Serve 1 cup of the soup with three 1-ounce slices cooked turkey bacon or similar vegetarian protein (see Equivalents Table, page 49), and a side of salad greens and chopped raw vegetables tossed with 1 to 2 teaspoons Greek Dressing (page 285). **For Dessert:** 1 cup blueberries.

Calories: 593; Carbohydrate: 24%; Protein: 23%; Fat: 54%

Phase 2 Meal: Use the Phases 2 and 3 Variation. Serve 1 cup of the soup with three 1-ounce slices cooked turkey bacon or similar vegetarian protein (see Equivalents Table, page 49), and a side of salad greens tossed with chopped raw vegetables, ¼ cup Cooked Quinoa (page 231), a small diced pear, and 1 to 2 teaspoons Cashew Balsamic Dressing (page 286).

Calories: 606; Carbohydrate: 33%; Protein: 23%; Fat: 44%

Phase 3 Meal: Use the Phases 2 and 3 Variation. Serve 1 cup of the soup with two 1-ounce slices cooked turkey bacon or similar vegetarian protein (see Equivalents Table, page 49), and a side of salad greens tossed with chopped raw vegetables, ½ cup cooked white rice, a small diced pear, and 1 to 2 teaspoons Cashew Balsamic Dressing (page 286).

Calories: 593; Carbohydrate: 39%; Protein: 19%; Fat: 42%

Basic Miso Soup (All Phases)

Easy to make and comforting to eat. Miso contains fermentation products linked to a wide range of health benefits. Add sea vegetables to the mix to create a mineral-rich first course for most any East Asian meal. To get the maximum benefit from your miso, be sure to buy it from the refrigerated section, rather than dried soup packets.

Preparation time: 5 minutes

Total time: 20 minutes

Makes 4 servings (about 8 cups)

- 3 to 4 inches wakame or alaria seaweed
- 6 cups water
- 1 small stalk celery, diced
- 1 cup diced or thinly sliced daikon radish or other root vegetable
- 4 ounces extra-firm tofu, drained, pressed with an absorbent towel, and diced into small pieces (optional)
- 3 to 6 tablespoons miso paste (any type)
- 1 scallion, thinly sliced

Break the seaweed into small pieces or soak it in the water until soft enough to cut with a knife. Place the water and seaweed in a pot and bring to a boil over medium heat.

Add the vegetables and tofu. Reduce the heat to medium and cook until the vegetables are just tender, 5 to 10 minutes.

Transfer about ½ cup of the broth to a small cup or bowl. Add 3 tablespoons of the miso and stir to dissolve.

Stir the dissolved miso into the soup. Turn off the heat and allow the miso to simmer in the hot broth for a couple of minutes. It will begin to form cloudy eruptions as it activates and will look like it is boiling in the water.

Taste and adjust the seasonings. If you're using lighter miso, you may need to add up to 3 tablespoons more to achieve the desired flavor (dissolve it in some of the broth separately before adding it), whereas you may not need to add any more if you're using a darker, heartier miso.

Serve the soup hot, garnished with the scallion.

Calories: 85
Carbohydrate: 8 g

Protein: 7 g
Fat: 3 g

Chef Dawn's Tasty Tip

Miso Magic

Like fine wine, miso varies widely in flavor and salt content. Lighter, golden-colored types require a shorter fermentation period, yielding a mellow flavor, with soft, sweet undertones. Heartier, darker miso delivers a robust flavor. Miso can substitute for salt, enhancing a variety of sweet or savory soups, sauces, and marinades. Some of my favorites are the lighter miso added to Creamy Millet Vegetable Soup (page 255), or a combination of lighter and heartier misos added to Split Pea Soup (page 251), Chicken Soup on a Budget (page 243), or any of the bean dishes. Experiment yourself to create a simple, exquisite meal.

SALADS

Greek Salad (All Phases)

Our zesty Greek Dressing adds extra liveliness to crisp vegetables and tangy feta. This classic salad is easy enough to enter the regular rotation.

Preparation time: 5 minutes

Total time: 5 minutes

Makes 4 servings

- 6 cups lettuce or salad greens of your choice
- 1 large tomato, diced
- 1 large cucumber, diced
- ½ small red onion, halved and sliced into thin half-moons, or ¼ cup Pickled Red Onions (page 69)
- 10 to 12 Kalamata olives, pitted
- 1 cup cooked chickpeas (see Do-It-Yourself Beans, page 74) or canned chickpeas, drained and rinsed
- 4 ounces feta cheese
- 2 to 3 tablespoons Greek Dressing (page 285)

Toss all the ingredients together in a large bowl.

Calories: 252
Carbohydrate: 19 g

Protein: 10 g
Fat: 16 g

Variations

For Phases 2 and 3: Add 1⅓ cups Cooked Quinoa (page 231).

Phase 1 Meal: Add ¼ avocado and ½ cup Shredded Chicken (page 110). Serve with 1 cup Minestrone Soup (page 248). **For Dessert:** 1 Chocolate Truffle (page 314).

Calories: 667; Carbohydrate: 26%; Protein: 26%; Fat: 48%

Phase 2 Meal: Use the Phase 2 and 3 Variation, and add Beef, Bison, or Turkey Meatballs (page 149). **For Dessert:** 1 cup blueberries.

Calories: 688; Carbohydrate: 37%; Protein: 22%; Fat: 41%

Phase 3 Meal: Serve with a 4-inch whole wheat pita drizzled with 1 teaspoon olive oil, and 1 cup Sicilian Fava Bean Soup (page 244). **For Dessert:** Apple Pie Parfait (page 319).

Calories: 652; Carbohydrate: 42%; Protein: 16%; Fat: 42%

Jicama, Clementine, and Avocado Salad (All Phases)

A perfect salad for warm summer nights. Jicama has a sweet, fruity flavor similar to a pear, with the crunch of a crisp apple. Give this simple salad a try to see just how satisfying jicama can be!

Preparation time: 10 minutes

Total time: 10 minutes

Makes 4 servings

- 1 small jicama, peeled and diced (about 2 cups)
- 2 avocados, diced
- 3 medium clementines or mandarins, peeled, sectioned, and cut into pieces
- 1 ounce fresh cilantro, stems and leaves minced (about ½ cup)
- Juice of 1 lime

Combine all the ingredients in a bowl, making sure to cover the avocado well with the lime juice to keep it from browning. Serve immediately, or cover and refrigerate for up to 3 days. (See photo insert page 13.)

Calories: 180
Carbohydrate: 22 g

Protein: 3 g
Fat: 11 g

Variation

For Phase 3 or when serving with higher-fat recipes, use only 1 avocado.

The Perfect Cucumber-Tomato Salad (All Phases)

This refreshing salad is designed to complement higher-fat meals. Crisp vegetables and tangy lemon will leave you feeling refreshed after a rich entrée. Choose thin-skinned, low-seed cucumbers like English or Persian. If you've made them ahead of time, Pickled Red Onions enhance the flavor of these simple ingredients.

Preparation time: 5 minutes

Total time: 5 minutes

Makes 4 servings

- ½ small red onion, thinly sliced
- ½ teaspoon salt or 1 to 2 tablespoons umeboshi vinegar (see page 64)
- 1 pound cucumber (about 2 Persian or 1 English hothouse cucumber), diced (see Tip)
- 1 large ripe tomato, diced
- ¼ cup packed, chopped fresh parsley or cilantro, stems and leaves
- 1 tablespoon fresh lemon or lime juice

Combine onions and salt in a large bowl. Massage the salt into the onions until the onions become soft and release their liquid, about 1 minute. Stir in the cucumber, tomato, parsley, and lemon juice until well combined. Taste and adjust the seasonings. Serve immediately or refrigerate for up to 3 days.

Tip: If using large cucumbers with heavy or tough seeds and thick skin, seed and peel them.

Calories: 25   Protein: 2 g
Carbohydrate: 5 g   Fat: 0 g

Variation

Substitute ¼ to ½ cup Pickled Red Onions (page 69) for the sliced onions, and adjust the salt to taste.

Fresh Quinoa Salad with Pomegranates (Phases 2 and 3)

Fresh vegetables with zesty lemons, garlic, and pomegranate seeds turn simple quinoa into a bright burst of flavor.

Preparation time: 10 minutes plus 1 hour resting time

Total time: 10 minutes

Makes 4 servings

- 1 cup Cooked Quinoa (page 231), cooled
- 1 medium tomato, finely diced
- 1 medium carrot, shredded
- ¼ cup pomegranate seeds
- ¼ cup Gremolata (page 299)
- 1 to 3 teaspoons fresh lemon juice, or to taste
- ¼ teaspoon salt, or to taste
- ¼ teaspoon ground black pepper, or to taste

Toss all the ingredients together in a large bowl. Set aside for at least 1 hour or make a day ahead to allow the flavors to develop. Taste and adjust the seasonings. Serve.

Store in an airtight container in the refrigerator for up to a few days.

Calories: 79
Carbohydrate: 15 g
Protein: 3 g
Fat: 1 g

Variation

Add 1 to 2 tablespoons olive oil when serving with lower-fat meals.

Texas Caviar (Black-Eyed Pea Salad) (All Phases)

This refreshing take on black-eyed pea salad makes a creative use for leftover beans. You can substitute any small beans that hold together well when cooked, like French lentils or adzuki beans. Make it ahead to allow the flavors time to fully develop.

Preparation time: 10 minutes plus 1 hour resting time

Total time: 1 hour 10 minutes

Makes 4 to 6 servings

- 2 cups cooked black-eyed peas, French lentils, or mung beans, or 1½ cups adzuki beans (see Do-It-Yourself Beans, page 74; start with ⅔ to ¾ cup dried beans), or equivalent drained and rinsed canned beans
- ¼ cup Pickled Red Onions (page 69), or ½ small red onion, minced
- ½ small red, yellow, or green bell pepper, finely diced
- ½ cup packed, chopped fresh cilantro or parsley, stems and leaves
- 2 to 3 tablespoons Creamy Peppercorn Vinaigrette (page 286)

Toss all the ingredients together in a large bowl. Cover and refrigerate for at least 1 hour or make a day ahead to allow the flavors to develop.

Store in an airtight container in the refrigerator for up to 1 week.

Based on 4 servings	Carbohydrate: 20 g	Fat: 6 g
Calories: 156	Protein: 7 g	

Variation

For a spicy salad, add a small can of green chiles, or a few tablespoons minced fresh chile like jalapeño, serrano, or poblano, or to taste.

BUDDHA BOWLS

Chef Dawn's Tasty Tip

Buddha Bowls

A trendy name for a layered or sectioned, full-meal bowl that each person builds themselves is the Buddha bowl. Everything (veggies, beans, protein, etc.) is put over a base, usually greens or grains. Then a signature sauce is poured on top and...voilà! A personalized meal for everyone at the table.

First, you need a base, something hearty and delicious, to create cohesiveness in your Buddha bowl: fresh or steamed greens, whole kernel grains, or root vegetables.

Next choose your toppings. Beans are not necessary in every Buddha bowl, but they add nice flavor, texture, color, and some extra protein; some other good-quality carbs; and some fat. Any beans will work (black, pinto, chickpeas, etc.—see Do-It-Yourself Beans, page 74), whole or pureed, like Refried Beans (page 225), and sometimes seasoned (simple or spicy—salt, pepper, garlic powder, cumin, ground chile, or even a bit of fresh salsa cooked into them). Even a bit of hummus will do.

Then choose any protein you like: chicken, beef, pork, seafood, or vegetarian proteins.

In addition to other toppings, sauté or roast some onions, bell peppers, mushrooms, zucchini, or other favorite vegetables to round out the bowl, or simply use leftover vegetable side dishes from the previous night's dinner. Higher-fat toppings such as cheese, sour cream, or avocado, or fresh toppings like shredded carrots, onions, cabbage, or lightly pickled vegetables (see Do-It-Yourself Pickles, pages 62 to 71) are also nice in these Buddha bowls.

Finally, the sauce brings your Buddha bowl together. From a simple drizzle of oil to an elaborate and flavorful sauce or a squeeze of lemon, each bowl will call for a different sauce to make it shine. Buddha bowls are also an efficient way to use leftovers.

Japanese Buddha Bowl (Phases 2 and 3, with Phase 1 Variation)

Make the components ahead of time and assemble this Asian-flavored bowl for an impressive lunch or dinner when you are traveling or won't have time to cook.

Preparation time: 5 minutes

Total time: 10 minutes

Makes 1 serving

- 1 teaspoon toasted sesame oil
- ½ cup broccoli florets
- 1 small carrot, shredded or cut into matchsticks (⅓ to ½ cup)
- 6 to 8 snow peas or snap peas
- 1 tablespoon water
- ½ cup cooked brown rice
- 6 ounces Marinated Baked Tofu (page 175) in Spicy Asian Marinade (page 294) or other favorite sauce
- 1 serving Seasoned Shiitake Mushrooms (page 217)
- 2 teaspoons Ginger Tahini Dressing (page 288)
- 1 tablespoon toasted sesame seeds

Heat the sesame oil in a skillet over medium heat. Add the broccoli and carrots. Cook, stirring, for 3 to 5 minutes, or until vegetables become tender-crisp and are still bright in color. Add the peas and water. Cover and steam gently for 1 minute to lightly cook the peas.

Place the brown rice in the bottom of a bowl.

Layer or section the vegetables, tofu, and mushrooms in the bowl, and top with the dressing and sesame seeds. Serve or pack for a to-go meal.

Calories: 608   Protein: 35 g
Carbohydrate: 56 g   Fat: 28 g

Variations

Substitute On-a-Budget Marinated Chicken (page 116, baked in Spicy Asian Marinade, page 294) for the tofu.

For Phase 1: Substitute ½ cup shelled edamame for the brown rice; add a tangerine, peeled and sectioned; and use the Spicy Asian Marinade (page 294; without honey).

For Phase 3: Substitute 1½ ounces cooked udon or soba noodles for the brown rice.

Phase 1 Meal: Use the Phase 1 Variation.

Calories: 588; Carbohydrate: 24%; Protein: 28%; Fat: 48%

Phase 2 Meal: Serve as per the recipe.

Calories: 608; Carbohydrate: 36%; Protein: 23%; Fat: 41%

Phase 3 Meal: Use the Phase 3 Variation.

Calories: 626; Carbohydrate: 37%; Protein: 24%; Fat: 39%

Grilled Salmon Buddha Bowl (All Phases)

Simple and flavorful, this bowl will rival any grab-and-go prepared food at a lower cost and with higher-quality ingredients. Serve with warm salmon fresh from the oven or grill, or chilled leftovers from the refrigerator.

Preparation time: 5 minutes

Total time: 5 minutes

Makes 1 serving

- 1 cup mixed lettuces
- Handful of sprouts of your choice
- ½ cup thinly shredded cabbage
- ½ small carrot or other vegetable, such as daikon radish, shredded (⅓ to ½ cup)
- 4 to 5 ounces cooked salmon, such as Easy Dijon Salmon (page 128) or Teriyaki Salmon (page 141; Phases 2 and 3 only)
- 1 small tangerine, peeled and sectioned
- ½ avocado
- ¼ recipe Sautéed Bok Choy and Shiitake (page 213) or other sautéed vegetables
- 2 to 3 tablespoons Ginger Tahini Dressing (page 288)

Arrange all the ingredients, except the dressing, in a bowl, either layered or in sections. Top with or toss with the dressing. (See photo insert page 4.)

Tip: Start with 6 ounces raw fish to yield about 4½ ounces cooked.

Calories: 581   Protein: 44 g
Carbohydrate: 36 g   Fat: 32 g

Phase 1 Meal: Use Easy Dijon Salmon (page 128) or any grilled or broiled salmon. **For Dessert:** 1 Chocolate Truffle (page 314).

Calories: 684; Carbohydrate: 25%; Protein: 25%; Fat: 50%

Phase 2 Meal: Use Teriyaki Salmon (page 141). Substitute ½ cup Cooked Quinoa (page 231) for the tangerine. **For Dessert:** 2 Chocolate-Dipped Strawberries (page 313).

Calories: 687; Carbohydrate: 34%; Protein: 27%; Fat: 39%

Phase 3 Meal: Use a smaller portion of Teriyaki Salmon (page 141). Substitute 1 ounce soba noodles, cooked, for the tangerine. **For Dessert:** ½ apple, cored and sliced, topped with 1½ tablespoons Coconut Cardamom Macadamia Butter (page 57).

Calories: 675; Carbohydrate: 38%; Protein: 22%; Fat: 40%

Greek Salad Buddha Bowl (All Phases)

Nothing like a Greek salad for zesty, fresh, satisfying flavors. Adding falafel and chicken rounds out this bowl, creating a complete meal that will leave you satisfied.

Preparation time: 10 minutes

Total time: 10 minutes

Makes 1 serving

- 1 teaspoon tahini
- 1 teaspoon fresh lemon juice
- 1 cup mixed salad greens
- 1 small tomato, diced
- ½ cup diced cucumber
- ¼ cup thinly sliced red onion
- ⅓ cup cooked chickpeas (see Do-It-Yourself Beans, page 74) or canned chickpeas, drained and rinsed
- A few Kalamata olives, pitted
- 3 to 4 ounces cooked chicken, such as ½ cup Shredded Chicken (page 110) or store-bought rotisserie chicken, or equivalent vegetarian protein (see Equivalents Table, page 49)
- 2 tablespoons crumbled feta cheese (about ½ ounce)
- 1 tablespoon Greek Dressing (page 285)
- ⅓ serving (about 2 patties) Falafel (page 178)

Combine the tahini and lemon juice in a small bowl, adding a bit of water to reach a thinner consistency, if desired. Set aside.

In a large bowl, toss the greens, tomato, cucumber, red onion, chickpeas, olives, chicken, and feta with the dressing. Arrange the falafel on top and spread or drizzle the tahini-lemon mixture on the falafel.

Calories: 605   Protein: 38 g
Carbohydrate: 37 g   Fat: 36 g

Phase 1 Meal: For Dessert: 2 Chocolate-Dipped Strawberries (page 313).

Calories: 658; Carbohydrate: 26%; Protein: 23%; Fat: 51%

Phase 2 Meal: Omit the tahini and lemon juice. Add ⅓ cup Cooked Quinoa (page 231) and reduce the feta to 1 tablespoon. **For Dessert:** ½ cup blueberries.

  Calories: 663; Carbohydrate: 35%; Protein: 23%; Fat: 42%

Phase 3 Meal: Omit the tahini and lemon juice. Reduce the feta to 1 tablespoon. Serve with a 4-inch whole wheat pita. **For Dessert:** ½ cup blueberries.

  Calories: 663; Carbohydrate: 36%; Protein: 22%; Fat: 41%

French Salad Niçoise Buddha Bowl
(Phases 2 and 3, with Phase 1 Variation)

Transport yourself to the South of France with these timeless flavors. Elegant simplicity.

Preparation time: 10 minutes

Total time: 15 minutes

Makes 1 serving

- ½ cup green beans
- ½ cup cooked brown rice
- 3 ounces canned tuna
- 1 egg, hard-boiled and sliced
- A few Kalamata olives or other olives of your choice, pitted
- 1 small tomato, diced
- ½ red bell pepper, diced
- 1 tablespoon capers
- 1 cup mixed lettuces
- 1 to 2 tablespoons Creamy Peppercorn Vinaigrette (page 286)
- A few anchovies, for garnish (optional)

Place about 2 inches of water into a small pot and bring to a boil over high heat. Immerse the green beans in the boiling water for 15 seconds, until they are tender-crisp and still bright. Remove with a mesh skimmer or slotted spoon and set aside in a colander or on a plate covered with a bamboo sushi mat to drain.

Arrange all the ingredients except the vinaigrette and anchovies in a large bowl. Toss with the vinaigrette and top with the anchovies, if desired.

Calories: 535
Carbohydrate: 43 g

Protein: 37 g
Fat: 25 g

Phase 1 Meal: Substitute ⅓ cup cooked cannellini beans for the brown rice, double the number of olives, and use the higher amount of dressing or add a drizzle of olive oil. **For Dessert:** 2 Chocolate-Dipped Strawberries (page 313).

Calories: 619; Carbohydrate: 25%; Protein: 25%; Fat: 50%

Phase 2 Meal: For Dessert: 1 tangerine.

Calories: 575; Carbohydrate: 36%; Protein: 26%; Fat: 38%

Phase 3 Meal: Substitute 1 cup diced boiled Yukon Gold potatoes for the brown rice. **For Dessert:** 1 tangerine.

Calories: 587; Carbohydrate: 39%; Protein: 25%; Fat: 36%

My *Always Delicious* Story

For much of my life, I was literally always hungry and needed to eat every two hours or so. If I didn't eat frequently, I would get all sorts of symptoms, including the shakes, chest pain, cold sweats, and nausea. No matter how much I ate, I was still constantly hungry. Nothing seemed to satisfy the cravings for long. But the more I ate, the more I gained… and the worse I felt. I'd go to bed earlier every evening, wake up every couple hours, and start the day dead tired. Afternoon naps became necessary just to function. As a single mother of three, I simply couldn't keep it up. I was losing a battle, but against an unknown adversary—and it frustrated me terribly.

Reading *Always Hungry?* was a long-awaited wakeup call. At first, I was amazed how much food I was supposed to eat, but ate it I did, and I regretted nothing! After just a few days, I felt better than I had in years. My symptoms, which I had attributed to stress, disappeared so quickly that I realized they were in fact linked to food. Afternoon naps and dead-tired mornings soon became a thing of the past! I'm now up early, rested, and functional the entire day! My cravings are easily satisfied with fresh fruit and nuts. Even my greatest nemesis, potato chips, no longer taste all that great anymore. I wish I had known about this program years ago, instead of wasting so much time on those unsustainable low-calorie diets.

—*Solweig B., age 52, Edmonton, Alberta, Canada*

CHAPTER 10

Snacks & Appetizers

Spinach Onion Pakoras with Tamarind Dipping Sauce (Phases 2 and 3, with Phase 1 Variation)

Pakoras are a popular Indian street food, typically served fresh from the sizzling oil. Dip them in our sweet tamarind sauce for a crowd-pleasing appetizer. We recommend a trip to your local Indian market or online ordering for the tamarind concentrate or tamarind paste. Personalize the pakoras with your favorite curry mixture in place of the spices listed, or add your own favorite spice combinations.

Preparation time: 20 minutes

Total time: 30 minutes

Makes 6 servings (about 30 pakoras)

Tamarind Sauce

- 2 small dates, pitted
- ¼ cup raisins
- ¾ cup water
- 1 to 2 teaspoons minced mild to medium chile, such as serrano or jalapeño
- 5 or 6 sprigs cilantro, stems and leaves coarsely chopped
- 2 teaspoons chopped fresh mint
- 1 tablespoon tamarind concentrate or 3 tablespoons tamarind paste
- ¼ teaspoon garam masala (see Tip, page 182)
- ⅛ teaspoon salt

Pakoras

- ¼ cup water
- 1 (½-inch) piece fresh ginger, peeled and sliced into rounds
- 1 medium onion, cut into thin half-moons
- 8 ounces baby spinach, coarsely chopped (4 to 5 cups packed)
- ¼ teaspoon salt
- 1 to 2 teaspoons minced mild to medium chile, such as serrano or jalapeño
- ½ teaspoon garlic powder
- ½ to 1 teaspoon ground cumin
- ½ to 1 teaspoon ground coriander
- ½ to 1 teaspoon ground turmeric
- ⅛ teaspoon cayenne pepper or other powdered chile (optional, for a spicier pakora)
- 1½ cups chickpea flour (see Tip, page 91)
- ½ teaspoon baking powder.
- ½ cup neutral-tasting oil, such as high-oleic safflower or avocado oil

Make the sauce: Place all the sauce ingredients in a wide-mouthed glass jar or cup that will fit an immersion blender without splashing. Blend until smooth. Taste and adjust the seasonings. Place a lid on the jar. For best results, set aside for at least 1 hour to allow the flavors to develop. The sauce will keep in the refrigerator for up to 2 weeks.

Make the pakoras: Place water and ginger into a wide-mouthed glass jar or cup that will fit an immersion blender without splashing. Blend, working the blender into the ginger until the pieces are finely shredded. Set aside.

Place the onion, spinach, and salt in a large bowl. Rub the vegetables together with your hands for a few minutes until the juices begin to release. Stir in the chiles, garlic powder, cumin, coriander, turmeric, cayenne (if using), and the pureed ginger mixture.

Combine the chickpea flour and baking powder. Add to the vegetable mixture and stir until the flour is evenly distributed and has been completely absorbed.

To panfry the pakoras, heat the oil in a 12-inch cast-iron skillet. To deep-fry, heat 2 to 3 inches of oil in a deep fryer, heavy-bottomed pot, or wok to 325 to 350°F. Drop about 2 tablespoons of the batter at a time into the hot oil, working in batches to avoid crowding the pan, and cook, turning, until golden brown on all sides. Use a slotted spoon to transfer the pakoras to a plate lined with paper towels or covered with a bamboo sushi mat to drain. Having the oil at the right temperature is the key to browning the pakoras without leaving them soggy, so be sure not to crowd the pan and take time to let the oil come back to temperature between batches (see Chef Dawn's Tasty Tip on page 167 for more on deep-frying).

Keep the pakoras warm in the oven until ready to serve. Serve with the tamarind sauce for dipping.

Calories: 239 (with sauce)	Carbohydrate: 30 g Protein: 7 g	Fat: 11 g
Calories: 23 (Tamarind sauce per tablespoon)	Carbohydrate: 6 g Protein: 0 g	Fat: 0 g

Variations

For Phase 1, serve the pakoras without the tamarind sauce, or use your favorite Phase 1 sauce for dipping.

Chef Dawn's Tasty Tip

Spice It Up

Although I usually limit ingredients for everyday cooking to those easily available at most grocers, a few are worth a little extra effort. Tamarind is one of them. A common ingredient in Indian and Thai cooking, tamarind's unique sour flavor makes it an excellent addition to sauces and marinades. Although available in many forms, the dark syrupy concentrate and the thick paste are my favorites, and both provide a wealth of flavor with just a touch. Typically, 1 tablespoon of concentrate equals about 3 tablespoons of paste. Dilute either with water. Add tamarind to raisins and spices for a sweet-and-sour dipping sauce like Tamarind Sauce (see page 270) or to add depth to a savory flavoring like Sugar-Free Worcestershire Sauce (page 284). It's an ingredient worth trying.

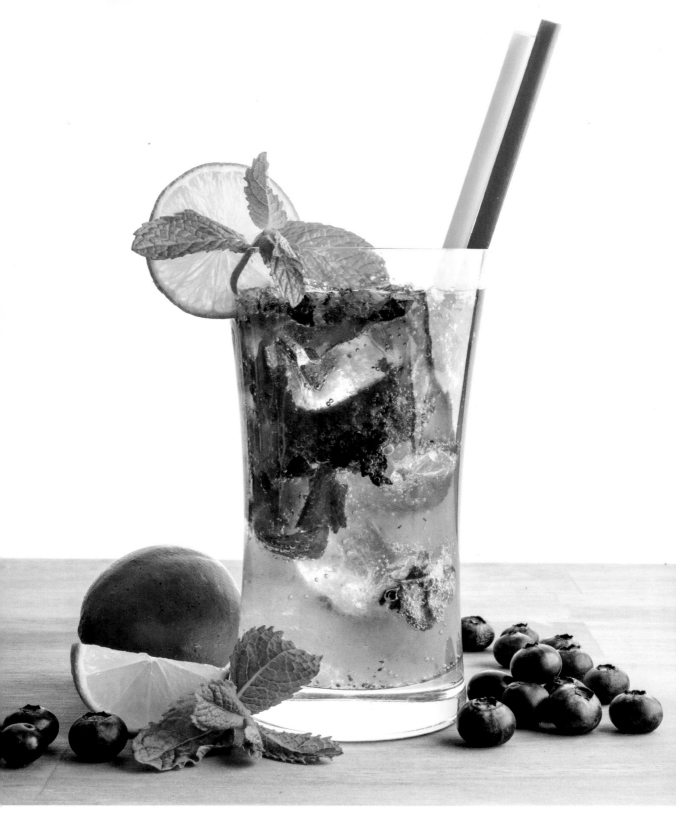

Blueberry Lime Mint Fizz, page 308

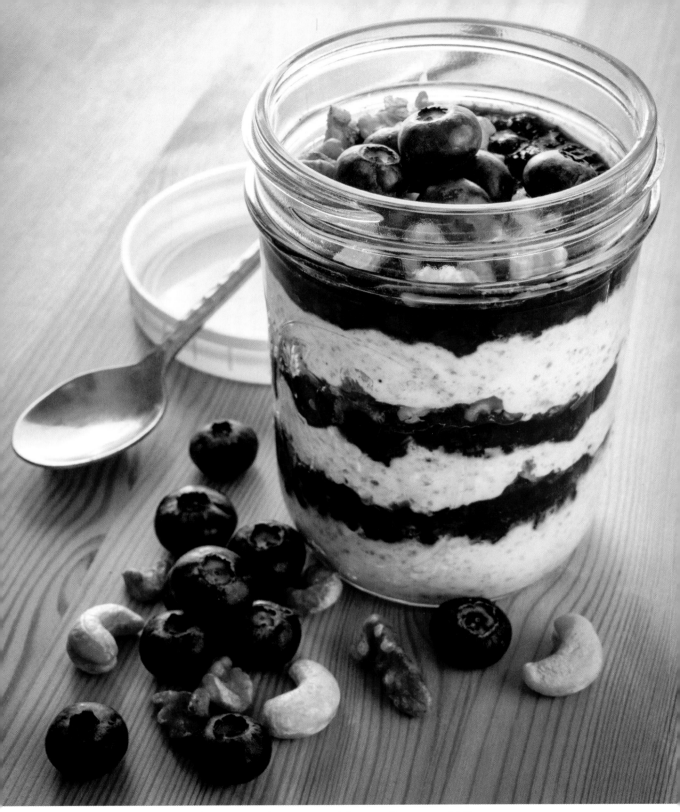

On-the-Go Breakfast Parfait, page 106

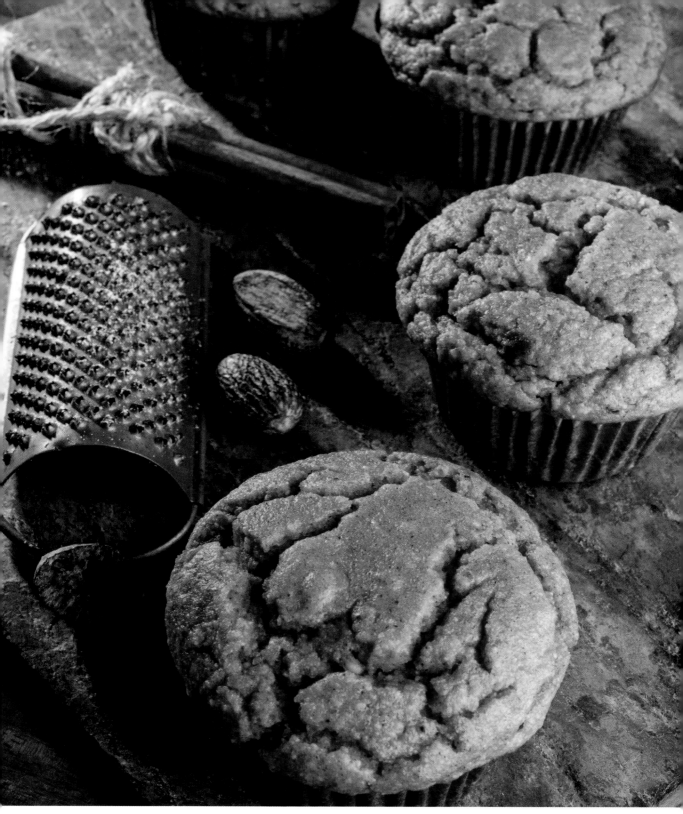

Grain-Free Pumpkin Spice Muffins, page 90

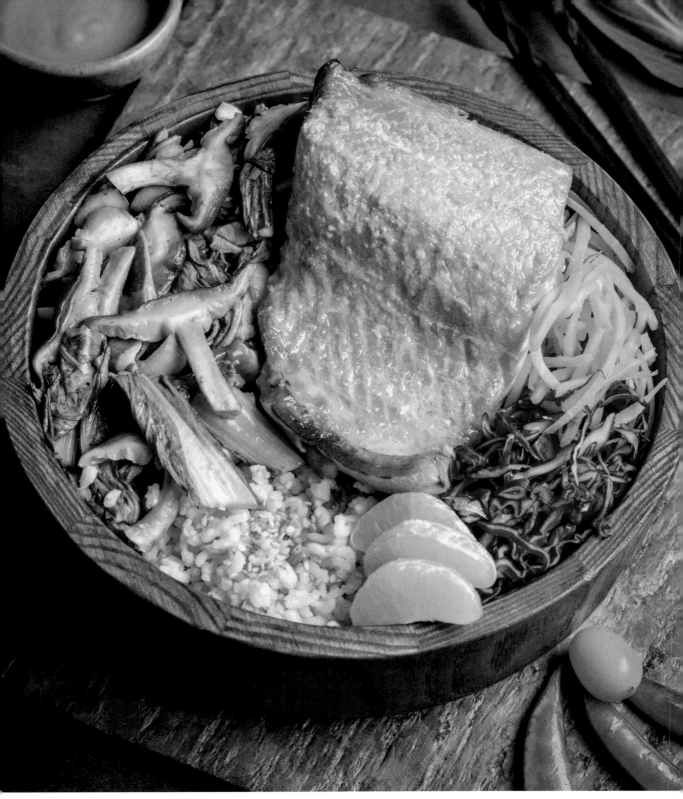

Grilled Salmon Buddha Bowl, page 266, with Teriyaki Salmon, page 141,
Sautéed Bok Choy and Shiitake, page 213, and Ginger Tahini Dressing, page 288

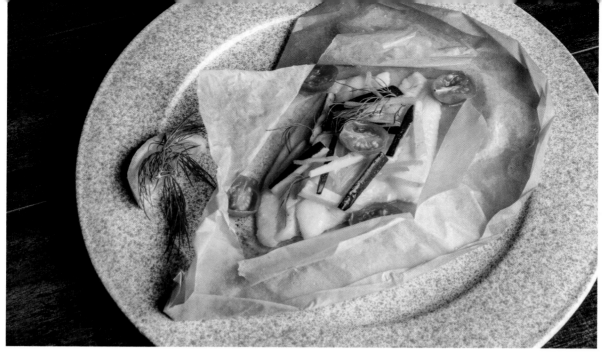

Parchment-Baked Fish (Fish en Papillote), page 138

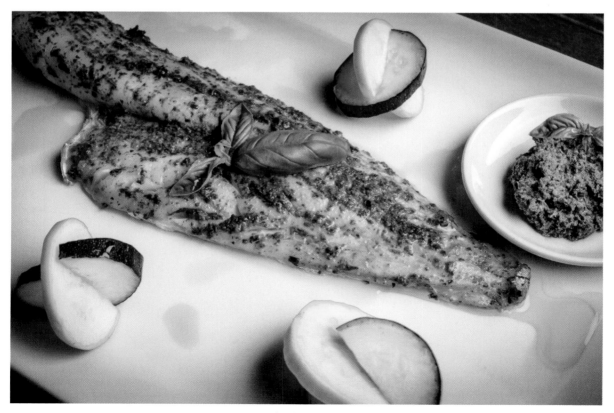

Pesto Baked Fish, page 143

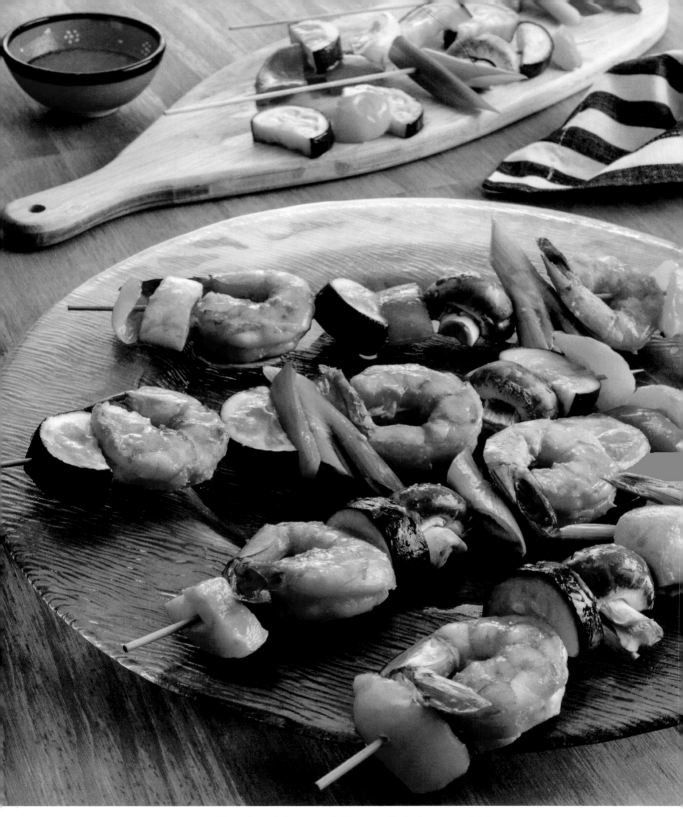

Drunken Marinated Shrimp Kebabs, page 144

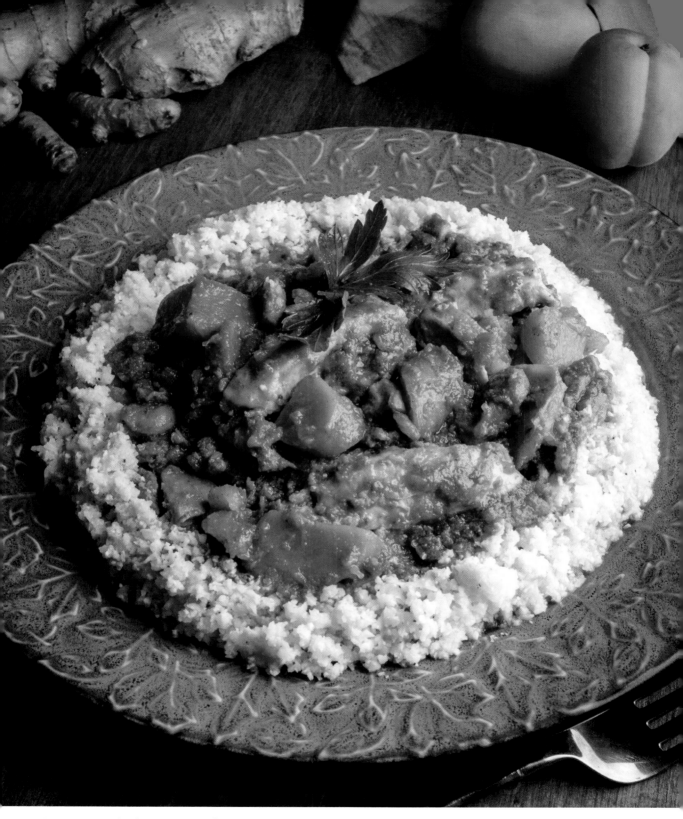

Moroccan Chicken Stew with Apricots, page 133, served with Cauliflower Couscous, page 211

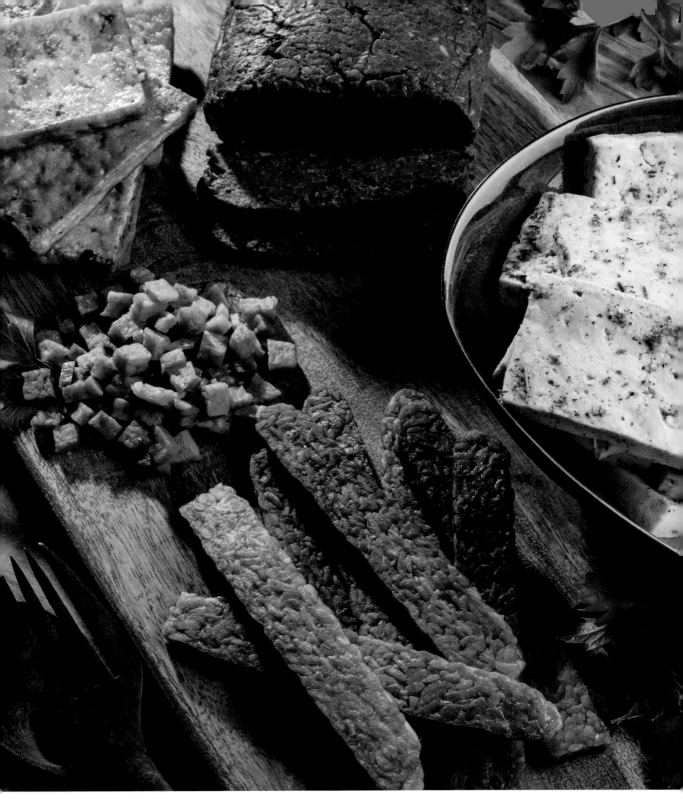

Smoke-Dried Tomato Seitan, page 73, Panfried Tofu and Tempeh, page 193,
Crumbled Tempeh, page 192, Marinated Baked Tofu, page 175, in Lemon Thyme Marinade, page 296

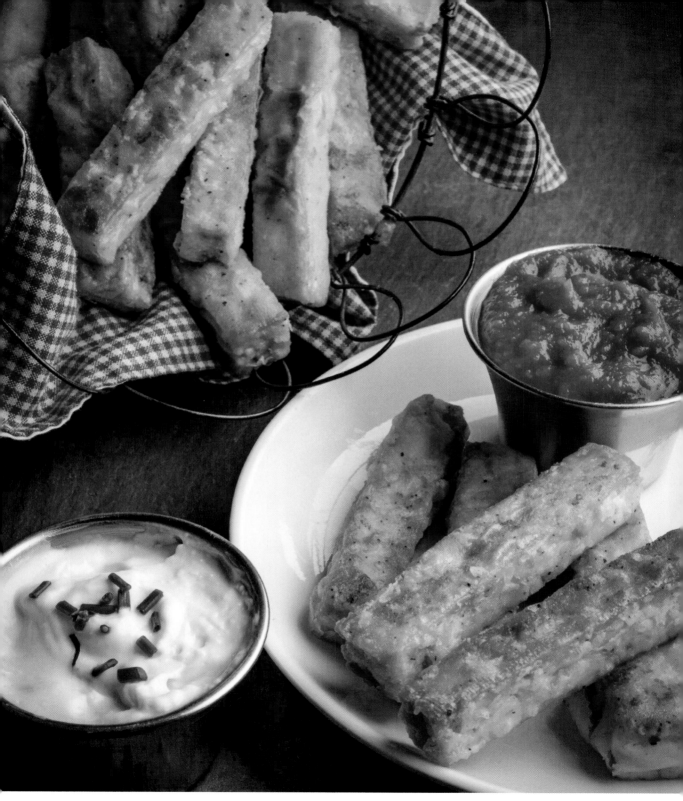

Crispy Tofu Fries, page 173, with Smoked Paprika Ketchup, page 291, and Lemon Aioli, page 298

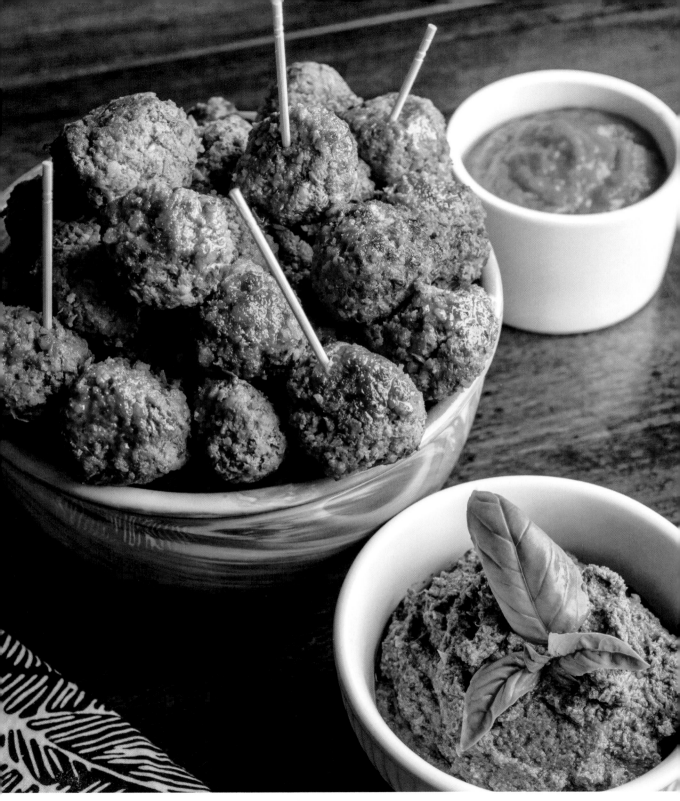

Beef, Bison, or Turkey Meatballs, page 149, with Smoked Paprika Ketchup, page 291, and Basil Walnut Pesto, page 297

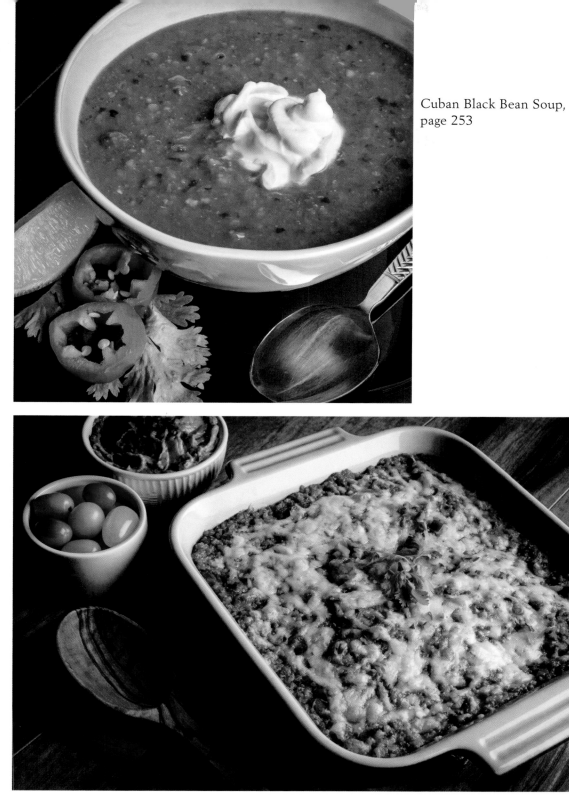

Cuban Black Bean Soup, page 253

Quinoa Enchilada Casserole, page 183

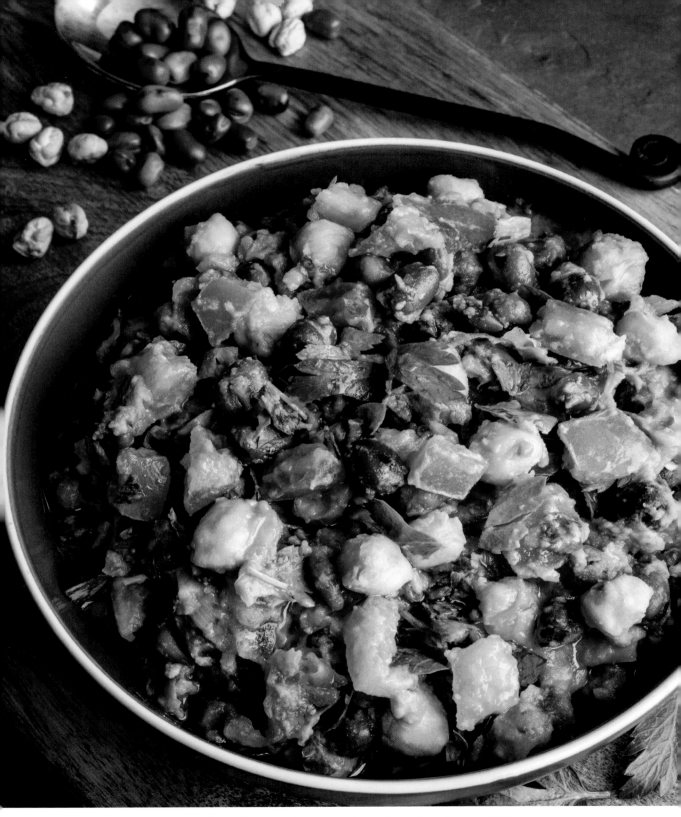

Ful Mudammas (Egyptian Fava Bean Stew), page 222

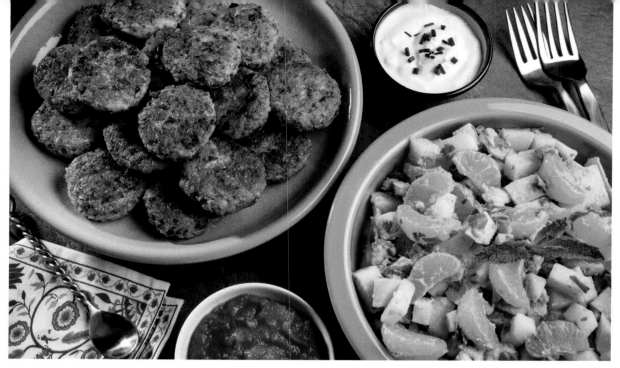

Quinoa Croquettes, page 232, with Lemon Aioli, page 298, and Smoked Paprika Ketchup, page 291, dipping sauces, and Jicama, Clementine, and Avocado Salad, page 260

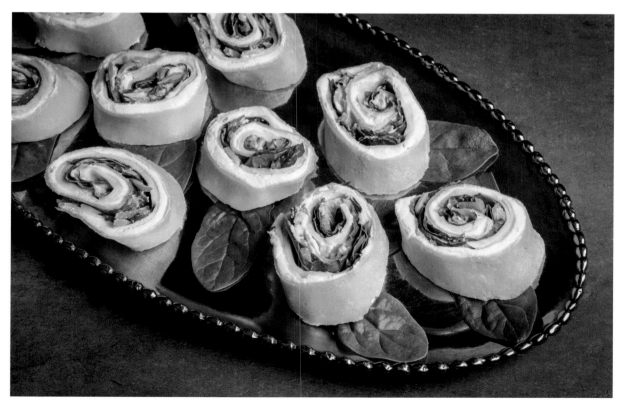

Socca Pinwheels, page 273

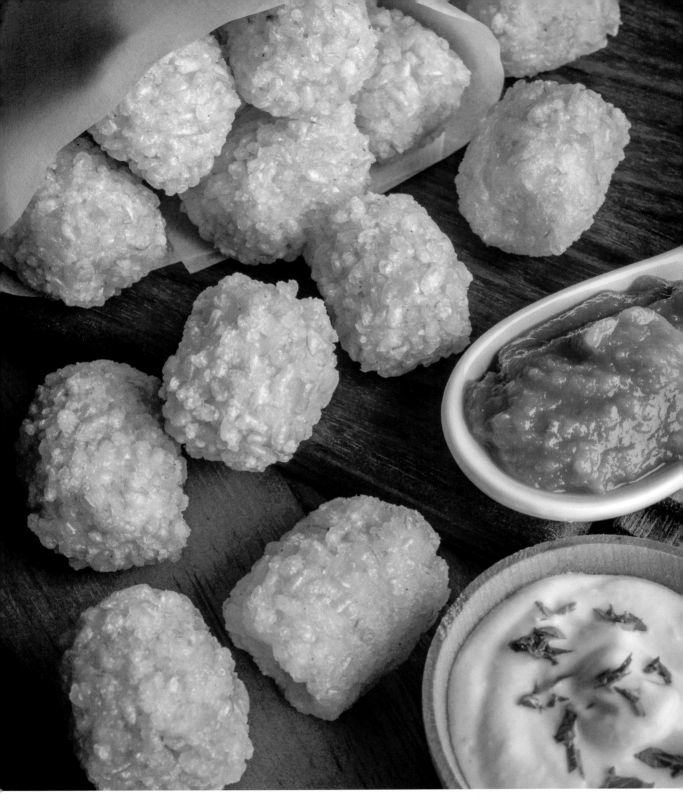

Brown Rice "Tater" Tots, page 228, with Lemon Aioli, page 298, and Smoked Paprika Ketchup, page 291, dipping sauces

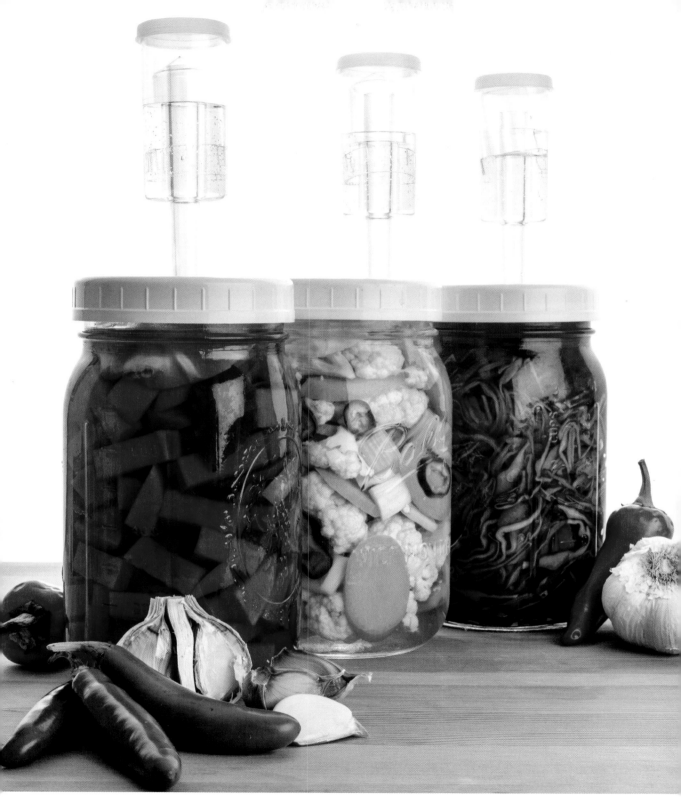

Do-It-Yourself Pickles, page 62—Middle Eastern Pickled Turnips, page 67,
Spicy Pickled Vegetables (Escabeche), page 68, and Easy Pickled Cabbage, page 66

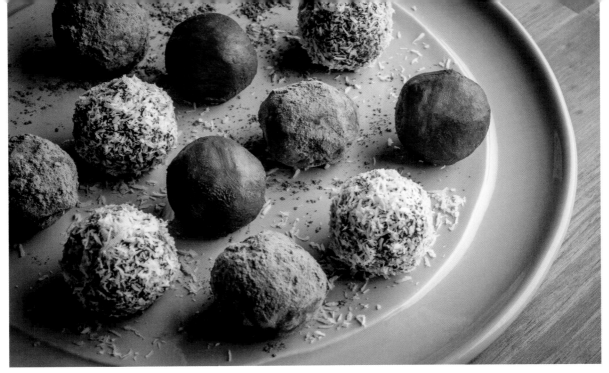

Chocolate Truffles, page 314

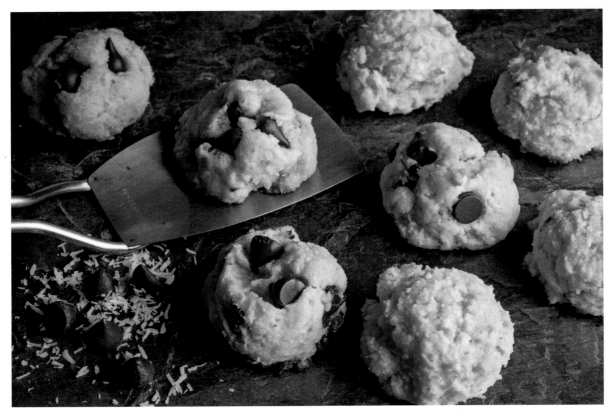

Almond Coconut Macaroons, page 312

Socca Pinwheels (All Phases)

The ultimate retro snack with a modern twist, these attractive little roll-ups are a great choice for potlucks, parties, or snack boxes. They may become your new go-to delicious finger food.

Preparation time: 10 minutes

Total time: 10 minutes

Makes 4 to 6 servings

- 4 ounces sliced deli meat or smoked salmon
- 4 ounces deli-sliced cheese or spreadable goat cheese
- 2 Basic Socca Wraps (page 198)
- 2 ounces arugula or spinach, chopped (about 1 cup packed)
- 2 tablespoons Lemon Aioli (page 298)
- ¼ cup shredded carrots

Layer the meat and sliced cheese on the wraps, distributing them evenly between the two. Toss the arugula and carrots with the aioli and spread it evenly over the top of the sliced cheese.

Starting on one edge, roll the wrap into a log as tightly as you can. Cut the roll crosswise into ½- to 1-inch-thick slices (cut them on an angle for a nice presentation), leaving the end pieces a bit thicker to keep them from falling apart. (See photo insert page 13.)

Based on 4 servings
Calories: 232

Carbohydrate: 5 g
Protein: 15 g

Fat: 16 g

Variations

Substitute hummus, Basil Walnut Pesto (page 297), Lime Cilantro Pesto (page 298), or another favorite dressing for the Lemon Aioli.

Black Bean Pâté (All Phases)

Packed with rich flavors, this pâté closely resembles the texture of a traditional meat pâté, making it versatile enough to serve to a meat-eating or vegetarian crowd. Make it a few days ahead and refrigerate to allow the flavors to fully meld, and serve as an easy but impressive appetizer for parties, potlucks, and entertaining.

Preparation time: 5 minutes

Total time: 1 to 1½ hours

Makes 6 to 8 servings

- 1 teaspoon extra-virgin olive oil or olive oil spray, for the pan
- 1 medium onion, cut into large chunks
- 2 cloves garlic
- 6 large scallions, coarsely chopped, plus 1 scallion, sliced, for garnish
- 10 to 12 sprigs cilantro
- 2 teaspoons green or black peppercorns, coarsely ground (about 1½ teaspoons ground pepper)
- 3 cups cooked black beans (see Do-It-Yourself Beans, page 74) or drained and rinsed canned beans
- 6 tablespoons tahini
- 2 tablespoons red miso or other hearty or dark-colored miso paste
- ¼ teaspoon salt, or to taste
- ¾ cup hulled pumpkin seeds, lightly toasted (see Guide to Roasting Nuts, page 334)
- 1 scallion, thinly sliced

Preheat the oven to 350°F. Rub an 8 x 4-inch loaf pan with the olive oil or coat with olive oil spray.

Combine the onion, garlic, scallions, and cilantro in a food processor and pulse until finely chopped. Add the ground peppercorns, beans, tahini, and miso and process until smooth. Taste and add the salt, using more or less as needed, depending on the saltiness of the beans; remember that the flavor will come together as the pâté bakes or sets in the refrigerator. Add the pumpkin seeds and process until just coarsely broken down.

Spread the bean mixture evenly into the prepared loaf pan and cover with foil. Bake until a golden crust surrounds the edges, 1½ to 2 hours. Remove the foil for the last 15 minutes. The loaf will rise as it bakes. For a denser texture, remove the pan from the oven, place a piece of parchment paper directly on top of the loaf, and nestle a second loaf pan or a jar on top to press the pâté as it cools.

Let cool, then remove from the pan, transfer to a serving plate, and smooth the sides as if you're frosting a cake.

Garnish with the sliced scallion. Serve as a spread with crudités or Socca Crackers (page 202) or sliced as a side dish. Refrigerate for up to 1 week or freeze for up to 3 months.

Based on 6 servings	Carbohydrate: 31 g	Fat: 18 g
Calories: 349	Protein: 19 g	

Mushroom Pâté (All Phases)

When we were challenged to create a vegan mock chopped liver, this spread was the result! It packs a deep umami flavor that is sure to please. Get creative with herbs or spices to make it your own. Serve as a simple dip or a fancy pâté for any occasion, with lightly blanched vegetable rounds like daikon or carrots (see Guide to Cooking Vegetables, page 329), crackers, or raw leafy vegetables like Belgian endive or radicchio leaves.

Preparation time: 10 minutes

Total time: 75 to 80 minutes

Makes 8 servings

- 1 to 2 tablespoons extra-virgin olive oil
- Olive oil spray (optional)
- ¼ cup dried red lentils (green or brown lentils work, if you don't have red)
- ¾ cup spring water or filtered water
- ¼ teaspoon ground black pepper, plus more as needed
- ¾ teaspoon salt, plus more as needed
- 1 medium yellow onion, diced
- 1 clove garlic, minced or pressed
- 1 pound baby bella/cremini mushrooms, sliced
- 1 cup walnuts, lightly toasted (see Guide to Roasting Nuts, page 334)
- 1 tablespoon dark miso paste
- Scallions or fresh herbs, chopped, for garnish

Preheat the oven to 375°F. Rub an 8 x 4-inch loaf pan with 1 tablespoon of the oil or spray with olive oil spray.

Rinse the lentils in cold water a few times and drain. Transfer the lentils to a pot with the water. Bring the water to a boil over medium-high heat. Skim off any foam that rises to the top with a mesh skimmer or spoon. Add the pepper. Reduce the heat to low. Cover and simmer for 20 minutes, or until the lentils are well cooked and all the water has been absorbed. (Alternatively, use ½ to ⅔ cup cooked lentils in place of the dried lentils and water.) Stir in ½ teaspoon of the salt.

Heat the remaining 1 tablespoon olive oil in a large skillet over medium heat. Add the onion and garlic and cook, stirring, until translucent, 3 to 5 minutes. Add the mushrooms and remaining ¼ teaspoon salt. Cook, stirring, until the mushrooms are well cooked and the onion begins to caramelize, about 15 minutes. Remove from the heat.

Place the mushroom mixture, cooked lentils, walnuts, and miso in a food processor and process until smooth. (Alternatively, place in a deep bowl and blend with an immersion blender until smooth.) Taste and adjust the seasoning with salt and pepper.

Spread the mushroom mixture evenly into the prepared pan. Bake, uncovered, for 45 minutes to 1 hour until the edges and top form a golden crust. Remove from the oven and let cool.

Gently remove the pâté from the pan, transfer to a serving plate, and smooth the edges as if you're frosting a cake. Garnish with scallions or fresh herbs, cover, and refrigerate until completely cool before serving.

Tip: This recipe is best made a day ahead to allow the flavors to fully meld.

Calories: 148
Carbohydrate: 10 g

Protein: 5 g
Fat: 11 g

Variation

Blending it smooth with an immersion blender or in a high-powered blender, instead of baking, will create a lighter mousse consistency.

Spinach Artichoke Snack Bites (All Phases)

We've taken this familiar appetizer and converted it to an easy bite-size morsel. Mess-free and no chips for dipping required. These flavorful bites are perfect for tailgates, business luncheons, or lazy Sunday dinners.

Preparation time: 10 minutes

Total time: 30 to 40 minutes

Makes 4 to 8 servings

- 8 ounces frozen chopped spinach, thawed
- ½ (14.5-ounce) can artichoke hearts, drained and chopped
- ¼ cup 4% small-curd cottage cheese, or about 2 ounces extra-firm tofu, drained, pressed with an absorbent towel, and crumbled
- ¼ cup grated Parmesan or crumbled feta cheese (2 ounces)
- ¼ cup Chickpea Bread Crumbs (page 196)
- 1 egg, beaten
- ¼ to ½ teaspoon salt, or to taste
- ⅛ teaspoon ground black pepper
- Lemon Aioli (page 298), for dipping

Preheat the oven to 350°F. Line a baking sheet with parchment paper.

Drain the spinach and squeeze out excess liquid. Transfer to a large bowl and add the artichokes, cottage cheese, Parmesan, chickpea bread crumbs, egg, salt to taste, and pepper.

Form the spinach mixture into 1-inch balls by packing it into a rounded tablespoon or a 1- to 1½-inch ice cream scoop. Place the balls about 1 inch apart on the prepared baking sheet. Bake for 20 to 30 minutes, until the egg is set.

Serve alone or with Lemon Aioli (page 298) for dipping.

Based on 4 servings Calories: 116	Carbohydrate: 10 g Protein: 9 g	Fat: 5 g
Based on 4 servings, with 2 tablespoons Lemon Aioli per serving	Calories: 248 Carbohydrate: 11 g Protein: 9 g	Fat: 19 g

Arugula, Beet, and Goat Cheese Snack Bites (Phases 2 and 3)

A favorite salad combination in one simple appetizer bite. These grab-and-go morsels are perfect for everything from a snack on the run to delicate appetizers at an elegant dinner party. A little tofu quietly introduces some plant-based protein.

Preparation time: 15 minutes

Total time: 35 to 45 minutes

Makes 6 servings

- 3 ounces arugula (about 1½ packed cups)
- ½ pound beets (1 medium beet), cut into large chunks
- 3.5 ounces extra-firm tofu, drained, pressed with an absorbent towel, and cut into 1-inch chunks
- ⅓ cup Chickpea Bread Crumbs (page 196)
- ½ cup walnuts, raw or lightly toasted
- 4 ounces goat cheese, crumbled
- 1 egg, beaten
- 1 tablespoon fresh lemon juice
- ½ teaspoon salt, or to taste
- ¼ teaspoon ground black pepper

Fig-Balsamic Reduction

- ½ cup balsamic vinegar
- 1 dried fig

Preheat the oven to 350°F. Line a baking sheet with parchment paper.

Place the arugula, beets, tofu, bread crumbs, and walnuts in a food processor. Process to the consistency of small crumbs. Combine in a large bowl with the goat cheese, egg, lemon juice, salt, and pepper.

Form the beet mixture into small bites by packing it into a rounded tablespoon or a 1- to 1½-inch ice cream scoop. Place about 1 inch apart on the prepared baking sheet. Bake for 20 to 30 minutes, until the egg is set.

Make the fig-balsamic reduction: Place the vinegar and fig in a wide-mouthed mason jar or cup that will fit an immersion blender without splashing. Puree until smooth. Transfer to a small saucepan and heat until bubbling around the edges. Reduce the heat to medium-low and simmer, uncovered, until reduced to ⅓ cup.

Drizzle the snack bites lightly with the reduction.

With 1 teaspoon sauce per serving	Calories: 198 Carbohydrate: 12 g	Protein: 10 g Fat: 13 g

Variation

Use cottage cheese in place of the tofu.

Mint Chocolate Power Balls (All Phases)

The wait is over! For years, readers have asked for a Phase 1 power bar substitute that's quick to make. These little gems provide a balanced ratio of macronutrients without any preservatives or refined sugar—a snack you can feel good about. Get creative with other extracts or spices to create a variety of flavor options, like orange or cinnamon. You'll need a food processor and a little patience, but they're well worth the effort.

Preparation time: 5 minutes

Total time: 5 minutes

Makes 8 servings (16 balls)

- 1½ cups cashews
- 3 ounces dark chocolate (at least 70% cacao), broken into small chunks
- ½ to 1 teaspoon pure peppermint extract, or 3 or 4 drops food-grade peppermint essential oil
- 2½ servings unsweetened, unflavored 100% whey protein powder (check the package nutritional info—1 serving should yield 22 g protein)

Place all the ingredients in a food processor and process for 4 to 5 minutes, scraping the sides and bottom regularly until completely incorporated and the mixture forms a smooth ball. This takes a bit of patience. The chocolate will begin to soften as the friction of the food processor warms it a bit. Just as with homemade nut butters, the mixture will go through stages: coarsely chopped, finely chopped, then the beginnings of a paste, then it will form into a cohesive ball that is completely mixed.

Remove from the processor and form into 16 equal-sized (1½- to 2-inch) balls. Store in an airtight container in the cupboard for up to a few weeks.

Calories: 219 Carbohydrate: 12 g (22%)	Protein: 11 g (21%) Fat: 14 g (57%)

Variations

For Orange Chocolate Power Balls: Substitute orange extract or food-grade orange essential oil for the peppermint.

For Chocolate Vanilla Power Balls: Substitute 1 to 2 teaspoons pure vanilla extract for the peppermint.

Tamari Roasted Almonds (All Phases)

Leave the expensive premade tamari almonds at the store! This is one of the most convenient snacks to have around, and it's so easy to make at home. Always fresh, delicious, and ready to eat.

Preparation time: 1 minute

Total time: 15 minutes

Makes 4 servings

- 1 tablespoon soy sauce or wheat-free tamari
- 1 tablespoon water
- Herbs or spices of your choice (optional)
- 1 cup raw almonds

Preheat the oven to 350°F.

Combine the soy sauce, water, and herbs or spices (if using) in a small bowl or cup and set aside.

Spread the almonds in a single layer on a rimmed baking sheet. Bake for 10 minutes. Remove from the oven and immediately pour into a large bowl. Pour the soy sauce mixture over the hot almonds and stir until they are evenly coated.

Spread the almonds back on the baking sheet. Bake for 3 to 8 minutes more, stirring regularly, until the soy sauce has dried on the almonds.

Remove from the heat and let cool completely. Store at room temperature in a glass jar or other container with a tight-fitting lid for up to 2 weeks.

Calories: 187
Carbohydrate: 7 g
Protein: 7 g
Fat: 15 g

Cucumber Vegetable Rolls (All Phases)

For their *Always Hungry?* book project, George Brown College culinary students Gia An Tiet and Ziyang Lai used presentation to turn a few simple ingredients into a gourmet appetizer worthy of a fine Japanese restaurant.

Preparation time: 10 minutes

Total time: 10 minutes

Makes 4 servings

- 2 cucumbers (thinner-skinned, low-seed varieties like English cucumbers work best)
- 7 ounces smoked salmon slices or cubes
- 2 teaspoons wasabi powder
- ½ avocado, sliced
- 1 medium carrot, thinly sliced
- 1 cup Swiss chard, frisée, or other decorative lettuce or green vegetable
- 4 to 6 spears asparagus, thinly sliced

Dipping Sauce

- 2 to 4 teaspoons wasabi powder
- 1 tablespoon soy sauce
- 1 tablespoon fresh lemon juice

Shave the cucumber lengthwise with a vegetable peeler to form long, thin sheets. The wider pieces work best to form the roll.

Coat the salmon with the wasabi powder. Place a small amount of salmon, avocado, carrot, Swiss chard, and asparagus at the end of each cucumber slice (perpendicular) so that the top of the asparagus and other ingredients extend past one side of the cucumber, and the bottoms of each ingredient line up with the other side. Roll the cucumber gently around the stuffing, with the ingredients sticking out one side (the top of the finished product) and flat on the other side (the bottom). Stand each roll up on a platter with the vegetables peeking out the top.

Make the dipping sauce: Combine the wasabi powder, soy sauce, and lemon juice in a small bowl. Mix well.

Serve the rolls with the dipping sauce.

Calories: 136
Carbohydrate: 10 g
Protein: 12 g
Fat: 5 g

My *Always Delicious* Story

I'm a pediatrician and have been on this *Always Hungry?* journey with my husband, my friend Amy, and her husband, Tim, for the past six months. We have together lost over sixty pounds. My husband's cholesterol has normalized for the first time in years, and Amy has had resolution of her lifelong kidney stones. I try every day to carry the message of mindful eating and disease prevention to my patients and their families.

Kim M., age 44, Colleyville, Texas

CHAPTER 11

Sauces, Rubs & Marinades

All-Purpose Seasoned Salt (All Phases)

Seasoned salt adds a quick depth of flavor to almost everything and saves time as you are cooking. Unfortunately, store-bought seasoned salts often have anticaking agents, MSG, and other additives. Making them on your own is easy, though. This simple spice mixture works well on everything from meat or fish to vegetables and grains.

Preparation time: 5 minutes

Total time: 5 minutes

Makes about ½ cup

- 1½ to 2 tablespoons salt
- 2 teaspoons ground black pepper
- 4 teaspoons paprika
- 2 teaspoons garlic powder
- 2 teaspoons onion powder or dried minced onions
- 2 teaspoons dried thyme
- 2 teaspoons red pepper flakes, or ¼ teaspoon cayenne pepper
- 1 teaspoon ground coriander

Combine all the ingredients in a small jar. Cover and shake well until well mixed. Store in a cool, dry place.

Tip: Make a double or triple batch to have around whenever you need it.

Calories: 16 (Per 1 tablespoon)   Protein: 1 g
Carbohydrate: 3 g   Fat: 0 g

Sugar-Free Worcestershire Sauce (All Phases)

A sauce doesn't stick around for two hundred years as a classic favorite unless it is really good. This one tastes just like the Worcestershire you get from the store, only without the added sugar, preservatives, and anchovies. We use it in many of the recipes in this book—make a batch soon to keep around. This recipe works with lemon juice in place of tamarind until you can find that traditional ingredient at a specialty (Asian or Indian) market (see Chef Dawn's Tasty Tip, page 272).

Preparation time: 5 minutes

Total time: 5 minutes

Makes 1 cup

- ⅓ cup apple cider vinegar
- 2 large cloves garlic
- Dash of cayenne
- ⅓ cup soy sauce
- Dash cloves
- ½ teaspoon tamarind concentrate (or 1 teaspoon lemon juice)
- ¼ teaspoon black pepper

Place all ingredients in a wide-mouthed mason jar or cup that will fit an immersion blender without splashing. Blend until smooth. The mixture will be frothy and then settle as the sauce rests in the jar.

Place a lid on the jar. For best results, set aside for at least 1 hour to allow the flavors to develop. Store in a cool, dry cabinet or in the refrigerator. The sauce will keep for up to 3 months.

Use in recipes that call for Worcestershire sauce.

Calories: 2 (Per 1 teaspoon)   Protein: 0
Carbohydrate: 0   Fat: 0

Greek Dressing (All Phases)

This classic Greek dressing is perfect for all your favorite summer salads. Its tangy lemon flavor also works well as a marinade for meats or tofu.

Preparation time: 5 minutes

Total time: 5 minutes

Makes about 1 cup

- 3 tablespoons fresh lemon juice (from 1 large lemon)
- 1 tablespoon red wine vinegar
- 1¼ teaspoons dried oregano
- ½ teaspoon salt
- ¼ teaspoon ground black pepper
- 3 cloves garlic
- 3 Kalamata olives, pitted
- ⅔ cup olive oil

Place all the ingredients in a wide-mouthed mason jar or cup that will fit an immersion blender without splashing. Blend, working the blender in the jar until the olives and garlic are in tiny pieces.

Place a lid on the jar. For best results, set aside for at least 1 hour to allow the flavors to develop. The dressing will keep in the refrigerator for 1 to 2 weeks.

Calories: 84 (Per 1 tablespoon)   Protein: 0
Carbohydrate: 1   Fat: 9 g

Creamy Peppercorn Vinaigrette (All Phases)

Spicy black peppercorns with creamy Parmesan and a bold burst of mustard liven up fresh greens, vegetables, or salads.

Preparation time: 5 minutes

Total time: 5 minutes

Makes about 1¼ cups

- 2 tablespoons brown mustard
- 2 tablespoons red wine vinegar
- 1 clove garlic
- 1 to 2 teaspoons whole black peppercorns
- 2 tablespoons grated Parmesan cheese
- ¾ cup olive oil

Combine all the ingredients in a wide-mouthed mason jar or cup that will fit an immersion blender without splashing. Blend, working the blender in the jar until garlic and peppercorns are coarsely ground.

Place a lid on the jar. For best results, set aside for at least 1 hour to allow the flavors to develop. The dressing will keep in the refrigerator for 1 to 2 weeks.

Calories: 76 (Per 1 tablespoon)   Protein: 0 g
Carbohydrate: 0 g   Fat: 9 g

Cashew Balsamic Dressing (Phases 2 and 3)

You won't believe how a few simple ingredients can come together to create a dressing this delectable. Sweet and tangy balsamic, creamy cashews, and just enough saltiness. The sum is definitely greater than the parts!

Preparation time: 5 minutes

Total time: 5 minutes

Makes about 1 cup

- 2½ tablespoons soy sauce
- 1½ tablespoons balsamic vinegar

- 2 tablespoons water
- ½ cup neutral-tasting oil, such as high-oleic safflower or avocado oil
- ¼ cup cashews

Place all the ingredients in a wide-mouthed mason jar or cup that will fit an immersion blender without splashing. Pulse a few times to blend until the cashews are in small pieces but still chunky.

Place a lid on the jar. For best results, set aside for at least 1 hour to allow the flavors to develop. The dressing will keep in the refrigerator for 1 to 2 weeks.

Calories: 75 (Per 1 tablespoon)   Protein: 0 g
Carbohydrate: 1 g   Fat: 8 g

Creamy Sun-Dried Tomato Dressing (All Phases)

The bold flavor of sun-dried tomatoes paired with creamy Parmesan creates a rich, savory dressing for salads or vegetables. Omit the Parmesan for a vegan dressing and a lighter, more intense tomato flavor.

Preparation time: 5 minutes

Total time: 5 minutes

Makes about 1½ cups

- 5 unsalted sun-dried tomatoes (about ½ ounce)
- ½ cup boiling water
- 2 tablespoons red wine vinegar
- ¼ teaspoon salt
- ½ teaspoon ground black pepper
- 2 tablespoons grated Parmesan cheese (optional)
- 1 tablespoon tahini
- ½ cup extra-virgin olive oil

Place all the ingredients in a wide-mouthed mason jar or cup that will fit an immersion blender without splashing. Blend until smooth. Add additional water as needed to reach the desired consistency.

Place a lid on the jar. For best results, set aside for at least 1 hour to allow the flavors to develop. The dressing will keep in the refrigerator for 1 to 2 weeks.

Tip: If you can't find unsalted sun-dried tomatoes, use salted and adjust the amount of salt to taste; or use sun-dried tomatoes packed in oil and reduce the oil in the recipe by about 1 tablespoon.

Calories: 47 (Per 1 tablespoon with Parmesan)   Carbohydrate: 1 g   Fat: 5 g
Protein: 0 g

Variation

Soak the sun-dried tomatoes in the water overnight before using in the recipe.

Ginger Tahini Dressing (All Phases)

The sharp bite of ginger mellowed by tahini and white miso make this dressing a delightful topper for fresh salads, vegetables, whole grains, or Buddha Bowls (pages 263 to 269).

Preparation time: 5 minutes

Total time: 5 minutes

Makes about 1 cup

- ¼ cup tahini
- 2 tablespoons white miso paste
- 1 (2-inch) piece ginger, peeled and thinly sliced
- 2 teaspoons rice vinegar
- 1 teaspoon soy sauce
- ½ cup warm water

Place all the ingredients in a wide-mouthed mason jar or cup that will fit an immersion blender without splashing. Blend, working the blender into the pieces of ginger until smooth. Add additional water as needed to reach the desired consistency.

Place a lid on the jar. For best results, set aside for at least 1 hour to allow the flavors to develop. The dressing will keep in the refrigerator for 1 to 2 weeks. (See photo insert page 4.)

Calories: 27 (Per 1 tablespoon)   Protein: 1 g
Carbohydrate: 2 g   Fat: 2 g

Chef Dawn's Tasty Tip

Fresh Ginger—The Star of the Show

Fresh ginger, a favorite ingredient of mine, adds a bright kick of flavor to many recipes. That flavor, however, is not easily replicated with the ground version. Here are a few tips on how to prep and store fresh ginger for easy use anytime.

1. Peeling ginger: Scrape the skin off fresh ginger using a spoon. This method is easy and wastes less of the precious ginger flesh compared to using a knife.
2. For pureed sauces or soups: Peel and slice the ginger, then puree with the other ingredients.
3. For ginger juice: Peel 3 to 4 inches fresh ginger and cut into slices. Add ¼ cup water, then blend with an immersion blender. Use immediately with its pulp, or strain through a fine-mesh strainer for just the juice. Store in the refrigerator until ready to use, up to 1 week. Stir or shake well before using.
4. For longer storage, especially with fresh, plump, juicy ginger: Peel the ginger and place the whole piece in a zip-top freezer bag (young ginger has a very thin skin that doesn't require peeling). When ready to use, grate the frozen ginger using a sharp, fine-toothed grater or zester like a Microplane. The ginger can be grated into a bowl or directly into soups, stir-fries, or other recipes. The sharp zester easily cuts the frozen pulp fibers, so there is no need to juice or strain it. Frozen ginger will keep for several months.
5. Or use a few drops of food-grade ginger essential oil in place of fresh ginger. It adds that bright flavor and keeps well for quick use anytime.

Barbecue Sauce (Phases 2 and 3)

A sweet-and-spicy barbecue sauce without high-fructose corn syrup is difficult to find in the store. This recipe uses apples and honey to achieve the desired flavor, and the smoky ingredients give any dish that just-off-the-grill taste.

Preparation time: 5 minutes

Total time: 35 minutes

Makes 4 cups

- 1 medium Fuji or other sweet apple, cored and diced
- 1 (14.5-ounce) can fire-roasted or regular diced tomatoes
- 1 (6-ounce) can tomato paste
- 1 tablespoon powdered red chile, such as New Mexican, ancho, or chile de árbol (optional)
- 1 tablespoon onion powder
- 1 tablespoon garlic powder
- 1½ teaspoons ground cumin
- ¼ teaspoon ground chipotle chile (optional—spicy but smoky)
- 2 tablespoons apple cider vinegar
- 2 to 3 tablespoons honey
- 3 to 4 tablespoons liquid smoke, or 1 tablespoon smoked paprika
- 1 teaspoon salt
- ¼ teaspoon smoked paprika

Place all the ingredients in a large wide-mouthed mason jar that will fit an immersion blender without splashing. Blend until smooth. (Alternatively, use a high-speed blender.)

Transfer to a saucepan and bring to a simmer over medium heat, then reduce the heat to low, cover, and simmer, stirring very frequently to avoid burning or sticking, especially toward the end of the cooking time, until the mixture looks darker and smoother, about 30 minutes.

If desired, let cool and blend to a smoother consistency. Cool and store in an airtight container in the refrigerator for up to 2 weeks.

Calories: 10 (Per 1 tablespoon)   Protein: 0 g
Carbohydrate: 2 g   Fat: 0 g

Smoked Paprika Ketchup (Phases 2 and 3)

Whoever thought ketchup was best out of a bottle and laden with sugar was sorely mistaken! This recipe is perfect with our Meat Loaf (page 152) or Walnut Lentil Loaf (page 168) or as a dipping sauce for Tofu Fries (page 173) or Brown Rice "Tater" Tots (page 228).

Preparation time: 3 minutes

Total time: 30 minutes

Makes about 1¼ cups

- 1 tablespoon extra-virgin olive oil
- 1 large onion, diced
- 1 (6-ounce) can tomato paste
- 1 (14.5-ounce) can diced tomatoes
- ¾ teaspoon salt
- 1 tablespoon red wine vinegar
- 3 tablespoons honey
- 1½ teaspoons Sugar-Free Worcestershire Sauce (page 284)
- 1 teaspoon smoked paprika

Heat the oil in a saucepan over medium heat. Add the onion and cook until it begins to caramelize, 10 to 15 minutes.

Add the tomato paste, diced tomatoes with their juices, salt, vinegar, honey, Worcestershire, and smoked paprika. Bring to a boil, then reduce the heat to low and simmer, stirring occasionally, for 10 minutes.

Puree directly in the pot with an immersion blender, then simmer for 2 to 3 minutes more. (If the sauce is not deep enough to fully immerse the blender and prevent splattering, carefully transfer the sauce to a deep bowl or jar to blend. Return to the pan after blending.) Taste and adjust the seasonings.

Remove from the heat and let cool. Store in a glass jar in the refrigerator for up to 2 weeks. (See photo insert page 9.)

Calories: 36 (Per 1 tablespoon)   Protein: 1 g
Carbohydrate: 7 g   Fat: 1 g

Moroccan Sauce (All Phases)

Although traditional spice mixes rely on ground ginger and turmeric, the fresh roots add a bright flavor that can't be matched (see Chef Dawn's Tasty Tip on prepping and storing ginger, page 289). The combination of sweet and savory in this sauce makes it a great companion to almost any protein.

Preparation time: 5 minutes

Total time: 7 minutes

Makes ⅔ to ¾ cup

- 1 (2-inch) piece fresh ginger, peeled and sliced into thin rounds
- 3 medium cloves garlic
- 1 (3- to 4-inch) piece fresh turmeric, peeled, or 1 teaspoon ground turmeric (optional)
- 2 teaspoons paprika
- 1 teaspoon ground cumin
- 1 teaspoon ground coriander
- ½ teaspoon ground cinnamon
- ¼ teaspoon ground cloves
- Dash of freshly grated nutmeg
- ¼ teaspoon ground white or black pepper
- 9 or 10 sprigs cilantro, stems and leaves coarsely chopped
- ¼ cup extra-virgin olive oil
- ¼ cup water
- ½ teaspoon salt
- Dash of cayenne pepper, or to taste (optional)

Place all the ingredients in a wide-mouthed mason jar or cup that will fit an immersion blender without splashing. Blend, working the blender in the jar until the garlic, ginger, and turmeric are smooth.

Place a lid on the jar. For best results, set aside for at least 1 hour to allow the flavors to develop. The sauce will keep in the refrigerator for up to 2 weeks.

Calories: 45 (Per 1 tablespoon)   Protein: 0 g
Carbohydrate: 1 g   Fat: 5 g

Citrus Teriyaki Sauce (Phases 2 and 3)

A popular sauce used in Japanese cuisine, teriyaki is most often loaded with sugar and cornstarch. This recipe, however, provides all the sweetness you need to satisfy your teriyaki cravings. The pulp from the citrus, ginger, and garlic help to thicken the sauce without the need for cornstarch (see Chef Dawn's Tasty Tip on prepping and storing ginger, page 289).

Preparation time: 5 minutes

Total time: 5 to 15 minutes

Makes about 1⅓ cups

- ¼ cup soy sauce
- ¼ cup water
- 2 medium or 4 mini mandarins or tangerines, or 1 orange, peeled and seeded
- 2 tablespoons honey
- 1 (¾-inch) piece fresh ginger, peeled and thinly sliced
- 2 cloves garlic

Place all the ingredients in a wide-mouthed glass mason jar or cup that will fit an immersion blender without splashing. Blend, working the blender into the larger pieces to grind them down (the texture will remain somewhat pulpy).

If using as a marinade for a protein that will be cooked, use as is. If using as a sauce at the end of cooking, transfer the teriyaki to a small saucepan. Bring to a boil, then reduce the heat to low and simmer for 5 to 10 minutes, or until the sauce reduces and thickens slightly. The sauce will keep in the refrigerator for 1 to 2 weeks.

Calories: 13 (Per 1 tablespoon)   Protein: 0 g
Carbohydrate: 3 g   Fat: 0 g

Spicy Asian Marinade or Salad Dressing
(Phases 2 and 3, with Phase 1 Variation)

Just enough kick to wake you up. Adjust the level of spiciness to your own preference by increasing or decreasing the chiles and ginger (see Chef Dawn's Tasty Tip on prepping and storing ginger, page 289). Use as a salad dressing, stir-fry sauce, or marinade.

Preparation time: 5 minutes

Total time: 5 minutes

Makes about 1 cup

- ½ cup water
- 1 (3-inch) piece fresh ginger, peeled and thinly sliced
- 3 or 4 cloves garlic
- ½ to 1 small fresh hot chile, such as Thai, serrano, poblano, jalapeño, or cayenne
- 1 tablespoon toasted sesame oil
- 2 to 3 tablespoons soy sauce
- ½ teaspoon salt
- 1½ tablespoons honey (optional)
- ⅛ teaspoon ground white or black pepper

Place all the ingredients in a wide-mouthed mason jar or cup that will fit an immersion blender without splashing. Blend until smooth, working the blender into the thicker pieces of ginger, garlic, and chile until they are finely minced.

Place a lid on the jar. For best results, set aside for at least 1 hour to allow the flavors to develop. The marinade will keep in the refrigerator for 1 to 2 weeks.

Calories: 17 (Per 1 tablespoon)   Protein: 0 g
Carbohydrate: 2 g   Fat: 1 g

Variations

If using this sauce with tofu or tempeh, double the quantities of the chiles, ginger, and salt, as these proteins will soak up more flavor than other forms of protein.

For Phase 1: Omit the honey.

Fresh Turmeric Garlic Marinade (All Phases)

Curious how to use fresh turmeric? This simple marinade can be made in a snap. A family favorite at the Ludwig home. It's especially good when used in the On-a-Budget Marinated Chicken (page 116) or Marinated Baked Tofu (page 175) recipes.

Preparation time: 5 minutes

Total time: 5 minutes

Makes about ½ cup

- 1 (3-inch) piece fresh turmeric, peeled
- 3 or 4 cloves garlic
- ½ to 1 teaspoon salt
- ¼ cup water
- 2 tablespoons extra-virgin olive oil

Place all the ingredients in a wide-mouthed mason jar or cup that will fit an immersion blender without splashing. Blend until smooth.

Place a lid on the jar and refrigerate. The marinade will keep in the refrigerator for up to a few weeks.

Tip: Use a spoon to peel the outer skin from the fresh turmeric as you would with fresh ginger (see Chef Dawn's Tasty Tip on prepping and storing ginger, page 289).

Calories: 33 (Per 1 tablespoon)   Protein: 0 g
Carbohydrate: 1 g   Fat: 4 g

Lemon Thyme or Tarragon Marinade (All Phases)

A bright citrus marinade with the familiar flavor of thyme, this versatile marinade goes well with most proteins.

Preparation time: 5 minutes

Total time: 5 minutes

Makes about ½ cup

- 2 cloves garlic
- 1½ tablespoons fresh lemon juice (1 small lemon)
- ½ teaspoon dried thyme or tarragon or other favorite herbs
- 1 teaspoon salt
- ¼ teaspoon ground black pepper
- 2 tablespoons extra-virgin olive oil
- ¼ cup water or dry white wine

Place all the ingredients in a wide-mouthed mason jar or cup that will fit an immersion blender without splashing. Blend until smooth.

Place a lid on the jar. The marinade will keep in the refrigerator for up to a few weeks.

Calories: 32 (Per 1 tablespoon)   Protein: 0 g
Carbohydrate: 0 g   Fat: 4 g

Variation

Increase the black pepper and omit the herbs for a lemon-pepper sauce.

Basil Walnut Pesto (All Phases)

Pesto in a breeze! Expensive pine nuts can make pesto a pricey investment, so this simple version uses toasted walnuts instead. Their nutty flavor and fat content give the right level of richness to this versatile spread. Use this recipe to extend the life of your basil—it keeps much longer in this paste form (freeze it in ice cube trays for even longer storage).

Preparation time: 5 minutes

Total time: 5 minutes

Makes about 1 cup

- 2 to 2½ ounces fresh basil, tough bottom stems removed, leaves and smaller stems coarsely chopped (about 1 cup packed)
- 1 ounce fresh parsley, tough bottom stems removed, leaves and smaller stems coarsely chopped (½ cup packed)
- ⅓ cup walnuts, toasted
- 1 small clove garlic
- ¼ cup extra-virgin olive oil
- 1 tablespoon water, or more as needed
- ⅛ to ¼ teaspoon salt
- 1 to 2 teaspoons fresh lemon juice
- 2 tablespoons grated Parmesan cheese

Place all the ingredients in a wide-mouthed mason jar or cup that will fit an immersion blender without splashing. Puree to a thick paste, working the leaves and larger chunks with the blender to grind them down.

If desired, add water 1 tablespoon at a time to create a creamier pesto.

Place a lid on the jar. For best results, set aside for at least 1 hour to allow the flavors to develop. The pesto will keep in the refrigerator for up to 2 weeks. (See photo insert page 10.)

Calories: 50 (Per 1 tablespoon)   Protein: 1 g
Carbohydrate: 1 g   Fat: 5 g

Variation

Dairy-free version: Omit the Parmesan and season with a bit more salt or umeboshi vinegar (see page 64) to replace the taste of the cheese.

Lime Cilantro Pesto (All Phases)

This light, refreshing pesto variation adds zing to steamed vegetables, taco salads, or wraps. Spread it on fish or chicken and bake to create flavorful, restaurant-quality meals in minutes.

Preparation time: 5 minutes

Total time: 5 minutes

Makes about 1 cup

- 3 tablespoons fresh lime juice
- 1 cup packed cilantro, stems and leaves coarsely chopped (2 ounces)
- 1 cup packed flat leaf parsley, stems and leaves coarsely chopped (2 ounces)
- ½ teaspoon salt
- 1 tablespoon tahini
- 1 tablespoon water, plus more as needed
- 2 tablespoons extra-virgin olive oil

Place all the ingredients in a wide-mouthed mason jar or cup that will fit an immersion blender without splashing. Puree, working the blender into the leaves to create a thick paste.

If desired, add more water 1 tablespoon at a time to create a creamier pesto.

Place a lid on the jar. For best results, set aside for at least 1 hour to allow the flavors to develop. The pesto will keep in the refrigerator for up to 2 weeks.

Calories: 22 (Per 1 tablespoon)   Protein: 0 g
Carbohydrate: 1 g   Fat: 2 g

Lemon Aioli (All Phases)

Tangy citrus combined with bright garlic. This aioli is one of a kind, and so satisfying that you'll be tempted to eat it right off the spoon. The vegan version is just as rich and creamy as the one with whole milk, and fits well alongside any meals.

Preparation time: 5 minutes

Total time: 5 minutes

Makes about 1¼ cups

- ¼ cup unsweetened soy milk or whole milk
- ½ teaspoon salt
- 2 or 3 large cloves garlic
- 2 to 3 teaspoons fresh lemon juice (from about ½ small lemon)
- ¼ teaspoon white wine vinegar
- ⅔ cup neutral-tasting oil, such as high-oleic safflower or avocado oil

Place the milk, salt, garlic, lemon juice, and vinegar in a wide-mouthed glass jar or cup that will fit an immersion blender without splashing. Blend, working the blender into the garlic until it is finely minced.

With the blender running, pour the oil into the jar in a steady stream and blend until the aioli is thick and all the oil has been incorporated.

Place a lid on the jar. Set aside in the refrigerator for at least 1 hour to allow the flavors to fully develop. The marinade will keep in the refrigerator for up to 2 weeks. (See photo insert page 9.)

Calories: 68 (Per 1 tablespoon)   Protein: 0 g
Carbohydrate: 0 g   Fat: 8 g

Variations

Use a room-temperature egg in place of the milk. *Caution:* Raw egg is not recommended for infants, the elderly, pregnant women, or people with weakened immune systems.

Decrease the amount of garlic and add dill or any other fresh herbs of your choice to make an interesting herbed mayo.

Gremolata (All Phases)

Italian restaurants traditionally brighten braised meats with this simple condiment. You can also toss it with whole grains or vegetables to add a zesty kick to any meal.

Preparation time: 5 minutes

Total time: 5 minutes

Makes about ¼ cup

- 2 teaspoons lemon zest
- 1 large clove garlic, minced or pressed
- ¼ cup minced, fresh flat-leaf parsley

Combine all the ingredients in a small bowl or jar.

Leave as is, or if you have a mortar and pestle (a bowl and the end of a rolling pin can also work), grind the ingredients together into a thick, chunky paste. Set aside on the counter until ready to serve so the flavors can develop. Store in the refrigerator for up to 1 week.

Spoon onto fish, meat, or other protein as a marinade, sauce, or in the last 5 to 10 minutes of cooking. Or serve as a finish on top of warm protein.

Calories: 2 (Per 1 tablespoon)   Protein: 0 g
Carbohydrate: 1 g   Fat: 0 g

Cilantro Chimichurri (All Phases)

This traditional Latin American–style chimichurri can be used raw as a garnish or cooked as a marinade or sauce. It goes especially well with fatty meats. Adding a few garnish-style sauces to your table is an easy way to accommodate a wide range of tastes and preferences.

Preparation time: 5 minutes

Total time: 5 minutes

Makes about 1 cup

- 3 or 4 cloves garlic, minced
- 1 cup packed cilantro, stems and leaves minced (2 ounces)
- 1 cup packed fresh flat-leaf parsley, thick bottom stems removed, leaves and smaller stems minced (2 ounces)
- 1 to 2 teaspoons minced mild to medium chile, such as serrano or jalapeño (optional)
- 2 teaspoons fresh lime juice
- ¼ teaspoon salt
- ⅛ teaspoon ground black pepper
- 1 teaspoon fresh oregano, or ½ teaspoon dried Mexican, spicy, or regular oregano
- ⅓ cup extra-virgin olive oil

Combine all the ingredients in a small bowl or jar. Use as is or, if you have a mortar and pestle (a bowl and the end of a rolling pin can also work), grind the ingredients together into a thick, chunky paste.

Set aside for at least 1 hour so flavors can develop before serving. Place a lid on the jar and store in the refrigerator for 1 to 2 weeks.

Spoon onto fish, meat, or other protein in the last 5 to 10 minutes of cooking. Or serve as a finish on top of warm protein.

Calories: 42 (Per 1 tablespoon)   Protein: 0 g
Carbohydrate: 0 g   Fat: 5 g

Parsley Chimichurri (All Phases)

A European twist on the Latin American favorite. Use as a garnish for meats, soups, whole grains, or vegetables. Also works well as a marinade for your favorite proteins.

Preparation time: 5 minutes

Total time: 5 minutes

Makes about 1 cup

- 4 or 5 cloves garlic, minced
- 4 ounces fresh flat-leaf parsley, thick bottom stems removed, leaves and smaller stems minced (2 cups)
- 1 teaspoon white wine vinegar
- 1 teaspoon fresh oregano, or ½ teaspoon dried
- ⅓ cup extra-virgin olive oil

Combine all the ingredients in a small bowl or jar. Use as is or, if you have a mortar and pestle (a bowl and the end of a rolling pin can also work), grind the ingredients together into a thick, chunky paste. Set aside for at least 1 hour so the flavors can develop before serving. Place a lid on the jar and store in the refrigerator for 1 to 2 weeks.

Spoon onto fish, meat, or other protein in the last 5 to 10 minutes of cooking. Or serve as a finish on top of warm protein.

Calories: 43 (Per 1 tablespoon)   Protein: 0 g
Carbohydrate: 1 g   Fat: 5 g

Fresh Salsa (All Phases)

This recipe is inspired by a Texas friend who always had the perfect salsa ready to go for any party using (shush) canned tomatoes! A shockingly first-rate salsa that adds a light, refreshing bite to any dish any time of year. Adjust the level of spiciness to fit your taste. Serve as a side sauce or as a seasoning in recipes like Slow Cooker Chili (page 249) or to spice up soups, beans, meats, vegetables, or grains.

Preparation time: 5 minutes

Total time: 5 minutes

Makes 3 cups

- 2 or 3 cloves garlic
- 1 medium onion, cut into large chunks
- ½ to 1 cup packed cilantro, leaves and stems coarsely chopped (1 to 2 ounces)
- Juice of 1 lime
- 1 to 2 jalapeños or other chiles of your choice, or to taste
- ½ teaspoon salt
- 1 (14.5-ounce) can diced tomatoes

Place the garlic, onion, cilantro, lime juice, jalapeño, and salt in a food processor. Process until finely chopped.

Add the tomatoes. Pulse to a finely chopped salsa consistency.

Transfer to a glass mason jar with a lid. Store in the refrigerator for 2 to 3 weeks.

Calories: 4 (Per 1 tablespoon) Protein: 0 g
Carbohydrate: 1 g Fat: 0 g

Indian Raita (All Phases)

Spicy Indian dishes are often served with a yogurt-and-mint sauce to balance the many flavors of the meal. It's a cool and refreshing way to enjoy vegetables and get your probiotics at the same time.

Preparation time: 10 minutes

Total time: 10 minutes

Makes 4 servings (about 2 cups)

- ½ pound cucumber (about 2 large Persian or 1 English cucumber; see Tip, page 261)
- ¼ teaspoon salt, plus more for sprinkling
- 1 cup plain whole-milk Greek yogurt
- 1½ teaspoons fresh lime juice
- ⅛ teaspoon ground coriander
- ¼ teaspoon ground cumin
- ⅛ teaspoon ground black pepper
- ¼ cup minced red onion
- 10 to 12 large mint leaves or more, to taste

Grate the cucumber, sprinkle with a pinch of salt, stir, and place it in a mesh strainer or colander. Press against the cucumber to drain the liquid. (Alternatively, place the grated cucumber in a doubled layer of cheesecloth or a muslin towel, twist the top, and squeeze out the juice.)

Combine the drained cucumber, yogurt, lime juice, coriander, cumin, salt, pepper, red onion, and mint. Mix well. Store in an airtight container in the refrigerator for at least 1 hour to allow flavors to develop. It will keep for up to a week in the refrigerator.

Calories: 73
Carbohydrate: 5 g

Protein: 6 g
Fat: 3 g

Variations

For a soupier consistency, grate the cucumbers but don't squeeze out the juice.

Add other vegetables like shredded carrots.

Tzatziki (All Phases)

This traditional Greek condiment is often served alongside grilled meats to add a fresh, zesty touch to the meal.

Preparation time: 10 minutes

Total time: 10 minutes

Makes 4 to 6 servings (about 2 cups)

- ½ pound cucumber (about 2 large Persian or 1 English cucumber; see Tip, page 261)
- ½ teaspoon salt, plus more for sprinkling
- 1½ cups plain whole-milk Greek yogurt, or ¾ cup Dairy-Free Sour Cream (page 306)
- 1 tablespoon fresh lemon juice
- 1 clove garlic, minced or pressed
- ¼ teaspoon ground black pepper
- ¼ cup fresh dill, chopped, or more to taste

Grate the cucumber, sprinkle with a pinch of salt, stir, and place it in a mesh strainer or colander. Press against the cucumber to drain the liquid. (Alternatively, place the grated cucumber in a doubled layer of cheesecloth or a muslin towel, twist the top, and squeeze out the juice.)

Combine the drained cucumber, yogurt, lemon juice, garlic, salt, pepper, and dill in an airtight container. Mix well. Cover and refrigerate for at least 1 hour to allow the flavors to develop. It will keep for up to 1 week in the refrigerator.

Based on 6 servings Calories: 68 (Yogurt)	Carbohydrate: 4 g Protein: 6 g	Fat: 3 g
Based on 6 servings Calories: 19 (Dairy-Free Sour Cream)	Carbohydrate: 2 g Protein: 2 g	Fat: 1 g

Green Chile Cream Sauce (All Phases)

This crowd-pleasing sauce makes use of blended white beans to create its luscious texture. The addition of green chiles lends a smoky flavor with just enough kick, making this a sauce that works well with almost any protein. Use as a topping on your favorite proteins like chicken or fish or to create rich, creamy casseroles like Creamy Green Chile Chicken (page 124) or Creamy Green Chile Casserole (page 187). Definitely a keeper!

Preparation time: 5 minutes

Total time: 25 minutes

Makes about 5½ cups

- ¼ cup neutral-tasting oil, such as high-oleic safflower or avocado oil
- 1 medium onion, diced
- 1 large clove garlic
- ¼ cup chickpea flour (see Tip, page 91)
- ½ teaspoon salt
- ⅛ teaspoon ground black pepper
- 1 cup cooked white beans measured with cooking liquid (see Do-It-Yourself Beans, page 74) or drained and rinsed canned beans measured with water
- 2 cups whole milk or unsweetened soy milk
- 3 (4-ounce) cans roasted green chiles, chopped

Heat the oil in a deep skillet or pot over medium heat. Add the onion and garlic. Cook, stirring, until translucent, 3 to 5 minutes.

Add the chickpea flour, salt, and pepper. Cook, stirring, until the flour starts to turn golden brown, about 5 minutes.

Stir in the beans and milk. Puree directly in the pot with an immersion blender until smooth and creamy.

Add the chiles and cook, stirring regularly, until the sauce thickens, 5 to 10 minutes.

Use immediately for your favorite recipes or store in an airtight container in the refrigerator for up to a week.

Calories: 14 (Per 1 tablespoon)   Protein: 0 g
Carbohydrate: 1 g   Fat: 1 g

Dairy-Free Sour Cream (All Phases)

Store-bought dairy-free sour cream usually has a multitude of emulsifiers and other artificial additives. And doesn't it always seem to go bad before you can finish it? This simple version is delicious, easy to make, and all-natural. The secret ingredient, umeboshi vinegar (see page 64), gives it a tangy depth of flavor that replicates real sour cream.

Preparation time: 5 minutes

Total time: 5 minutes

Makes about 1¾ cups

- 1 (16-ounce) package soft or silken tofu, drained if packed in water
- 3 tablespoons apple cider vinegar
- 2 tablespoons umeboshi vinegar (see page 64) or ½ teaspoon salt
- 1 scallion, chopped
- ⅓ cup neutral-tasting oil, such as high-oleic safflower or avocado oil

Place all the ingredients in a wide-mouthed mason jar or cup that will fit an immersion blender without splashing. Blend until smooth.

Place a lid on the jar. For best results, set aside for at least 1 hour to allow the flavors to develop. This will keep in the refrigerator for 1 to 2 weeks.

Calories: 29 (Per 1 tablespoon)   Protein: 1 g
Carbohydrate: ½ g   Fat: 3 g

Variations

Substitute 8 ounces extra-firm tofu and ½ cup unsweetened soy milk for the soft or silken tofu.

Dairy-Free French Onion Dip: Add 1 to 2 tablespoons dried minced onion, 3 tablespoons onion powder, ½ teaspoon garlic powder, ¼ teaspoon ground black or white pepper, or to taste, ¼ teaspoon paprika, and ½ cup chopped fresh parsley. Stir or blend well and refrigerate to allow flavors to fully develop for at least 1 hour.

My *Always Delicious* Story

One of the most powerful tools I've gained from *AH* is the recognition of the profound influence of food choices on my eating behaviors. I've learned that the foods I eat can either support or obscure satiety, hunger, and cravings. It's been a relief to learn that my previous failures at weight loss weren't due to personal lack of willpower! It really was about the foods I was eating. My big "aha" has been that focusing on *what* I'm eating has a far bigger influence on my weight, health, cravings, and hunger than focusing on *how much* I'm eating.

Jen S., age 46, Duxbury, Massachusetts

CHAPTER 12

Beverages & Desserts

Blueberry Lime Mint Fizz (All Phases)

The syrupy sweetness of colas and other sugary drinks can be a challenge for some people to eliminate from their diets. Luckily, there's an even more satisfying way to get your fizzy fix. Sparkling water, a few favorite fruits, and herbs make a delicious—and much healthier—alternative.

Preparation time: 5 minutes

Total time: 5 minutes

Makes 2 servings

- ¼ cup blueberries
- 8 to 10 fresh mint leaves
- 2 to 3 teaspoons fresh lime juice
- ½ cup ice or more, as desired
- 20 ounces sparkling water

Evenly distribute the blueberries, mint, and lime juice at the bottom of two large glasses. Mash with a wooden spoon or pestle to release the flavors. (In bartending, this is called muddling.) Add ice to each glass and fill with the sparkling water. Stir gently, taste, and add more lime or mint as needed. Serve immediately. (See photo insert page 1.)

Calories: 12   Protein: 0 g
Carbohydrate: 3 g   Fat: 0 g

Variations

Add ¼ cup of the sparkling water to a large glass jar with the berries and mint. Pulse a few times with an immersion blender. Stir in the lime juice and remaining sparkling water. Pour over ice, and serve immediately.

Herb-flavored mocktail: Use strawberries, 4 or 5 fresh large basil leaves, and fresh lemon juice in place of the blueberries, mint, and lime juice.

Blend 1 (½-inch) piece fresh ginger, peeled and sliced with ¼ cup water and strain into any drink, to taste (see Chef Dawn's Tasty Tip on prepping and storing fresh ginger, page 289).

Peppermint Hot Chocolate (All Phases)

Hot chocolate doesn't have to come in a packet! So rich and creamy, this beverage makes a great warm-up on winter mornings. A cool burst of peppermint complements the smooth chocolate. Feel free to experiment with other extracts or essential oils to find your favorite flavor.

Preparation time: 5 minutes

Total time: 10 minutes

Makes 1 serving

- 1 cup whole milk or unsweetened soy or almond milk
- 1 ounce dark chocolate (at least 70% cacao)
- A few drops of food-grade peppermint essential oil, or a splash of pure peppermint extract

Heat the milk in a small saucepan over medium heat. Be careful not to walk away for long, as milk can come to a boil explosively.

Stir in the chocolate and peppermint oil and whisk until the chocolate melts. If desired, pulse directly in the pot with an immersion blender to fully incorporate the chocolate and the milk. Pour into a mug and serve hot.

Calories: 318 (Whole milk)   Protein: 10 g
Carbohydrate: 25 g   Fat: 20 g

Calories: 250 (Soy milk)   Protein: 9 g
Carbohydrate: 17 g   Fat: 16 g

Fruity Coconut Ice Pops (Phases 2 and 3, with Phase 1 Variation)

Want ice pops that are more than just frozen sugar? The key to a creamy pop is starting with a thick, nearly frozen base before adding it to the molds. Coconut milk or Greek yogurt and frozen fruit are the perfect combination for a cool and refreshing summer treat.

Preparation time: 5 minutes

Total time: 5 minutes

Makes 4 servings

- 1 cup unsweetened canned coconut milk
- ¾ cup frozen berries
- 1 teaspoon honey (optional, omit for Phase 1 variation)

Place the coconut milk, berries, and honey (if using) in a wide-mouthed mason jar or cup that will fit an immersion blender without splashing. Blend until smooth and creamy.

Transfer immediately into a four-well ice pop mold and freeze. Serve frozen.

Calories: 134 (With honey)   Protein: 1 g
Carbohydrate: 7 g   Fat: 12 g

Calories: 129 (Without honey) Protein: 1 g
Carbohydrate: 6 g   Fat: 12 g

Variations

Substitute plain whole-milk Greek yogurt for half or all the coconut milk.

For a sweeter pop, add ½ frozen banana.

Calories: 147   Protein: 2 g
Carbohydrate: 11 g   Fat: 12 g

Mango Lassi (Phases 2 and 3)

This traditional Indian drink makes a delicious dessert. It's rich and fruity without being too heavy. The extra protein from the Greek yogurt complements a protein-light meal or makes a balanced snack anytime.

Preparation time: 5 minutes

Total time: 5 minutes

Makes 2 servings

- ⅔ cup frozen mango
- 1 cup plain whole-milk Greek yogurt
- ¼ cup whole milk or unsweetened soy milk
- 1 teaspoon honey
- ⅛ teaspoon ground cardamom, or more to taste

Place all the ingredients in a blender. Blend until smooth. Pour into 2 glasses and serve immediately.

Calories: 205   Protein: 14 g
Carbohydrate: 19 g   Fat: 9 g

Variations

Pour into 4 to 8 ice pop molds, depending on the size of the molds, to make 4 to 8 frozen desserts.

For a smaller dessert, serve a half portion to each person.

Almond Coconut Macaroons (Phases 2 and 3)

These fluffy macaroon cookies make a satisfying substitute for the standard sugary version. Add a few dark chocolate chips to create a perfect, homey dessert.

Preparation time: 5 minutes

Total time: 15 minutes

Makes 8 to 12 servings (24 cookies)

- 1½ cups almond flour
- 1 cup unsweetened finely shredded coconut
- ¼ teaspoon salt
- ½ teaspoon baking soda
- 6 tablespoons avocado oil
- ¼ cup honey
- 1 egg, beaten
- 1 teaspoon pure vanilla extract

Preheat the oven to 350°F. Line a baking sheet with parchment paper.

Combine the almond flour, coconut, salt, and baking soda in a large bowl until well mixed.

In a separate bowl, whisk together the oil, honey, egg, and vanilla.

Mix the wet ingredients into the dry ingredients with a spatula until well combined.

Using a round tablespoon or small ice cream scoop, spoon 1 heaping tablespoon of the dough onto the prepared baking sheet; repeat to make 24 cookies, spacing them ½ to 1 inch apart. Distribute any remaining dough among the cookies.

Bake for 7 to 9 minutes, or until the tops are golden brown. (See photo insert page 16.)

Calories: 104 (Per cookie)   Protein: 2 g
Carbohydrate: 6 g   Fat: 9 g

Variations

Vegan version: Omit the egg and increase oil to ½ cup.

Chocolate Chip Cookies: Add ¼ cup (about 1½ ounces) dark chocolate chips (at least 70% cacao) to the batter before scooping.

Snickerdoodles: Add 1 teaspoon ground cinnamon.

Add other spices like ground cardamom or essential oils or citrus zest like lemon, orange, or tangerine.

Chocolate-Dipped Fruit (All Phases)

An elegant dessert the whole family will love. At the store, chocolate-covered fruit might be too expensive to incorporate into your regular routine, but you can make these at home anytime at a fraction of the cost! Get creative with various fruits and toppings to create a showstopping dessert in minutes.

Preparation time: 10 minutes

Total time: 30 minutes

Makes 6 to 12 servings

- 1 pound medium strawberries
- 3 ounces dark chocolate (at least 70% cacao), broken into pieces

Wash the strawberries, leaving the stems on, and pat dry or set on a towel to dry. Make sure the berries are dry before dipping. If water gets into the chocolate, it will cause the chocolate to become grainy and ruined for dipping.

Place a large piece of parchment paper on a baking sheet or cutting board to hold the strawberries after dipping.

Put the chocolate in the top pot of a double boiler. Bring the water in the bottom pot to a boil.

Once chocolate is melted, make sure the strawberries are dry and then dip them in the chocolate one at a time, holding them by the green leafy parts to cover the berry with chocolate. Leave a small space around the green leaves and stem. Let any excess drip off the berry, then place it on the prepared baking sheet to cool and set.

Leave on the counter to cool for a few hours or place in the refrigerator for 30 minutes or until the chocolate has hardened. Remove and serve at room temperature.

Reheat any remaining chocolate and drizzle onto the berries in a zigzag pattern. (Alternatively, make a few Coconut Clusters with the remaining chocolate: Add shredded coconut and nuts to the remaining melted chocolate and stir well to completely cover. Scoop the mixture into small clusters on parchment paper and set aside to cool.)

Calories: 27 (Per strawberry)   Protein: 0 g
Carbohydrate: 3 g   Fat: 2 g

Variations

Peel and separate wedges of tangerine or cut other fruits like pear or apple slices. Dip them into the melted chocolate to completely cover, using a toothpick to hold them, or to halfway cover, allowing a small portion of the fruit to show.

Sprinkle the chocolate-covered fruit with shredded coconut or finely chopped nuts before it dries for a fun texture and interesting additional flavor.

For an impressive fruit kebab: Thread cut fruit onto bamboo skewers. Hold the skewer at a 45-degree angle with the bottom end touching a large piece of parchment paper. Drizzle chocolate over the fruit in a slow, steady stream, twisting the skewer while pouring. Let any excess drip off, then place the skewer on the parchment paper to cool. Cubed pears work nicely here as well.

For Phases 2 and 3: Bananas are also nice, thickly sliced, used fresh or frozen, then dipped into chocolate, or place a wooden chopstick in the end of a whole banana, freeze, and dip into melted chocolate and freeze again until ready to eat.

For Phases 2 and 3: Substitute dried fruit like apricots or other dried fruit in place of the strawberries.

Chef Dawn's Tasty Tip

Melting Chocolate

Although we don't typically recommend them, microwaves make for an easy way to melt chocolate without needing a double boiler. Follow the manufacturer's instructions for melting chocolate.

Chocolate Truffles (All Phases)

The most difficult step in most chocolate recipes is melting your chocolate without overcooking. In this simple recipe, we've eliminated that step by allowing small pieces of chocolate to melt naturally in hot milk. No double boiler required. Play around with the type and amount of milk to create the right texture for your taste.

Preparation time: 5 minutes plus cooling time

Total time: 3 hours

Makes 6 to 8 servings

- 5 to 6 tablespoons half-and-half or heavy cream
- ¼ teaspoon pure vanilla extract
- 3 ounces dark chocolate (at least 70% cacao), cut into small pieces
- 1 tablespoon unsweetened cocoa powder

Place the half-and-half in a small saucepan and heat over medium-low heat, stirring regularly, until it is bubbling at the edges. Turn off the heat. Add the vanilla.

Add the chocolate and let stand for 30 seconds. Stir or whisk gently, beginning in the middle, until the half-and-half and chocolate begin to emulsify and look smooth. Continue stirring in a wider circle, gently incorporating the chocolate, until all chocolate is incorporated and the mixture is smooth and creamy.

Transfer the chocolate to a bowl with a lid. Set aside to cool on the counter overnight or cover and cool in the refrigerator for 2 to 3 hours.

Spread the cocoa powder on a small plate or place in a shallow bowl and set aside. Line a baking sheet with parchment paper.

Once the chocolate is cool and firm enough to work with, use a small 1-inch ice cream scoop to form it into six to eight 1-inch balls. Roll the balls smooth between your hands (your hands will slightly melt the outside of the chocolate ball, making them easier to coat in toppings), then roll the chocolate balls in the cocoa powder until covered and place them on the prepared baking sheet. (See photo insert page 16.)

Store in an airtight container on the counter for a few days or in the refrigerator for 1 to 2 weeks. Serve at room temperature.

Tips: Cooking with chocolate can be affected by the climatic conditions, including humidity in the air. Cool, dry climates are best for making chocolate truffles. If you live in a warm or humid climate, use an air conditioner or dehumidifier to improve conditions before cooking. In extra-dry climates, a bit more dairy may be used to create a creamier texture.

Be sure to use dry utensils, as small drops of liquid can cause chocolate to become grainy. If your chocolate becomes grainy from water droplets or overcooking, add a tablespoon or two of hot dairy to it and stir as described above until it becomes smooth. If the end result is a truffle that is too soft, freeze individual truffles for 30 minutes, then dip them in melted chocolate to create a hard outer shell (see Chef Dawn's Tasty Tip for melting chocolate, page 314).

| Based on 6 servings | Carbohydrate: 8 g | Fat: 7 g |
| Calories: 103 | Protein: 2 g | |

Variations

Use whole milk or unsweetened almond, soy, or canned coconut milk in place of the half-and-half or heavy cream. With the less-fatty milks, you may need up to ½ cup to get the texture right. To test the final texture, place a small amount on a spoon in the freezer for 5 minutes to completely cool it.

Add a drop of your favorite food-grade essential oil to the batter. Peppermint, orange, or sweet spices like cinnamon or cardamom work especially well. You can even add a dash of cayenne for a spicy kick like Mexican-style chocolate.

Roll the truffles in finely crushed nuts, seeds, or unsweetened shredded coconut instead of cocoa powder.

Dip the truffles into melted chocolate and set on parchment paper to cool to create a hard outer layer instead of rolling them in cocoa powder.

Coconut BonBons (Phases 2 and 3)

These dark chocolate beauties are as delectable as their name suggests. Each creamy bite will end even a mundane meal on a luxurious note. Just one is surprisingly satisfying.

Preparation time: 25 minutes

Total time: 35 minutes

Makes 6 servings

- ½ cup unsweetened canned coconut milk
- 1 to 2 teaspoons honey
- ½ teaspoon pure vanilla extract
- ½ cup unsweetened finely shredded coconut
- 3 ounces dark chocolate (at least 70% cacao)

Place the coconut milk and honey in a small pot. Bring to a boil. Reduce the heat to medium-low. Simmer, uncovered, stirring regularly, for 10 to 15 minutes to reduce the liquid by about one-third.

Transfer the liquid to a glass bowl. Stir in the vanilla and shredded coconut. Refrigerate for 5 to 10 minutes or until cool enough to handle. The mixture should be thick enough to scoop and dip in chocolate. If not, then refrigerate or freeze until thick enough to handle.

Line a plate or baking sheet with parchment paper. Using a 1-inch ice cream scoop, scoop a heaping tablespoon of the coconut to make a ball or bonbon shape with a rounded top and flattened bottom. Repeat to make 6 pieces. Place the bonbons in the freezer for 10 minutes.

Melt the chocolate in a double boiler (see Chef Dawn's Tasty Tip for melting chocolate, page 314). Roll each frozen bonbon in chocolate to completely cover, and set aside on the prepared baking sheet to cool. Spoon or drizzle any remaining chocolate on top of the cooling bonbons until all chocolate has been used.

Refrigerate for 1 hour or up to overnight before serving. Store in the refrigerator in an airtight container for up to 2 weeks.

Tip: Finely shredded coconut is necessary for the liquid to absorb and create a nougat consistency. Coarsely shredded coconut will create a mixture that is too liquid to scoop. If this happens, place the coconut mixture in the freezer before spooning it out.

Calories: 167   Protein: 2 g
Carbohydrate: 12 g   Fat: 13 g

Vegan Orange Chocolate Pudding (Phases 2 and 3)

Rich, creamy avocados make the perfect base for this versatile pudding. A hint of citrus lends a sophisticated flavor that both kids and adults will love.

Preparation time: 5 minutes plus chilling time

Total time: 1 hour

Makes 4 servings (1 cup)

- 2 ripe avocados, pitted and peeled
- ¼ cup unsweetened cocoa powder
- 2 tablespoons unsweetened soy or almond milk or whole milk
- 2 tablespoons pure maple syrup, or 2 dates, pitted
- 1 teaspoon pure vanilla extract
- 1 teaspoon orange or tangerine zest, or 1 drop food-grade orange essential oil

Place all the ingredients in a wide-mouthed mason jar or cup that will fit an immersion blender without splashing. Blend until smooth and creamy. Spoon the pudding evenly into four ramekins or small bowls.

Although this pudding can be eaten right away, it is better when placed in the refrigerator for at least 1 hour to allow the flavors to fully integrate before serving.

Calories: 160   Protein: 3 g
Carbohydrate: 16 g   Fat: 11 g

Variation

Omit the orange and add 2 tablespoons Cold-Brewed Coffee Concentrate (page 62), espresso, or strong-brewed coffee, or 1 tablespoon instant coffee grounds.

Chef Dawn's Tasty Tip

Don't Get Stuck on Sweetness

When using honey or maple syrup, rub your measuring spoons or cups with oil to keep the sweeteners from sticking, or simply measure the oil first, then measure the sweetener in the oiled container before rinsing it.

Chocolate Custard (All Phases)

George Brown College culinary students Iman Faddoul and Metti Hambisa wowed us with this traditional dark chocolate custard as part of their *Always Hungry?* book class project. It brings all the rich chocolate flavor you need without the added sugar.

Preparation time: 5 minutes plus chilling time

Total time: 35 minutes

Makes 4 servings

- ½ cup whole milk or unsweetened soy milk
- 3 large eggs
- 3½ ounces dark chocolate (at least 70% cacao), broken into small pieces
- 1 medium peach, pitted and sliced, or about 1 cup other seasonal fruit, for garnish

Heat the milk in a small saucepan over medium heat, stirring regularly, until tiny bubbles form on the side of the pan. Remove from the heat.

In a small bowl, whisk the eggs and set aside.

Melt the chocolate in a double boiler, then remove from the heat (see Chef Dawn's Tasty Tip for melting chocolate, page 314).

While whisking, slowly add the milk 3 tablespoons at a time to the melted chocolate, whisking until all the milk has been added.

While whisking continuously, slowly add the whisked eggs to the melted chocolate mixture. Place back on the double boiler or over very low heat and cook, stirring regularly, for 5 minutes, or until the mixture thickens.

Remove from the heat and pour the mixture into four small ramekins. Refrigerate for 20 minutes or until fully cooled.

Garnish the custards with the peach slices.

Calories: 234	Protein: 8 g
Carbohydrate: 17 g	Fat: 15 g

Apple Pie Parfait (Phases 2 and 3, with Phase 1 Variation)

This spicy parfait packs a combination of exciting textures in each bite. Bursting with crunchy nuts and chewy dried fruit, interspersed with layers of smooth Greek yogurt, this is an apple pie that's perfect all year.

Preparation time: 10 minutes

Total time: 70 minutes

Makes 8 servings (2 cups)

- 1½ ounces unsweetened dried apples, chopped (about ⅓ cup packed)
- 4 large dried figs, chopped (about 2 ounces)
- 2 large unsweetened dates, pitted and chopped (about 1½ ounces)
- 1 medium apple or pear, cored and cut into small dice (leave the peel on)
- 2 cups water
- 1 cinnamon stick, or ½ teaspoon ground cinnamon
- ½ cup slivered almonds, cashews, or sunflower seeds
- Pinch of salt
- ½ teaspoon pure vanilla extract
- 2½ cups plain whole-milk Greek yogurt

Place the dried apples, figs, dates, fresh apple, water, cinnamon, slivered almonds, and salt in a saucepan. Bring to a boil over medium heat. Cover the pan, reduce the heat to low, and simmer, stirring occasionally, for 45 minutes to 1 hour, or until the liquid has been absorbed and the fruit has thickened to a compote consistency. (Alternatively, after bringing it to a boil, transfer the fruit mixture to a slow cooker and cook on low for 4 to 5 hours.) Stir in the vanilla. Remove from the heat and allow to cool slightly or chill for later. Or make ahead and store in the refrigerator for up to a couple of weeks.

In a parfait cup or glass (wineglasses work beautifully for this), layer 2 tablespoons of yogurt followed by 2 tablespoons of the fruit compote, and repeat for a four-layer parfait. Top with a heaping tablespoon of yogurt.

Calories: 181   Protein: 9 g
Carbohydrate: 21 g   Fat: 7 g

Variations

Use any other unsweetened dried fruit to equal about ¾ cup packed.

For Phase 1: Substitute 2 cups cooked fruit for the dried fruit and apple and cook until soft, and substitute ricotta for half the Greek yogurt.

Calories: 171   Protein: 10 g
Carbohydrate: 10 g   Fat: 11 g

Pear Cranberry Pie (Phases 2 and 3)

Our simple chickpea crust balances the sweet pears, tart cranberries, and touch of spicy ginger. Your guests will never know there's no added sugar in this pie.

Preparation time: 10 minutes

Total time: 1½ hours

Makes 10 to 12 servings (one 9-inch pie)

- 2 tablespoons raisins
- 4 large pears (about 2½ pounds), cored and diced (leave the peel on)
- ½ cup water
- 1 cup whole fresh or frozen cranberries (about 4 ounces)
- Pinch of salt
- ½ teaspoon tangerine or orange zest
- Squeeze of fresh tangerine juice (optional)

- ½ teaspoon finely grated ginger or ginger juice (optional; see Chef Dawn's Tasty Tip for prepping and storing fresh ginger, page 289)
- 2 recipes Grain-Free Piecrust dough (page 206)

Preheat the oven to 350°F.

Place the raisins, one of the pears, and water in a pot. If using frozen cranberries, add them now as well. Bring to a boil. Reduce the heat to maintain a simmer and cook for 10 minutes, or until the raisins and pears are soft.

Add the cranberries and salt. Bring back to a boil. Reduce the heat and simmer until the cranberries have popped, about 5 minutes, less if frozen cranberries were added at the beginning. Simmer for 5 to 10 minutes more to fully soften the cranberries.

Add the tangerine zest and juice (if using) and ginger to taste (if using). Pulse with an immersion blender to create a chunky sauce. Stir in the remaining pears.

Roll one round of the pie dough between sheets of parchment paper to fit into a 9-inch pie plate. Place the dough into the pie plate. If desired, prebake the bottom crust for 5 to 10 minutes. Meanwhile, roll out the top crust.

Pour the filling into the bottom crust and cover with the top crust, sealing the edges by crimping, fluting, or pressing them with the tines of a fork, then make a few slits in the middle to allow steam to escape.

Bake for 40 to 45 minutes, or until the crust is golden and the filling is bubbling. Cool for at least 15 minutes before serving. Serve warm or cool. The filling will thicken as it is completely cooled. Store in the refrigerator for up to a week.

Based on 10 servings	Carbohydrate: 34 g	Fat: 13 g
Calories: 284	Protein: 7 g	

Variation

Make 12 individual mini pies in a standard muffin tin. Follow the crust directions as described in Meat Pies (page 154).

Pumpkin Pie Tartlets (Phases 2 and 3)

These miniature pies are so sweet and creamy, and look beautiful when made in muffin tins. A low-sugar, gluten-free treat for the holidays.

Preparation time: 5 minutes

Total time: 1¼ hours

Makes 12 servings (12 muffin-size pies or one 9-inch pie)

- 4 cups large chunks peeled winter squash, such as kabocha, butternut, buttercup, etc. (3 cups packed, cooked)
- ¼ teaspoon salt
- ¼ cup neutral-tasting oil, such as high-oleic safflower or avocado oil
- 2 tablespoons pure maple syrup
- 2 tablespoons honey
- ½ cup unsweetened soy or almond milk, or whole milk
- 1½ teaspoons ground cinnamon
- ¼ teaspoon ground ginger or 1 teaspoon ginger juice (see page 289)
- ¼ teaspoon ground cloves
- ¼ teaspoon freshly grated nutmeg
- ¼ teaspoon ground allspice (optional)
- 1 teaspoon pure vanilla extract
- 2 eggs, or 8 ounces extra-firm tofu, or 2 tablespoons chia seeds, finely ground and mixed with ½ cup water
- Olive oil spray or oil for muffin tins
- ½ cup almond flour

Preheat the oven to 350°F.

Fit a steamer basket in a pot. Add 1 to 2 inches of water to the bottom of the pot, just under the level of the basket. Place the squash in the steamer basket and bring the water to a boil. Reduce the heat to medium-low and steam the squash until tender, about 15 minutes.

Transfer the cooked squash to a high-powered blender or food processor, add the remaining ingredients, and puree until smooth, or add the remaining ingredients directly to the pot and blend using an immersion blender. Rub or spray a standard muffin tin with oil. Sprinkle 2 teaspoons of almond flour into the bottom of each well, then fill with pie filling for a quick tartlet with a simple bottom crust and custard-like sides.

Bake for 50 to 60 minutes or until the filling is completely set and begins to crack on top. Cool for 30 minutes to an hour, then gently remove the tartlets from the tins by running a thin spatula or knife around the edge of the tartlet to release it from the tin. These can be served warm but are best after 1 to 2 days in the refrigerator when flavors have had time to fully meld and the filling becomes a bit more dense. Store in an airtight container in the refrigerator for up to 10 days.

Tip: Measure out your oil first and use the same utensil for the sweetener (see Chef Dawn's Tasty Tip, page 318).

Calories: 139   Protein: 3 g
Carbohydrate: 12 g   Fat: 9 g

Variation

Pie Variation: Use one Grain-Free Piecrust dough (page 206). Roll between parchment paper and press into a 9-inch pie plate or separate into 12 even pieces and roll individually to fit into the 12 muffin-tin wells. Prebake crust(s) for 5 to 7 minutes. Pour the blended filling into the prebaked piecrust(s) and bake for 50 to 60 minutes. Cool and store as indicated in the recipe.

Calories: 187   Protein: 5 g
Carbohydrate: 18 g   Fat: 11 g

Cashew Crème (Phases 2 and 3)

Simple ingredients whip together to create a luscious, creamy topping everyone will love. Naturally vegan, this crème is so smooth that you'll forget you started with whole nuts. Use it on top of fresh fruit, as a dip, or as an icing substitute.

Preparation time: 5 minutes

Total time: 5 minutes

Makes about 1 cup

- 1 cup raw cashews
- ½ cup boiling water
- 1 teaspoon pure vanilla extract
- 1 to 2 tablespoons pure maple syrup

Place all the ingredients in a blender. Blend until smooth and creamy. Set aside to cool before serving. Store in an airtight container in the refrigerator for up to 1 week.

Tip: This recipe works best in a high-powered blender or with an immersion blender. To make the process a bit easier, soften the cashews by soaking them overnight in ½ cup water. In this case, use the soaked cashews and any remaining soaking water in place of the raw cashews and boiling water.

Calories: 40 (Per 1 tablespoon)   Protein: 1 g
Carbohydrate: 3 g   Fat: 3 g

Cardamom Whipped Cream (All Phases)

Adding sweet spices like cardamom or cinnamon is a delicious way to "sweeten" up whipped cream without adding sugar.

Preparation time: 5 minutes

Total time: 5 minutes

Makes 6 to 12 servings (about ¾ cup)

- ⅓ cup heavy cream
- ¼ teaspoon ground cardamom, cinnamon, or other sweet spice

Pour the heavy cream into a deep bowl that will fit a handheld mixer or immersion blender with whisk attachment without splashing. Add the cardamom. Whip with a handheld mixer or using the whisk attachment of an immersion blender until the cream holds soft peaks. Serve immediately or store in the refrigerator until ready to use, or for up to 1 week.

Calories: 26 (Per 1 tablespoon)   Protein: 0 g
Carbohydrate: 0 g   Fat: 3 g

Candied Nuts (Phases 2 and 3)

A few of these are all you need to enliven simple desserts, or have a small handful for a scrumptious snack.

Preparation time: 2 minutes

Total time: 18 minutes

Makes 4 to 6 servings

- 1 cup whole nuts, such as walnuts, pecans, cashews, or other nuts or seeds of your choice
- 2 teaspoons pure maple syrup

Preheat the oven to 350°F.

Combine the nuts and maple syrup in a bowl and toss until the nuts are completely covered in syrup.

Spread into a shallow baking dish. Bake for about 15 minutes, stirring every 5 minutes, until the maple syrup is dried and sticking to the nuts.

Spread on parchment paper to cool. Once the nuts are completely cooled, store them at room temperature in a cupboard in a glass jar or container with a lid for up to a few weeks.

Calories: 50 (Per 1 tablespoon)   Protein: 1 g
Carbohydrate: 2 g   Fat: 5 g

Poached Pears (All Phases)

Spicy poached pears bring any dinner to an elegant conclusion. Bask in the warm flavors of cinnamon, nutmeg, and red wine as you savor each bite.

Preparation time: 10 minutes

Total time: 30 minutes

Makes 4 servings

- 4 medium pears, halved lengthwise and cored
- 4 to 6 dried plums or apricots (for Phases 2 and 3)
- ½ cup red wine
- ½ teaspoon ground cinnamon
- ¼ teaspoon freshly grated nutmeg
- Dash of salt

Arrange the pears cut-side up in a single layer in a shallow skillet with the dried fruit (if using) scattered around them. Pour the wine over the top so it covers the flesh of the pears. Sprinkle the spices over the fruit.

Bring to a boil over medium heat. Reduce the heat to medium-low, cover, and simmer for 10 to 15 minutes, or until the pears are soft. Remove from the heat. Serve warm.

Tip: Use a melon baller to core the pears and preserve as much of the flesh as possible.

Calories: 151 (With dried fruit)   Protein: 1 g
Carbohydrate: 35 g   Fat: 0 g

Calories: 123 (Without dried   Carbohydrate: 27 g   Fat: 0 g
  fruit)   Protein: 1 g

My *Always Delicious* Story

Every diet I've tried eventually failed. Some "worked" for a while, but the results were always the same—gaining the weight back and then some. Since the diets were different, I assumed the problem was me...my sweet tooth, my lack of willpower, my inability to exercise enough or eat less, and I didn't know how to change those things.

My original goal on *AH* was to reach the last weight at which I felt pretty good. But I didn't really believe that was achievable—I was going to be happy if I got halfway there. After just one week, I noticed that something was very different this time. I no longer felt ravenous all the time, and I wasn't craving any of the things that had always been my downfall. Everything tasted so good, yet I suddenly had willpower. Four months later, I'd hit that original goal weight and kept on losing! I realized that I wasn't waiting for this "diet" to be over. This was my way of life now. The things I want to eat are the things I should eat. I also just felt so much better. Pain in both shoulders that required cortisone shots was gone, debilitating nighttime leg cramps were gone, I didn't need to get up multiple times in the night to go to the bathroom, and I was just happier.

The reason those other diets failed wasn't *me*. It was the "nonfoods" and low-fat "diet food" that caused the failure. My body was protesting in every way possible, and I just didn't understand the language. In the past, it seemed like my body was working against me. It was hungry and craved things I knew I shouldn't eat but sometimes I just couldn't help myself. Now my body is no longer my enemy. It's working with me to let me know what it needs and rewards me in ways I never expected for treating it right. This plan has changed me in so many ways. Most important, it's changed what I do eat because it's changed what I want to eat. My mind and my body are now working together.

Linda P., age 70, Palm Desert, California

Acknowledgments

Upon publication of *Always Hungry?*, we received an outpouring of support and encouragement beyond anything we had imagined. Several dedicated readers helped us form a Facebook community and volunteered to moderate. Wow, what a difference they made! Today, our community is flourishing, thanks to our growing team of moderators and the enthusiastic participation of many thousands of readers. The community inspired us to write this cookbook.

We are forever grateful to our Rock Star moderators, recipe testers, and now friends Brian Baumgartner, Brian Goodhart, Carlisle Douglas, Cassandra Sample, Connie Hurlbut, Flo Bruehl, Gary Markley, Gloria Lindh, Heather Jinmaku-Brown, Ingrid Farnbach, Jan Adamczyk, Jenny Dufault, Jenny Knight, Jen Sullivan, Joanne Katzen-Jones, Julie Miller, Kate Sommers, Keri Mertens Rabe, Kimberly Cooper, Laura Norden, Leeann Maat, Linda Fischer Palmer, Lynne Thompson, Malvina Craig, Marilynn Slade, Michael Guy, Morgan Perkins, Nancy Boykin, Nikki Szegda Isakson, and Stephani Morancie. Thank you for your selfless work on our shared mission (and for making Dawn laugh before breakfast many times).

In addition to the moderators, other cooks and non-cooks provided feedback on the recipes, including Anne McKay, Cara Ebbeling, Craig Lambert, Jane Piercy, Peggy Falk, and Linda Steinberg (thanks for the yogic stretches); Becky Mozaffarian and Krystle Benedict and their families (thanks for the Friday recipe marathons); and Anna Merli and Natasha Novoselova (thanks for the countless hours together in the kitchen). Grandma Bettie Black was a loving presence in our home, supporting the family with childcare when Dawn was immersed in this project.

We are deeply grateful to Elizabeth Coyle for exceptional technical and editorial support. With her gentle, quiet, flexible, and compassionate demeanor, Elizabeth made a big project manageable and fun. She devoted many hours to inputting recipe data, calculating ratios, menu building, blogging, answering e-mails, and helping to translate Dawn's spoken words onto paper. We know that Elizabeth will go on to do great things in the food and publishing world. Thanks also to our dear friend Mariska van Aalst for editorial assistance and support.

Food pictures were taken by Scott and Donna Erb of Erb Photography, working with food stylist Dona Bourgery at That's a Wrap Design. It was a joy to work with this talented team.

We had the honor and pleasure of collaborating with the Culinary Management Nutrition faculty at the Centre for Hospitality and Culinary Arts at George Brown College, Toronto, to develop a course based on the *Always Hungry?* program. Several of the students' delicious and nutrient-compliant recipes are featured in this book. Thanks especially to Moira Cockburn, Tony Garcia, Sharon Booy, Candace Rambert, Patrick Secord, Ema Costantini, and their team and students. We look forward to much more together! Heartfelt thanks also to the sweet Heather Jinmaku-Brown, who provided several recipes to help round out the mix.

A thousand thanks to the team at Grand Central Publishing—our former editor Sarah Pelz (who's gone on to great new things), editorial director Karen Murgolo, assistant editor Morgan Hedden, publicity director Matthew Ballast, and the marketing trio of Brian McLendon, Amanda Pritzker, and Andrew Duncan. They make the agony and ecstasy of book writing more of the latter.

Our agent, Richard Pine, and his team at Inkwell Management, including Alexis Hurley and Eliza Rothstein, provided wise counsel, support, and friendship. These folks are as good as it gets!

The science for our nutritional approach is based in part on research findings from the New Balance Foundation Obesity Prevention Center at Boston Children's Hospital. We are grateful to the Center's current and former members (too numerous to mention by name here) and especially Center codirector Cara Ebbeling. Thanks also to Gary Taubes and Mark Friedman for stimulating discussions and critical feedback.

And finally, Dawn is indebted to all her teachers, students, and support teams who taught and inspired her along her professional and personal life's path. Special thanks to Carl and Julia Ferre; David and Cynthia Briscoe; Elizabeth Foster; Lino and Jane Stanchich; Warren Kramer; Michio Kushi, and the team at the Kushi Institute; Morgan Jones and the team at the Natural Epicurean Academy of Culinary Arts; and, last but most certainly not least, Adrienne Nikki Cobb.

Appendix

GUIDES TO PREPARING VEGETABLES, WHOLE GRAINS, NUTS, AND SEEDS

GUIDE TO COOKING VEGETABLES

Vegetables are a mainstay of the *Always Hungry* Solution—full of nutrition and a great vehicle for the rich sauces and dips used in all program phases. Get creative, and let this guide remove the guesswork.

Vegetable	Size and Prep	Cooking Time in Minutes				
		Sauté*	Steam	Boil	Blanch**	Roast
Arugula	Rinse well. Coarsely chop.	2 to 3	2 to 3	—	Less than 1	—
Asparagus	Cut away and discard tough ends.	4 to 6	7 to 8	6 to 8	1	8 to 10
Beets	To sauté: Peel and shred. To steam or boil: Peel and cut into 1-inch cubes. To blanch: Slice into thin rounds or half-moons. To roast: Place whole, unpeeled beets in a baking dish with ¼ cup water and cover tightly or wrap individually in foil; peel skin when they are done.	6 to 8	15 to 20	10 to 15	1 to 2	45 to 60 (depending on size)
Bell Peppers (Green, Red, Orange, or Yellow)	Remove and discard seeds. Cut into thin strips.	5 to 7	—	—	Less than 1	20 to 25

Vegetable	Size and Prep	Cooking Time in Minutes				
		Sauté*	Steam	Boil	Blanch**	Roast
Bok Choy, Tatsoi	Cut white parts into ½-inch slices, coarsely chop the leaves.	2 to 4	2 to 4	2 to 4	Less than 1	—
Broccoli	Peel or cut off hard outer part of the stem and cut into small sticks; separate tops into small florets.	4 to 6	6 to 8	6 to 8	1	20 to 25
Broccoli Rabe, Rapini, or Chinese Broccoli	Cut into ½-inch slices.	4 to 6	4 to 6	4 to 6	1	—
Cabbage (White, Green, or Red)	Remove and discard core. Shred thinly. To roast: Cut into 1½-inch-thick wedges.	5 to 7	8 to 10	8 to 10	1	20 to 25
Carrots	To sauté or blanch: Shred or cut into thin strips, rounds, or matchsticks. To steam, boil, or roast: Cut into thick rounds or chunks.	4 to 6	8 to 10	8 to 10	1 to 2	25 to 30
Cauliflower	Separate into small florets. Core diced.	4 to 6	7 to 9	7 to 9	1 to 2	15 to 18
Chard (Green or Red)	Rinse well. Cut the stems into ½-inch slices and coarsely chop the greens.	4 to 6— add stems first, then greens after 2 minutes	4 to 6 Stems on bottom	3 to 5	1 for stems, less for leaves	—
Collard Greens	Rinse well. Separate the stems from the leaves. Cut the stems into very thin rounds and coarsely chop the leaves.	5 to 8	5 to 8	3 to 5	1 to 2	—
Daikon or Other Types of Radish	Cut into thick chunks or leave small radishes whole. To sauté: Shred or cut into thin matchsticks. To blanch: Cut into thin rounds or half-moons.	4 to 6	4 to 6	5 to 8	1	15 to 20
Eggplant	Peel, if desired. Cut into 1-inch cubes or slices.	10 to 12	—	—	—	20 to 25
Fennel	Cut bulb and stems into thin rounds. To roast: Cut into quarters or chunks.	6 to 8	6 to 8	6 to 8	1 to 3	30 to 45
Green Beans	Trim off and discard tough ends or stems.	3 to 5	4 to 6	4 to 6	1 or less	8 to 10

Vegetable	Size and Prep	Cooking Time in Minutes				
		Sauté*	Steam	Boil	Blanch**	Roast
Kale	Rinse well. Separate the stems from the leaves. Cut the stems into very thin rounds and coarsely chop the leaves.	4 to 7	4 to 7	3 to 5	1 to 2	—
Leek	Cut in half lengthwise and thoroughly rinse all layers. Cut white and green parts into thin rounds. To roast: Cut into large chunks.	5 to 7	5 to 7	6 to 9	1 to 2	20 to 30
Mustard Greens	Rinse well. Separate the stems from the leaves. Cut the stems into very thin rounds and coarsely chop the leaves.	3 to 5	3 to 5	3 to 5	1	—
Napa or Chinese Cabbage	Cut the white parts into ½-inch slices and coarsely chop the leaves.	2 to 4	2 to 4	2 to 4	Less than 1	—
Onions (Sweet, Yellow, White, or Red)	Peel the tough outer skin. Slice in thin half-moons or dice. To roast: Cut into quarters or thick wedges.	8 to 10	10 to 12	8 to 10	2 to 3	20 to 25
Parsnips	Cut into ½-inch chunks. To sauté: Shred or cut into thin matchsticks. To blanch: Cut into thin rounds.	8 to 10	13 to 15	12 to 14	2	35 to 50
Rutabaga	Peel. Cut into ½-inch chunks. To sauté: Shred or cut into thin matchsticks. To blanch: Cut into thin rounds.	7 to 9	16 to 18	14 to 16	1 to 2	35 to 50
Snow Peas or Snap Peas	Trim off and discard tough ends or stems and peel the string down the edge.	2 to 3	2 to 3	2 to 3	Less than 1	—
Spinach	Rinse well. Coarsely chop.	2 to 3	2 to 3	3 to 5	Less than 1	—
Summer Squash (Yellow or Zucchini)	Cut into ¼-inch-thick slices or sticks.	5 to 10	5 to 7	5 to 7	1 to 2	15 to 20

Vegetable	Size and Prep	Cooking Time in Minutes				
		Sauté*	Steam	Boil	Blanch**	Roast
Sweet Potato	To sauté: Shred or cut into thin matchsticks. To steam or boil: Cut into 1-inch chunks or thick rounds. To blanch: Cut into thin rounds. To roast: Cut into 1-inch chunks or thick rounds, or leave whole.	8 to 10	8 to 10	10 to 12	2 to 3	45 to 60
Turnips	Cut into ½-inch chunks. To sauté: Shred or cut into thin matchsticks. To blanch: Cut into thin rounds.	6 to 8	12 to 14	10 to 12	1 to 2	30 to 40
Winter Squash (Buttercup, Butternut, Kabocha, or Acorn)	Cut in half. Remove and discard seeds. Cut into 1-inch chunks or thick wedges. The skin can be eaten unless very tough, like acorn. To blanch: Cut into thin half-moons.	—	14 to 16	12 to 14	2 to 3	30 to 40

* Olive oil is recommended, but other vegetable oils (for example, high-oleic safflower oil) and butter may be used.
** Immersing vegetables in cold water after blanching is not necessary.

GUIDE TO COOKING WHOLE GRAINS

Cooking whole grains may seem like a culinary mystery, but it really is quite simple: All you need is water, salt…and heat. Just bring to a boil, cover, and simmer for the time indicated. In Phase 2, we incorporate whole-kernel grains on a daily basis. Experiment with whole-kernel grains you might not have tried before—you'll likely find them more satisfying than the processed versions. Make extra to use for future meals. With cooked whole grains already made, meal preparation becomes quick and easy.

Whole Grain	Dry Amount	Water	Salt	Cooking Time	Approximate Yield
Presoaking Not Required					
Buckwheat (Kasha)	1 cup	1½ to 2 cups	⅛ teaspoon	15 to 20 minutes	3 cups
Cracked Wheat (Bulgur)	1 cup	1 to 1¼ cups boiling	⅛ teaspoon	5 minutes	2 cups
Farro	1 cup	2 cups	⅛ teaspoon	30 minutes	2 cups
Millet*	1 cup	2 to 4 cups boiling	⅛ teaspoon	30 minutes	3 to 5 cups
Pearl Barley	1 cup	3 cups	⅛ teaspoon	30 minutes	3 cups
Quinoa (rinse well)	1 cup	2 cups	⅛ teaspoon	20 minutes	3 cups
Steel-cut oats	1 cup	2 cups	Pinch	30 to 45 minutes	2 cups
Steel-cut oats (overnight version)	1 cup	4 cups	Pinch	Bring to a full boil, then let sit on the stove, covered, overnight. Or cool the oats and place in the refrigerator overnight. Serve cold or reheat before eating.	4½ cups
Presoaking Recommended (4 hours to overnight)**					
Brown Rice***	1 cup	1½ cups	⅛ teaspoon	50 minutes (cooking time will vary based on type of rice)	2 to 3 cups
Hulled Barley	1 cup	3 cups	⅛ teaspoon	1 hour or more	3 cups
Wheat Berries	1 cup	3 cups	⅛ teaspoon	1 hour or more	3 cups

   * For fluffy millet that separates nicely, use 2¼ cups boiling water; for soft, creamy millet, use 4 cups boiling water. The soft millet may also be cooled, cut, and pan-fried like polenta.

  ** Presoaking allows the grains to begin the process of germination, increasing nutrient value and also making for a richer, nuttier taste.

*** Short-grain rice will make a stickier rice. Long-grain and basmati rice will make a fluffier, separated grain.

GUIDE TO ROASTING NUTS AND SEEDS

Basic Cooking Instructions:

Preheat oven to 350°F. Spread raw nuts or seeds in a single layer onto a large baking sheet. Place in the oven and cook until lightly golden in color and the nutty aroma first begins to waft from the oven (see times listed below). Every oven is a bit different, so pay close attention, check them every few minutes, and avoid overcooking. Remove from the oven immediately when done and transfer to a large plate or serving tray to cool. Once cooled, store in a jar with a lid (wide mouth canning jars work nicely) or other airtight container.

Nuts or Seeds	Cooking Time
Almonds	10–12 minutes
Cashews	8–10 minutes
Macadamia	Use raw
Peanuts	10–12 minutes
Pecans	10–12 minutes
Pistachios	8–10 minutes
Pumpkin Seeds	6–8 minutes—done when they are golden and begin to puff up
Sesame Seeds	6–8 minutes—done when they are golden, fragrant, and begin to pop
Sunflower Seeds	5–7 minutes
Walnuts	8–10 minutes

Note: Toaster ovens cook much faster. Follow toaster oven directions or experiment with times for your toaster oven. Remember to let your nose guide you: The moment you smell the aroma, they're done!

CONVERTING TO METRICS

Volume Measurement Conversions

Cups	Tablespoons	Teaspoons	Milliliters
		1 tsp	5 ml
1/16 cup	1 tbsp	3 tsp	15 ml
1/8 cup	2 tbsp	6 tsp	30 ml
1/4 cup	4 tbsp	12 tsp	50 ml
1/3 cup	5 1/3 tbsp	16 tsp	75 ml
1/2 cup	8 tbsp	24 tsp	125 ml
2/3 cup	10 2/3 tbsp	32 tsp	150 ml
3/4 cup	12 tbsp	36 tsp	150 ml
1 cup	16 tbsp	48 tsp	250 ml

Weight Conversion Measurements

US	Metric
1 ounce	28.4 grams (g)
8 ounces	227.5 g
16 ounces (1 pound)	455 g

Cooking Temperature Conversions

Celsius/Centigrade	F = (C x 1.8) + 32
Fahrenheit	C = (F–32) x 0.5555

Zero degrees Celsius and 100°C are arbitrarily placed at the melting and boiling points of water, while Fahrenheit establishes 0°F as the stabilized temperature when equal amounts of ice, water, and salt are mixed. So, for example, if you are baking at 350°F and want to know that temperature in Celsius, the following calculation will provide it: C = (350–32) x 0.5555=176.66°C.

Notes

Chapter 1: Welcome to Always Delicious

1. **Heymsfield SB, et al.** "Why do obese patients not lose more weight when treated with low-calorie diets? A mechanistic perspective." *Am J Clin Nutr* 2007; 85:346–54.

2. **Kraschnewski JL, et al.** "Long-term weight loss maintenance in the United States." *Int J Obes* 2010; 34(11):1644–1654.

3. **Schwartz MB, et al.** "The influence of one's own body weight on implicit and explicit anti-fat bias." *Obesity* 2006; 14(3):440–7.

4. **Latner JD, et al.** "Getting worse: the stigmatization of obese children." *Obes Res* 2003; 11(3):452–6.

5. **Roehling MV, et al.** "Investigating the validity of stereotypes about overweight employees: the relationship between body weight and normal personality traits." *GOM* 2008; 33(4):392–424.

Chapter 2: The Science of Always Delicious

1. **Robson D.** "There really are 50 Eskimo words for 'snow.'" *Washington Post*, January 14, 2013. www.washingtonpost.com/national/health-science/there-really-are-50-eskimo-words-for-snow/2013/01/14/e0e3f4e0-59a0-11e2-beee-6e38f5215402_story.html?tid=ss_tw.

2. **Ludwig DS.** "The glycemic index: physiological mechanisms relating to obesity, diabetes, and cardiovascular disease." *JAMA* 2002; 287(18):2414–23.

3. **Mansoor N, et al.** "Effects of low-carbohydrate diets v. low-fat diets on body weight and cardiovascular risk factors: a meta-analysis of randomised controlled trials." *Br J Nutr* 2016; 115:466–016. **Mancini JG, et al.** "Systematic Review of the Mediterranean Diet for Long-Term Weight Loss." *Am J Med* 2016; 129:407–016; 129. **Sackner-Bernstein J, et al.** "Dietary Intervention for Overweight and Obese Adults: Comparison of Low-Carbohydrate and Low-Fat Diets. A Meta-Analysis." *PLoS One* 2015; 10:e0139817. **Tobias DK, et al.** "Effect of low-fat diet interventions versus other diet interventions on long-term weight change in adults: a systematic review and meta-analysis." *Lancet Diabetes Endocrinol* 2015; 3:968–015. **Bueno NB, et al.** "Very-low-carbohydrate ketogenic diet v. low-fat diet for long-term weight loss: a meta-analysis of randomised controlled trials." *Br J Nutr* 2013; 110:1178–013.

4. **Howard BV, et al.** "Low-fat dietary pattern and risk of cardiovascular disease: the Women's Health Initiative Randomized Controlled Dietary Modification Trial." *JAMA* 2006; 295(6):655–66.

5. **Look Ahead Research Group.** "Cardiovascular effects of intensive lifestyle intervention in type 2 diabetes." *N Engl J Med* 2013; 369:145–54.

6. **Bueno NB, et al.** "Very-low-carbohydrate ketogenic diet v. low-fat diet for long-term weight loss: a meta-analysis of randomised controlled trials." *Br J Nutr* 2013; 110:1178–87. **Sackner-Bernstein J, et al.** "Dietary Intervention for Overweight and Obese Adults: Comparison of Low-Carbohydrate and Low-Fat Diets. A Meta-Analysis." *PLoS One* 2015; 10:e0139817. **Mansoor N, et al.** "Effects of low-carbohydrate diets v. low-fat diets on body weight and cardiovascular risk factors: a meta-analysis of randomised controlled trials." *Br J Nutr* 2016; 115:466–79. **Maiorino MI, et al.** "Mediterranean diet cools down the inflammatory milieu in type 2 diabetes: the MÉDITA randomized controlled trial." *Endocrine* 2016; 54:634–641. **Jonasson L, et al.** "Advice to follow a low-carbohydrate diet has a favourable impact on low-grade inflammation in type 2 diabetes compared with advice to follow a low-fat diet." *Ann Med* 2014; 46:182–7. **Ryan MC, et al.** "The Mediterranean diet improves hepatic steatosis and insulin sensitivity in individuals with non-alcoholic fatty liver disease." *J Hepatol* 2013; 59:138–43. **Bozzetto L, et al.** "Liver fat is reduced by an isoenergetic MUFA diet in a controlled randomized study in type 2 diabetic patients." *Diabetes Care* 2012; 35:1429–35. **Wang DD, et al.** "Association of specific dietary fats with total and cause-specific mortality." *JAMA Intern Med* 2016; 176:1134–1145.

7. **Mayer-Gross W, et al.** "Taste and selection of food in hypoglycaemia." *Br J Exp Pathol* 1946; 27:297–305.

8. **Strachan MW, et al.** "Food cravings during acute hypoglycaemia in adults with Type 1 diabetes." *Physiol Behav* 2004; 80:675–82.

9. **Page KA, et al.** "Circulating glucose levels modulate neural control of desire for high-calorie foods in humans." *J Clin Invest* 2011 Oct; 121(10):4161–9.

10. **Ziauddeen H, et al.** "Is food addiction a valid and useful concept?" *Obes Rev* 2013; 14:19–28. **Pressman P, et al.** "Food Addiction: Clinical Reality or Mythology." *Am J Med* 2015; 128:1165–6. **Blundell JE, et al.** "Food addiction not helpful: the hedonic component—implicit wanting—is important." *Addiction* 2011; 106:1216–8. **Rogers PJ, et al.** "Food craving and food 'addiction': a critical review of the evidence from a biopsychosocial perspective." *Pharmacol Biochem Behav* 2000; 66:3–14.

11. **Lennerz BS, et al.** "Effects of dietary glycemic index on brain regions related to reward and craving in men." *Am J Clin Nutr* 2013; 98:641–7.

12. Entry for "satiety." Online Etymology Dictionary, accessed April 28, 2017. www.etymonline.com/index.php?term=satiety.

13. **Ludwig DS.** "Dietary glycemic index and obesity." *J Nutr* 2000; 130:280S–283S. **Roberts SB.** "High-glycemic index foods, hunger, and obesity: is there a connection?" *Nutr Rev* 2000; 58:163–9.

14. **Benton D, et al.** "The influence of the glycaemic load of breakfast on the behaviour of children in school." *Physiol Behav* 2007; 92:717–24.

15. **Ingwersen J, et al.** "A low glycaemic index breakfast cereal preferentially prevents children's cognitive performance from declining throughout the morning." *Appetite* 2007; 49:240–4.

16. **Benton D, et al.** "The delivery rate of dietary carbohydrates affects cognitive performance in both rats and humans." *Psychopharmacology* 2003; 166:86–90.

17. **Papanikolaou Y, et al.** "Better cognitive performance following a low-glycaemic-index compared with a high-glycaemic-index carbohydrate meal in adults with type 2 diabetes." *Diabetologia* 2006; 49:855–862.

18. **Breymeyer KL, et al.** "Subjective mood and energy levels of healthy weight and overweight/obese healthy adults on high- and low-glycemic load experimental diets." *Appetite* 2016; 107:253–259.

19. **Cheatham RA, et al.** "Long-term effects of provided low and high glycemic load low energy diets on mood and cognition." *Physiol Behav* 2009; 98:374–9.

20. **Gangwisch JE, et al.** "High glycemic index diet as a risk factor for depression: analyses from the Women's Health Initiative." *Am J Clin Nutr* 2015; 102:454–63.

21. **Walsh CO, et al.** "Effects of diet composition on postprandial energy availability during weight loss maintenance." *PLoS One* 2013; 8(3):e58172.

22. **Steiner JE.** "Facial expressions of the neonate infant indicating the hedonics of food-related chemical stimuli." In Weiffenbach JM, ed. "Taste and development: The genesis of sweet preference." U.S. Government Printing Office; Washington, DC: 1977, 173–188.

Index

addictions, 7, 16, 18–19
Addison's disease, 16–17
adzuki beans
    in Brown Rice Congee, 104–6
    DIY cooking, 74–77
    Savory Adzuki Beans, 223
Aioli, Lemon, **9**, 298–99
alcohol, 23, 48
All-Purpose Seasoned Salt, 283
Almond Butter, DIY, 55–57
Almond Coconut Macaroons, **16**, 312–13
almond flour, about, 195
almonds
    roasting guide, 334
    Tamari Roasted Almonds, 280
Always Delicious chef, 28–52
    composing a meal efficiently, 41–42
    cooking ruts, 46–47
    food substitutions, 39–41
    fresh and seasonal produce, 38–39
    kitchen tools, 36–38
    leftovers, 43–44
    meal planning, 29–30
    obstacles and if-then planning, 44–45
    Prep Day, 32–33
    presentation and food appeal, 45
    stocking and organizing kitchen, 34–36
    thinking like a chef, 28–29
Always Delicious science. *See* science
Always Delicious Victorious Cycle, 25, *26*
Always Hungry? (Ludwig), 1, 3, 4, 13
Always Hungry? Book Community, 5–8
Always Hungry Vicious Cycle, 24–25, *25*

appetizers, recipes, 270–81
Apple Cinnamon Muffins, 91
Apple Pie Parfait, 319–20
Apple Spice Pancakes, 96–97
artichoke hearts
    Artichoke Kalamata Olive Ragout, 220
    in Mediterranean Quinoa, 191–92
    Spinach Artichoke Snack Bites, 277
Artichoke Kalamata Olive Ragout, 220
artificial sweeteners, 17, 48
arugula
    Arugula, Beet, and Goat Cheese Snack Bites,
        278–79
    cooking guide, 329
    in Portobello or Baby Bella Pizzas, 176–77
    in Red Pepper Ring Omelets, 87–88
Arugula, Beet, and Goat Cheese Snack Bites,
    278–79
Asian Marinade or Salad Dressing, Spicy, 294
Asian Parchment-Baked Fish, 141
Asian spices, 35
Asian Stir-Fry, Spicy, 122–23
asparagus
    in Brown Rice Mushroom Risotto, 229–30
    cooking guide, 329
    Summer Grilled or Roasted Vegetables, 215
Avocado Salad, Jicama, Clementine, and, **13**,
    260–61

Baby Lima Beans in Creamy Shiitake Gravy, 224
Bacon-Cheddar Quiche, 94–95
Baked Chicken, Barbecue, 134–36
Baked Fish, Parchment-, **5**, 138–41

143–44
...ted, 175–76
...ns, 91
...late-Dipped, 314
...Pancakes, 97
...ked Chicken, 134–36
...Sauce, 290

cooking guide, 333
Make-Your-Own Whole-Grain Porridge, 101–3
Basic Miso Soup, 258
Basic Seitan, 72
Basic Socca Wrap, 198–99
basil, storing tips, 39
Basil Walnut Pesto, **10**, 297
beans. *See also specific types of beans*
  Brown Rice with Beans, 226
  in Buddha Bowls, 263–64
  canned, about, 74, 77
  DIY cooking, 74–77
  Prep Day, 33
  program foods summary, 48
  quick-cooking, 44, 74
  Refried Beans, 225
  side dishes, recipes, 221–25
  soups, recipes, 246–49, 253–54
beef
  Beef Meatballs, 149–51
  Beef Stroganoff, 158–59
  entrées, recipes, 148–61
  equivalents table, 49–50
  Grab-and-Go Meat Pies, 154–55
  Green Chile Beef Enchilada Casserole, 124–25
  Meat Loaf with Smoked Paprika Ketchup, 152–53
  program foods summary, 48
  Slow-Cooked Beef Chuck Pot Roast with
    Parsnips, 156–57
  Slow Cooker Barbecue Ribs, 159–61
  Slow Cooker Chili, 249–51
  Slow Cooker Shredded Beef, 148–49
Beef Stroganoff, 158–59
beets
  Arugula, Beet, and Goat Cheese Snack Bites,
    278–79
  cooking guide, 329
  in Polish White Borscht, 246–47
bell peppers
  cooking guide, 329
  Red Pepper Ring Omelets, 87–88

Summer Grilled or Roasted Vegetables, 215
belly fat, 43, 52
Berry Vanilla Coconut Shake, 83
beverages
  program foods summary, 48
  recipes, 308–11
  shakes, recipes, 82–85
biology vs. willpower, 11
biscuits. *See also* Rosemary Biscuits
  Breakfast Biscuit Stacks, 88–89
Bison Meatballs, **10**, 149–51
Bison Meat Loaf with Smoked Paprika Ketchup,
  152–53
Black Bean Pâté, 274–75
black beans
  Black Bean Pâté, 274–75
  Cuban Black Bean Soup, 253–54
  DIY cooking, 74–77
  Refried Beans, 225
black-eyed peas
  DIY cooking, 74–77
Black-Eyed Pea Salad (Texas Caviar), 262–63
blenders, 37
blood pressure, 6, 9, 15, 194
blood sugar, 6, 14, 17–18, 24
Blueberry Lime Mint Fizz, **1**, 308–9
Body Rub, 79
body weight science. *See* science
body weight set point, 4, 237
bok choy
  cooking guide, 330
  Sautéed Bok Choy and Shiitake, 213
  in Spicy Asian Stir-Fry, 122–23
Bone Broth, DIY, 58–61
bowls. *See* Buddha Bowls
brain, 16, 18–19
brain fog, 6, 26
Braised Cabbage with Apples, 218
Bread Crumbs, Easy Chickpea, 196–97
breakfast
  recipes, 81–109
  satiety and, 20–21
Breakfast Biscuit Stacks, 88–89
broccoli
  Broccoli Cheddar Soup, 256–57
  cooking guide, 330
  in Miso Pickles, 70–71
  in Spicy Asian Stir-Fry, 122–23
Broccoli Cheddar Soup, 256–57

broccoli rabe
  cooking guide, 330
  Garlicky White Beans with Broccoli Rabe, 221
brown rice
  Brown Rice Congee, 104–6
  Brown Rice Mushroom Risotto, 229–30
  Brown Rice "Tater" Tots, 228–29
  cooking guide, 333
  in Make-Your-Own Whole-Grain Porridge, 101–3
  Mexican Rice, 227
  Pressure-Cooked Brown Rice, 226–27
Brown Rice Congee, 104–6
Brown Rice Mushroom Risotto, 229–30
Brown Rice "Tater" Tots, **14**, 228–29
Brown Rice with Beans, 226
Brown Rice with Chestnuts, 227
Buddha Bowls, 45
  French Salad Niçoise, 268–69
  Greek Salad, 267–68
  Grilled Salmon, 266
  how to make, 263–64
  Japanese, 264–65
  recipes, 263–69
Butternut Sage Puree, 219

cabbage
  Braised Cabbage with Apples, 218
  Cabbage Kofta in a Tomato Tadka, 180–82
  cooking guide, 330, 331
  in Creamy Millet Vegetable Soup, 255
  Easy Pickled Cabbage, 66–67
  in Hot-and-Sour Soup, 240–41
  Sauerkraut, 65–66
  in Spicy Asian Stir-Fry, 122–23
  in Thai Coconut Fish Soup, 238–39
Cabbage Kofta in a Tomato Tadka, 180–82
calories in, calories out, 1–2
Candied Nuts, 324–25
canning jars, 38
carbohydrates
  insulin levels and, 13–14
  program foods summary, 47–48
Cardamom Coconut Macadamia Butter, 57
Cardamom Whipped Cream, 324
carrots
  cooking guide, 330
  Easy Pickled Carrots, 66–67
  Herb Roasted Root Vegetables, 214
Cashew Balsamic Dressing, 286–87

Cashew Butter, DIY, 55–58
Cashew Crème, 323–24
cashews
  Cashew Balsamic Dressing, 286–87
  Cashew Crème, 323–24
  in Mint Chocolate Power Balls, 279–80
  roasting guide, 334
casseroles
  Creamy Green Chile Casserole, 187–88
  Green Chile Chicken or Beef Enchilada
    Casserole, 124–25
  Prep Day, 33
  Quinoa Enchilada Casserole, 183–84
  Sage Walnut Lentil Loaf, 168–70
  Summer Squash Casserole, 185–86
cauliflower
  in Cabbage Kofta in a Tomato Tadka, 180–82
  Cauliflower Couscous, 211–12
  cooking guide, 330
  in Creamy Millet Vegetable Soup, 255
  Fennel Cauliflower Gratin, 190
  Spicy Pickled Vegetables (Escabeche), 68–69
  Summer Cauliflower Casserole, 186
Cauliflower Couscous, **7**, 211–12
celiac disease, 71
chard, cooking guide, 330
Cherry Chocolate Power Shake, 82
Chia Seed Pudding, 108–9
chia seeds, egg substitutes, 92
chicken
  Barbecue Baked Chicken, 134–36
  in Brown Rice Congee, 104–6
  Chicken Fingers, 114–15
  Chicken Parmesan, 126–27
  Chicken Soup on a Budget, 243–44
  Citrus Teriyaki Chicken Stir-Fry, 120–22
  Creamy Dijon Chicken and Mushrooms, 112–13
  Easy Dijon Chicken, 128–30
  entrées, recipes, 110–36
  equivalents table, 49–50
  Green Chile Chicken Enchilada Casserole,
    124–25
  Moroccan Chicken Stew with Apricots, 133–34
  No-Fuss Coq au Vin, 130–32
  On-a-Budget Marinated Chicken, 116–17
  Shredded Chicken, 110–11
  Shredded Chicken Quesadilla, 199–200
  Spicy Asian Stir-Fry, 122–23
  Teriyaki Chicken Kebabs, 141–42

15

126–27

18–20

n a Budget, 243–44

ddar Crisps, 200–201

ar

0, 195

le Spice Pancakes, 96–97

in asic Socca Wrap, 198–99

Chickpea Cheddar Crisps, 200–201

in Chile Cheese Fritters, 204–5

in Cornbread, 205–6

Easy Chickpea Bread Crumbs, 196–97

in Fried Fish Fillets or Chicken Fingers, 114–15

in Grain-Free Piecrust, 206–7

in Grain-Free Pizza, 208–10

in Grain-Free Pumpkin Spice Muffins, 90–91

recipes, 195–210

in Rosemary Biscuits, 203

in Smoke-Dried Tomato Seitan, 73–74

in Socca Cracker, 202

in Socca Crepes, 197–98

in Sweet Breakfast Crepe, 98–99

chickpeas

DIY cooking, 74–77

in Egyptian Fava Bean Stew, 222–23

in Falafel, 178–79

in Greek Salad, 259–60

in Shakshuka, 85–86

Chile Cheese Fritters, 204–5

chiles, 35–36. *See also* green chiles

Chili, Slow Cooker, 249–51

Chimichurri

Cilantro, 300–301

Parsley, 301

chocolate, melting tip, 314

Chocolate Chip Cookies, 312

Chocolate Custard, 318–19

Chocolate-Dipped Fruit, 313–14

Chocolate Mint Power Balls, 279–80

Chocolate Truffles, **16**, 314–16

Chocolate Vanilla Power Balls, 280

cholesterol, 15, 194, 282

Cilantro Chimichurri, 300–301

Citrus Teriyaki Chicken Stir-Fry, 120–22

Citrus Teriyaki Sauce, 293

clams, prep tip, 147

Coconut Almond Macaroons, **16**, 312–13

Coconut BonBons, 316–17

Coconut Cardamom Macadamia Butter, 57

Coconut Fish Soup, Thai, 238–39

coconut flour, about, 195

Coconut Ice Pops, Fruity, 310

Coconut Teff, Creamy, 103–4

coffee grinders, 37

Coffee Scrub, 78

Cold-Brewed Coffee Concentrate, DIY, 62

collard greens, cooking guide, 330

Community Supported Agriculture (CSA), 38, 46

compound butters, 47

Congee, Brown Rice, 104–6

Cooked Quinoa, 231

cooking ruts, 46–47

cooking videos, 47

Coq au Vin, No-Fuss, 130–32

Cornbread, 205–6

Couscous, Cauliflower, **7**, 211–12

cravings, 16–19

Creamy Cheese Sauce, 185

Creamy Coconut Teff, 103–4

Creamy Dijon Chicken and Mushrooms, 112–13

Creamy Green Chile Casserole, 187–88

Creamy Millet Vegetable Soup, 255

Creamy Peppercorn Vinaigrette, 286

Creamy Sun-Dried Tomato Dressing, 287–88

Creamy Vanilla Coffee Shake, 84–85

crepes, recipes, 98–100, 197–98

Crispy Tofu Fries, **9**, 173–74

Croquettes, Quinoa, **13**, 232–33

Crumbled Tempeh, **8**, 192–93

Cuban Black Bean Soup, **11**, 253–54

Cucumber Vegetable Rolls, 281

cucumbers

in Greek Salad, 259–60

in Indian Raita, 303

Perfect Cucumber-Tomato Salad, 261

in Tzatziki, 304

cutting boards, 37–38

dairy, program foods summary, 48

Dairy-Free Basil Walnut Pesto, 297

Dairy-Free Chia Seed Pudding, 108–9

Dairy-Free Chicken Potpie, 119

Dairy-Free Creamy Dijon Chicken and Mushrooms, 113

Dairy-Free Creamy Green Chile Casseroles, 125, 188

Dairy-Free Fennel Rutabaga Gratin, 190

Dairy-Free French Onion Dip, 306
dairy-free shakes, recipes, 82–85
Dairy-Free Sour Cream, 306
Deep-Fried Tofu or Tempeh, 170–71
deep-frying, about, 167
desserts
    Prep Day, 33
    recipes, 312–26
diabetes, 13, 15, 21
diet drinks, 48
do it yourself (DIY) recipes, 53–80
    Beans, 74–77
    Bone Broth, 58–61
    Cold-Brewed Coffee Concentrate, 62
    Greek Yogurt, 54–55
    Nut and Seed Butters, 55–58
    Pickles, 62–71
    Seitan, 71–74
    spa treatments, 77–79
Drunken Marinated Shrimp Kebabs, **6**, 144–46

Easy Chickpea Bread Crumbs, 196–97
Easy Dijon Chicken, 128–30
Easy Dijon Salmon, 128–30
Easy Pickled Cabbage or Carrots, **15**, 66–67
Easy Pizza Sauce, 208–10
eggplant
    cooking guide, 330
    in Souvlaki, 163–65
    Summer Grilled or Roasted Vegetables, 215
eggs
    Bacon-Cheddar Quiche, 94–95
    Red Pepper Ring Omelets, 87–88
    in Shakshuka, 85–86
    Spinach Feta Quiche, 92–94
egg substitutes, 92
Egg Yolk Face Mask, 79
Egyptian Fava Bean Stew (Ful Mudammas), **12**, 222–23
enchiladas, recipes, 124–25, 183–84
entrées, recipes, 110–94
    beef and pork, 148–61
    chicken, 110–36
    fish and seafood, 136–47
    lamb, 161–67
    vegetarian, 167–94
equivalents table, 49–51
Escabeche (Spicy Pickled Vegetables), **15**, 68–69

essential oils, 39
exercise, 2, 11

Facebook, *Always Hungry?* Book Community, 5–8
Falafel, 178–79
farro
    cooking guide, 333
    Make-Your-Own Whole-Grain Porridge, 101–3
fat, 14–15
    low-fat diets, 9, 24–25, *25*
fat cells, 3, 6, 13–15
fava beans
    DIY cooking, 74–77
    Egyptian Fava Bean Stew, 222–23
    Sicilian Fava Bean Soup, 244–45
fennel
    cooking guide, 330
    in Grab-and-Go Meat Pies, 154–55
Fennel Rutabaga Gratin, 189–90
feta
    in Greek Salad, 259–60
    Spinach Feta Quiche, 92–94
Fish and Mushrooms in Tarragon Cream Sauce, 136–38
fish and seafood
    Creamy Dijon Fish and Mushrooms, 113
    Drunken Marinated Shrimp Kebabs, 144–46
    Easy Dijon Salmon, 128–30
    entrées, recipes, 136–47
    equivalents table, 49–50
    Fish and Mushrooms in Tarragon Cream Sauce, 136–38
    Fried Fish Fillets, 114–15
    Grilled Salmon Buddha Bowl, 266
    Mussels in Garlic White Wine Broth, 146–47
    Parchment-Baked Fish, 138–41
    Pesto Baked Fish, 143–44
    Portuguese Seafood Stew, 241–42
    Teriyaki Salmon Kebabs, 141–42
    Thai Coconut Fish Soup, 238–39
Fish en Papillote (Parchment-Baked Fish), **5**, 138–41
flaxseeds, egg substitutes, 92
food addiction, 7, 16, 18–19
food allergies, 39–40
food appeal, 45
food cleanout, 36
food colors, 45
food containers, 45

food cravings. *See* cravings
food labels, 53
food leftovers, 43–44
food palatability, 22–24
food prep, 32–34, 41
food processors, 37
food ruts, 46–47
food stocking, 34–36
food substitutions, 39–41
  equivalents table, 49–51
Foot Soak, Relaxing, 77–78
French Onion Dip, Dairy-Free, 306
French Parchment-Baked Fish, 141
French Salad Niçoise Buddha Bowl, 268–69
French seasonings, 35
fresh produce, 38–39
Fresh Quinoa Salad with Pomegranates, 262
Fresh Salsa, 302
Fresh Turmeric Garlic Marinade, 295
Fried Fish Fillets, 114–15
Fruit Kebab, 314
Fruit Sauce, 106–7
fruits. *See also specific fruits*
  Chocolate-Dipped Fruit, 313–14
  equivalents table, 51
  fresh and seasonal, 38–39
  program foods summary, 48
Fruity Coconut Ice Pops, 310
Ful Mudammas (Egyptian Fava Bean Stew), **12**,
  222–23

garbanzo bean flour. *See* chickpea flour
garbanzo beans. *See* chickpeas
Garlicky White Beans with Broccoli Rabe, 221
Garlic White Wine Broth, Mussels in, 146–47
garnishes, 45
George Brown College (GBC), 8, 163, 171, 174,
  183, 211, 246, 281, 318
ginger
  in Citrus Teriyaki Sauce, 293
  Ginger Tahini Dressing, 288
  prepping and storing, 39, 289
  in Spicy Asian Marinade or Salad Dressing, 294
Ginger Tahini Dressing, **4**, 288
glucose, 13–14, 18
glutamate, 104
gluten-free, 29, 39, 53, 71, 92, 192, 195. *See also*
  chickpea flour
glycemic index (GI), 17*n*, 20–21

glycemic load (GL), 17, 17*n*
Grab-and-Go Meat Pies, 154–55
Grain-Free Piecrust, 206–7
Grain-Free Pizza, 208–10
Grain-Free Pumpkin Spice Muffins, **3**, 90–91
grains. *See* whole grains; *and specific grains*
Greek Dressing, 285
Greek Salad, 259–60
Greek Salad Buddha Bowl, 267–68
Greek Yogurt, DIY, 54–55
green beans
  cooking guide, 330
  in French Salad Niçoise Buddha Bowl, 268–69
Green Chile Chicken or Beef Enchilada Casserole,
  124–25
Green Chile Cream Sauce, 305
green chiles
  Chile Cheese Fritters, 204–5
  Creamy Green Chile Casserole, 187–88
  Green Chile Chicken or Beef Enchilada
    Casserole, 124–25
  Green Chile Cream Sauce, 305
Gremolata, 299–300
Grilled Salmon Buddha Bowl, **4**, 266
Grilled Vegetables, Summer, 215
gut microbiome, 62–63

Herbed Parchment-Baked Fish, 141
Herb-Flavored Mocktail, 309
Herb Roasted Root Vegetables, 214
herbs, 35–36
  growing your own, 39
  storing, 36, 39
high-fat diets, 14–15
Hot-and-Sour Soup, 240–41
Hot Chocolate, Peppermint, 309
hunger, 1, 3, 12–16
hypoglycemia, 17
hypothalamus, 16

Ice Pops, Fruity Coconut, 310
if-then planning, 44–45
Indian Raita, 303
Indian spices, 35
insulin, 3, 13–14
  cravings and, 17–18
  satiety and, 19–20
Italian Parchment-Baked Fish, 141
Italian seasonings, 35

Japanese Buddha Bowl, 264–65
Jicama, Clementine, and Avocado Salad, **13**, 260–61
jook (Brown Rice Congee), 104–6

kale
    cooking guide, 331
    in Grain-Free Pizza, 208–10
    in Portuguese Seafood Stew, 241–42
kebabs
    Drunken Marinated Shrimp Kebabs, 144–46
    Fruit Kebab, 314
    Teriyaki Salmon or Chicken Kebabs, 141–42
kitchen cleanout, 36
kitchen rules, 41–44
kitchen stocking, 34–36
kitchen tools, 36–38, 42
knives, 37
Kofta in a Tomato Tadka, Cabbage, 180–82
kombu, 104
    in Brown Rice Congee, 104–6

lamb
    entrées, recipes, 161–67
    equivalents table, 49–50
    Mustard Peppercorn Roasted Rack of Lamb, 166–67
    Slow-Cooked Moroccan Lamb Stew, 161–63
    in Souvlaki, 163–65
Lassi, Mango, 311
leeks, cooking guide, 331
leftovers, 43–44
legumes. *See* beans
Lemon Aioli, **9**, 298–99
Lemon Thyme or Tarragon Marinade, 296
lentils
    DIY cooking, 74–77
    Sage Walnut Lentil Loaf, 168–70
Life Supports, 4–5
lima beans
    Baby Lima Beans in Creamy Shiitake Gravy, 224
    DIY cooking, 74–77
Lime Cilantro Pesto, 298
Lime Mint Fizz, Blueberry, **1**, 308–9
low-calorie diets, failure of, 1–2
low-fat diets, 9, 24–25, *25*

Macadamia Nut Butter, DIY, 55–57
main entrées, recipes. *See* entrées, recipes

Make-Your-Own Whole-Grain Porridge, 101–3
Mango Lassi, 311
marinades, recipes, 283–306
Marinated Baked Tofu, 175–76
Marinated Chicken, On-a-Budget, 116–17
meal plans (planning), 29–30
    program foods summary, 47–48
    recipe planning worksheet, 31
meal prep, 32–34, 41
Meatballs, Beef, Bison, or Turkey, **10**, 149–51
Meat Loaf with Smoked Paprika Ketchup, 152–53
Meat Pies, Grab-and-Go, 154–55
Mediterranean Parchment-Baked Fish, 141
Mediterranean Quinoa, 191–92
metabolism, 3, 13, 21–22
Mexican Rice, 227
Mexican-style seasonings, 35
microplane zesters, 37
Middle Eastern Pickled Turnips, **15**, 67–68
Middle Eastern spices, 35
millet
    cooking guide, 333
    Creamy Millet Vegetable Soup, 255
    Make-Your-Own Whole-Grain Porridge, 101–3
    Millet Mashed Fauxtatoes, 236
    Millet Tabbouleh, 234–35
    Soft Millet-Corn Polenta, 236–37
Millet Mashed Fauxtatoes, 236
Millet Tabbouleh, 234–35
mind-set, prep ahead, 34
Minestrone Soup, 248–49
Mint Chocolate Power Balls, 279–80
miso
    about, 259
    Basic Miso Soup, 258
Miso Pickles, 70–71
Miso-Sake Marinade, 144
Miso-Scallion Condiment, 105
mood and food, 20–21
Moroccan Chicken Stew with Apricots, **7**, 133–34
Moroccan Lamb Stew, Slow-Cooked, 161–63
Moroccan Sauce, 292
Moroccan spices, 35
MSG, 104
muffins, recipes, 90–91
mung beans
    in Brown Rice Congee, 104–6
    DIY cooking, 74–77
Mushroom Pâté, 275–76

mushrooms
    in Artichoke Kalamata Olive Ragout, 220
    Baby Lima Beans in Creamy Shiitake Gravy, 224
    in Brown Rice Congee, 104–6
    Brown Rice Mushroom Risotto, 229–30
    Creamy Dijon Chicken and Mushrooms, 112–13
    Fish and Mushrooms in Tarragon Cream Sauce, 136–38
    Mushroom Pâté, 275–76
    Portobello or Baby Bella Pizzas, 176–77
    in Sage Walnut Lentil Loaf, 168–70
    Sautéed Bok Choy and Shiitake, 213
    Sautéed Mushrooms, 216
    Seasoned Shiitake Mushrooms, 217
    Spinach Mushroom Crepes, 99–100
Mushroom Seitan, 74
Mussels in Garlic White Wine Broth, 146–47
mustard greens, cooking guide, 331
Mustard Peppercorn Roasted Rack of Lamb, 166–67

No-Fuss Coq au Vin, 130–32
North African spices, 35
nucleus accumbens, 16, 18–19
Nut Butters, DIY, 55–58
nutrition labels, 53
nuts and seeds. *See also specific nuts*
    Candied Nuts, 324–25
    roasting guide, 334

oats
    cooking guide, 333
    Make-Your-Own Whole-Grain Porridge, 101–3
olives
    Artichoke Kalamata Olive Ragout, 220
    in Greek Salad, 259–60
Omelets, Red Pepper Ring, 87–88
On-a-Budget Marinated Chicken, 116–17
onions
    cooking guide, 331
    Quick Ume-Pickled Onions, 69–70
On-the-Go Breakfast Parfait, **2**, 106–7
Orange Chocolate Power Balls, 280
overeating, 1, 3, 11
oysters, prep tip, 147

Pakoras, Spinach Onion, with Tamarind Dipping Sauce, 270–72
palatability, 22–24

pancakes, recipes, 96–97
Panfried Tofu or Tempeh, **8**, 193–94
pantry cleanout, 36
pantry stocking, 34–36
Parchment-Baked Fish (Fish en Papillote), **5**, 138–41
Parfait, On-the-Go Breakfast, **2**, 106–7
Parmesan, Chicken, 126–27
Parsley Chimichurri, 301
parsnips
    cooking guide, 331
    Herb Roasted Root Vegetables, 214
    Slow-Cooked Beef Chuck Pot Roast with Parsnips, 156–57
passeggiata, 5
pâtés
    Black Bean, 274–75
    Mushroom, 275–76
Pear Cinnamon Cashew Butter, 58
Pear Cranberry Pie, 320–21
Pears, Poached, 325–26
Peppermint Hot Chocolate, 309
Perfect Cucumber-Tomato Salad, 261
pesto
    Basil Walnut Pesto, **10**, 297
    Lime Cilantro Pesto, 298
Pesto Baked Fish, **5**, 143–44
Phase 1 (Conquer Cravings), 4
    program foods summary, 47–48
Phase 2 (Retrain Your Fat Cells), 4
    program foods summary, 47–48
Phase 3 (Lose Weight Permanently), 4
    program foods summary, 47–48
Pickles, DIY, **15**, 62–71
    Easy Pickled Cabbage or Carrots, 66–67
    Middle Eastern Pickled Turnips, 67–68
    Miso Pickles, 70–71
    Quick Ume-Pickled Onions, 69–70
    Sauerkraut, 65–66
    Spicy Pickled Vegetables (Escabeche), 68–69
pickling primer, 63–64
Piecrust, Grain-Free, 206–7
pies
    Apple Pie Parfait, 319–20
    Pear Cranberry Pie, 320–21
    Pumpkin Pie Tartlets, 322–23
pizza
    Grain-Free Pizza, 208–10
    Portobello or Baby Bella Pizzas, 176–77

Poached Pears, 325–26
Polish White Borscht, 246–47
pork
    entrées, recipes, 148–61
    equivalents table, 49–50
    Mustard Peppercorn Roasted Rack of Pork,
        166–67
    Slow Cooker Barbecue Ribs, 159–61
    Slow Cooker Pulled Pork, 148–49
Porridge, Make-Your-Own Whole-Grain,
    101–3
Portobello or Baby Bella Pizzas, 176–77
Portuguese Seafood Stew, 241–42
Potpie, Chicken or Tofu, 118–20
Pot Roast with Parsnips, Slow-Cooked Beef Chuck,
    156–57
poutine, 174
Power Balls, 279–80
Prep Day, 32–33, 41, 45
Pressure-Cooked Brown Rice, 226–27
pressure cookers, 37
program foods summary, 47–48
proteins
    equivalents table, 49–50
    insulin levels and, 14
    Prep Day, 33
    ready-to-go, 45
puddings
    Chia Seed Pudding, 108–9
    Chocolate Custard, 318–19
    Vegan Orange Chocolate Pudding, 317–18
Pumpkin Pie Tartlets, 322–23
Pumpkin Spice Muffins, Grain-Free, **3**, 90–91
Pumpkin Spice Pancakes, 97

Quesadilla, Shredded Chicken, 199–200
quiches, recipes, 92–95
Quick Ume-Pickled Onions, 69–70
quinoa
    Cooked Quinoa, 231
    Fresh Quinoa Salad with Pomegranates, 262
    Mediterranean Quinoa, 191–92
    Quinoa Croquettes, 232–33
    Quinoa Enchilada Casserole, 183–84
    Quinoa Tabbouleh, 235
    in Red Pepper Ring Omelets, 87–88
Quinoa Croquettes, **13**, 232–33
Quinoa Enchilada Casserole, **11**, 183–84
Quinoa Tabbouleh, 235

radishes, cooking guide, 330
Raita, Indian, 303
recipe planning worksheet, 31
recipes
    beverages, 308–11
    breakfasts, 81–109
    Buddha Bowls, 263–69
    chickpea flour, 195–210
    desserts, 312–26
    do it yourself (DIY), 53–80
    entrées, 110–94
    salads, 259–63
    sauces, rubs and marinades, 283–306
    side dishes, 211–37
    snacks and appetizers, 270–81
    soups, 238–58
Red Pepper Ring Omelets, 87–88
Refried Beans, 225
Relaxing Foot Soak, 77–78
revisionist recipes, 40
    chickpea flour, 40, 195–210
rice. *See* brown rice
Risotto, Brown Rice Mushroom, 229–30
Roasted Root Vegetables, Herb, 214
Roasted Vegetables, 215
Rosemary Biscuits, 203
rubs, recipes, 283–306
rutabaga
    cooking guide, 331
    Fennel Rutabaga Gratin, 189–90

Sage Walnut Lentil Loaf, 168–70
salads, recipes, 259–63
    Fresh Quinoa Salad with Pomegranates, 262
    Greek Salad, 259–60
    Jicama, Clementine, and Avocado Salad, 260–61
    The Perfect Cucumber-Tomato Salad, 261
    Texas Caviar (Black-Eyed Pea Salad), 262–63
salmon, recipes, 128–30, 141–42, 266
Salsa, Fresh, 302
salt, cooking guidelines, 116
salt brine, for pickles, 64
salt cravings, 16–17
satiety, 19–22
sauces
    about, 33
    Prep Day, 32–33
    recipes, 283–306
Sauerkraut, 65–66

Sautéed Bok Choy and Shiitake, **4**, 213
Sautéed Mushrooms, 216
Savory Adzuki Beans, 223
Scallion-Miso Condiment, 105
science, 11–27
    from *Always Hungry* to *Always Delicious*, 24–26
    cravings, 16–19
    hunger, 12–16
    satiety, 19–22
    tastiness, 22–24
seafood. *See* fish and seafood
seasonal produce, 38–39
Seasoned Salt, All-Purpose, 283
Seasoned Shiitake Mushrooms, 217
Seed Butters, DIY, 55–58
seitan
    DIY, 71–74
    Mushroom Seitan, 74
    Smoke-Dried Tomato Seitan, **8**, 73–74
self-care, DIY, 77–79
set point, 4, 237
shakes, recipes, 82–85
Shakshuka, 85–86
sheet-pan dinners, 45, 129, 197
Shredded Chicken, 110–11
Shredded Chicken Quesadilla, 199–200
Shrimp Kebabs, Drunken Marinated, **6**, 144–46
Shrimp Stir-Fry, 121
Sicilian Fava Bean Soup, 244–45
side dishes, recipes, 211–37
    beans, 221–25
    vegetables, 211–20
    whole grains, 226–37
skillets, 37
Slow-Cooked Beef Chuck Pot Roast with Parsnips, 156–57
Slow-Cooked Moroccan Lamb Stew, 161–63
Slow-Cooked Moroccan Sweet Potato Stew, 162–63
Slow-Cooked Moroccan Vegetarian Stew, 162–63
Slow Cooker Barbecue Ribs, 159–61
Slow Cooker Chili, 249–51
Slow Cooker Shredded Beef or Pulled Pork, 148–49
Smoked Paprika Ketchup, **9**, 291
    Meat Loaf with, 152–53
Smoke-Dried Tomato Seitan, **8**, 73–74
snacks
    Prep Day, 33

program foods summary, 48
    recipes, 270–81
    stocking, 36
snap (or snow) peas
    in Citrus Teriyaki Chicken Stir-Fry, 120–22
    cooking guide, 331
    in Japanese Buddha Bowl, 264–65
Snickerdoodles, 312–13
Socca Cracker, 202
Socca Crepes, 197–98
Socca Pinwheels, **13**, 273
Socca Pizza Crust, 208–10
Socca Wrap, Basic, 198–99
Soft Millet-Corn Polenta, 236–37
soups
    Basic Miso Soup, 258
    Broccoli Cheddar Soup, 256–57
    Chicken or Turkey Soup on a Budget, 243–44
    Creamy Millet Vegetable Soup, 255
    Cuban Black Bean Soup, 253–54
    Hot-and-Sour Soup, 240–41
    Minestrone Soup, 248–49
    Polish White Borscht, 246–47
    Portuguese Seafood Stew, 241–42
    Prep Day, 33
    recipes, 238–58
    Sicilian Fava Bean Soup, 244–45
    Split Pea Soup, 251–52
    Thai Coconut Fish Soup, 238–39
Sour Cream, Dairy-Free, 306
Souvlaki, 163–65
soy, equivalents table, 49–50
spa treatments, DIY, 77–79
spatulas, 37
special diets, 39–41
spices, 35–36
    storing, 36, 39
Spicy Asian Marinade or Salad Dressing, 294
Spicy Asian Stir-Fry, 122–23
Spicy Pickled Vegetables (Escabeche), **15**, 68–69
spinach
    cooking guide, 331
    in Green Chile Chicken or Beef Enchilada Casserole, 124–25
    in Spicy Asian Stir-Fry, 122–23
Spinach Artichoke Snack Bites, 277
Spinach Feta Quiche, 92–94
Spinach Mushroom Crepes, 99–100

Spinach Onion Pakoras with Tamarind Dipping Sauce, 270–72
spiralizers, 37
Split Pea Soup, 251–52
squash
    Butternut Sage Puree, 219
    cooking guide, 332
    in Creamy Millet Vegetable Soup, 255
    Summer Squash Casserole, 185–86
stir-fries, 44
    Citrus Teriyaki Chicken Stir-Fry, 120–22
    Spicy Asian Stir-Fry, 122–23
stocking kitchen, 34–36
sugar, program foods summary, 48
Sugar-Free Worcestershire Sauce, 284
Summer Grilled or Roasted Vegetables, 215
Summer Squash Casserole, 185–86
Sun-Dried Tomato Dressing, Creamy, 287–88
Sweet Breakfast Crepe, 98–99
sweet potatoes
    cooking guide, 332
    Herb Roasted Root Vegetables, 214
    in Moroccan Chicken Stew with Apricots, 133–34
    in Slow-Cooked Moroccan Lamb Stew, 161–63
sweet spices, 36
symptom trackers, 40

Tabbouleh, 234–35
tamarind, about, 272
Tamarind Dipping Sauce, Spinach Onion Pakoras with, 270–72
Tamari Roasted Almonds, 280
Tarragon Cream Sauce, Fish and Mushrooms in, 136–38
tastiness, 22–24, 40
tatsoi, cooking guide, 330
teff
    Creamy Coconut Teff, 103–4
    Make-Your-Own Whole-Grain Porridge, 101–3
tempeh
    Crumbled Tempeh, 192–93
    Deep-Fried Tempeh, 170–71
    equivalents table, 50
    Grab-and-Go Pies, 155
    Meatballs, 150
    Panfried Tempeh, 193–94

in Portobello or Baby Bella Pizzas, 176–77
    in Souvlaki, 165
    Stroganoff, 159
Teriyaki Salmon or Chicken Kebabs, **4**, 141–42
Texas Caviar (Black-Eyed Pea Salad), 262–63
Thai Coconut Fish Soup, 238–39
Thai Parchment-Baked Fish, 141
toaster ovens, 37
tofu
    in Creamy Green Chile Casserole, 187–88
    Crispy Tofu Fries, 173–74
    Deep-Fried Tofu, 170–71
    egg substitutes, 92
    in Hot-and-Sour Soup, 240–41
    Marinated Baked Tofu, 175–76
    Panfried Tofu, 193–94
    in Summer Squash Casserole, 186
    Tofu Potpie, 118–20
    Tofu Vegetable Balls, 171–72
    in Vegan Citrus Teriyaki Stir-Fry, 121
    in Vegan Spicy Asian Stir-Fry, 123
    in Vegetarian Moroccan Stew with Apricots, 134
    in Vegetarian Mushrooms in Tarragon Cream Sauce, 136–38
    in Vegetarian Souvlaki, 165
Tofu Potpie, 118–20
Tofu Vegetable Balls, 171–72
Truffles, Chocolate, **16**, 314–16
Turkey Meatballs, **10**, 149–51
Turkey Meat Loaf with Smoked Paprika Ketchup, 152–53
Turkey Soup on a Budget, 243–44
Turmeric Garlic Marinade, Fresh, 295
turnips
    cooking guide, 332
    Middle Eastern Pickled Turnips, 67–68
Tzatziki, 304
    in Souvlaki, 163–65

umami, 104, 217, 223, 275
umeboshi vinegar, for pickles, 64

Vegan Citrus Teriyaki Stir-Fry, 121
Vegan Meat Pies, 155
Vegan Orange Chocolate Pudding, 317–18
Vegan Socca Crepes, 198
Vegan Spicy Asian Stir-Fry, 123

vegetables. *See also specific vegetables*
  cooking guide, 329–32
  equivalents table, 51
  fresh and seasonal, 38–39
  Prep Day, 32, 41
  program foods summary, 47–48
  side dishes, recipes, 211–20
  Spicy Pickled Vegetables, 68–69
Vegetarian Chili, Slow Cooker, 250–51
vegetarian entrées, recipes, 167–94
Vegetarian Green Chile Enchilada Casserole, 125
Vegetarian Meatballs, 150
Vegetarian Moroccan Stew with Apricots, 134
Vegetarian Mushrooms in Tarragon Cream Sauce,
    136–38
Vegetarian Parmesan, 127
Vegetarian Potpie, 118–20
Vegetarian Quesadilla, Shredded, 200
Vegetarian Souvlaki, 165
Vegetarian Stew, Portuguese, 242
Vegetarian Stroganoff, 159

Walnut Butter, DIY, 55–57
walnuts
  in Arugula, Beet, and Goat Cheese Snack Bites,
      278–79
  Basil Walnut Pesto, 297
  in Mushroom Pâté, 275–76
  roasting guide, 334
  Sage Walnut Lentil Loaf, 168–70
weight prejudice, 2
white beans
  DIY cooking, 74–77
  Garlicky White Beans with Broccoli Rabe, 221

  in Green Chile Cream Sauce, 305
  in Minestrone Soup, 248–49
  in Polish White Borscht, 246–47
whole grains. *See also specific grains*
  cooking guide, 333
  equivalents table, 51
  Make-Your-Own Whole-Grain Porridge,
      101–3
  Prep Day, 32, 33
  program foods summary, 47–48
  quick-cooking, 44
  side dishes, recipes, 226–37
  Whole-Grain Citrus Teriyaki Stir-Fry, 121
willpower vs. biology, 11
Women's Health Initiative (WHI), 14–15, 21
Worcestershire Sauce, Sugar-Free, 284

yogurt
  Greek Yogurt, DIY, 54–55
  in Indian Raita, 303
  in Mango Lassi, 311
  in Tzatziki, 304

zucchini
  cooking guide, 331
  in Creamy Green Chile Casserole, 187–88
  in Grain-Free Pizza, 208–10
  in Green Chile Chicken or Beef Enchilada
      Casserole, 124–25
  in Spicy Asian Stir-Fry, 122–23
  in Summer Squash Casserole, 185–86
  in Teriyaki Chicken Kebabs, 142
  Zucchini with Garlic and Greens, 212
Zucchini with Garlic and Greens, 212

About the Authors

David S. Ludwig, MD, PhD, is an endocrinologist and researcher at Boston Children's Hospital, professor of pediatrics at Harvard Medical School, and professor of nutrition at Harvard School of Public Health. Described as an "obesity warrior" by *Time* magazine, Dr. Ludwig appears frequently in national media, including the *New York Times*, NPR, ABC, NBC, CBS, and CNN. His last book, *Always Hungry?*, was a #1 *New York Times* bestseller.

Dawn Ludwig has devoted her career to helping people discover the fun, beauty, and delicious taste of natural foods. For fifteen years, she owned and directed the Natural Epicurean Academy of Culinary Arts in Austin, Texas, recognized as one of the top "Cutting Edge Cuisine" cooking schools in the United States. Dawn has written on the subjects of nutrition and health for a variety of publications, including *Whole Health Magazine*, *Natural Home*, *Austin Monthly*, *Austin Fit*, and others.